BEYOND NORMALITY: THE PREDICTIVE VALUE AND EFFICIENCY OF MEDICAL DIAGNOSES

BEYOND NORMALITY: THE PREDICTIVE VALUE AND EFFICIENCY OF MEDICAL DIAGNOSES

ROBERT S. GALEN, M.D., M.P.H.

S. RAYMOND GAMBINO, M.D.

Columbia University
College of Physicians and Surgeons

A Wiley Biomedical Publication

JOHN WILEY & SONS, New York • London • Sydney • Toronto

Copyright © 1975 by John Wiley & Sons, Inc.

All rights reserved. Published simultaneously in Canada.

No part of this book may be reproduced by any means, nor transmitted, nor translated into a machine language without the written permission of the publisher.

Library of Congress Cataloging in Publication Data:

Galen, Robert S.
    Beyond normality.

    (A Wiley biomedical publication)
    Bibliography: p.
    Includes indexes.
    1.   Diagnosis—Statistical methods.
2. Medicine, Clinical.   3. Function tests
(Medicine) I. Gambino, S. Raymond, joint author.
II. Title. [DNLM: 1. Diagnosis.   2. Preventive
medicine.   WA100 G153b]

RC71.3.G34   616.07′5′013   75-25915
ISBN 0-471-29047-5

Printed in the United States of America

10 9 8 7 6 5 4 3

PREFACE

How does a book come into being? The key ingredient is an idea—yet most ideas do not result in books. Where did our idea come from? In 1972, Bob Galen was a resident in Clinical Pathology under Ray Gambino. Bob was also taking courses at the School of Public Health. It was there, in an epidemiology seminar led by Professor Mervyn Susser, that he first heard the words sensitivity, specificity, and predictive value. When the predictive value model was presented by Professor Susser, Bob became upset and excited in the same instant—upset with what we were doing in the clinical laboratory and excited by the prospect of leaving normal ranges and Gaussian statistics behind. Later that day we met and it was clear that the predictive value model could not be left behind in a classroom. We spent hours discussing the model and ultimately became convinced that this was a story that needed to be told.

This book is divided into three main sections. The text chapters discuss the predictive value model and demonstrate its application to a variety of laboratory problems. The appendices describe statistical methods for analyzing predictive value data in the laboratory. And, finally, tables of predictive value and efficiency appear at the end of the book, based on sensitivity, specificity, and prevalence. It is our intention to provide physicians and other health workers with the intellectual scaffolding and statistical tables necessary to go beyond the simple concepts of normal and abnormal. We hope the reader will become facile in applying this model to laboratory tests, and that new tests will be evaluated in the predictive value format.

Many recent writers have influenced our thinking. Among them are Thorner, Remein, Murphy, Vecchio, Sunderman, Henry, Werner, Whitehead, and others that are referenced in this book. What was lacking in all prior expositions, however, were examples of the model applied to *actual* tests and diseases. Therefore, in writing this book we decided to include many examples, culled from medical journals, that illustrate the way in which the model can be used to make decisions regarding laboratory tests. In addition, we present a general discussion of the model as well as a detailed presentation of the mathematical basis for the model.

Finally, there is frequent discussion of other new statistical methods for interpreting data. These new methods include discriminant analysis and correlation-regression analysis of multiple variables. However, since the final output of any complex data analysis is *a single* decision, the predictive value model must be applied to the output of *any* complex statistical manipulation of clinical or laboratory data.

No matter where the test is done, or how it is done, or how it is analyzed—the predictive value model should be applied to the final output.

ROBERT S. GALEN
S. RAYMOND GAMBINO

New York, New York
September 1975

ACKNOWLEDGMENT

We wish to acknowledge the help of the following individuals.

Our secretaries: Mrs. Sophie Eskanazy and Miss Barbara Heck for manuscript preparation.

Our laboratory supervisors: Mrs. Joan Alvarez, Miss Ivelice Fonseca, and Miss Grace Peguero for their technical assistance in the laboratory.

Our medical students: Dr. James A. Rothendler for programming the predictive value and efficiency tables; Mr. Melvin P. Rosenwasser and Mr. Howard Taylor for technical assistance in carrying out the myocardial infarction study; Dr. Daniel J. Fink and Mr. Jerry Sebag for data processing support in the myocardial infarction study.

R. S. G.

S. R. G.

CONTENTS

Predictive Value and Efficiency Tables   **167**

Index   **235**

PREDICTIVE VALUE AND EFFICIENCY TABLES

**Predictive Value of a Positive Result
for the Following Prevalences:**

Prevalence (per 100,000)	1–	167
	2–5	168
	10–40	170
	50–300	172
	400–2000	174
	3000–10,000	176
	15,000–50,000	178

**Predictive Value of a Positive Result
for the Following Sensitivities:**

Sensitivity (%)	50–60	180
	70–80	182
	85–90	184
	91–92	186
	93–94	188
	95–96	190
	97–98	192
	99–100	194

**Predictive Value of a Positive Result
for the Following Specificities:**

Specificity (%)	50–80	196
	90–95	198
	97–99.3	200
	99.5–99.91	202
	99.92–99.95	204
	99.6–99.99	206
	100–	

BEYOND NORMALITY: THE PREDICTIVE VALUE AND EFFICIENCY OF MEDICAL DIAGNOSES

CHAPTER 1

BEYOND NORMALITY

I S this test result normal?—a simple question which common sense suggests should have a simple answer. However the usual answers are misleading because the concept of normality is itself inadequate for the proper interpretation of test results.

THE SEMANTICS OF NORMALITY

Part of the problem is semantic. The concept of normality has multiple meanings. Dr. Edmond Murphy, for example, has listed seven different meanings for "normal" and has arranged them in order of increasing abstraction. He also suggests terms that he believes to be preferable (Table 1).

Table 1. Murphy's seven meanings for "normal"

Paraphase	Where used	Preferable term
1. Probability function (Bell-shaped curve)	Statistics	Gaussian
2. Most representative of its class	Descriptive sciences	Average, median, modal
3. Commonly encountered in its class	Descriptive sciences	Habitual
4. Most suited to survival	Genetics, operations research	Optimal, "fittest"
5. Carrying no penalty	Clinical medicine	Innocuous, harmless
6. Commonly aspired to	Politics, sociology	Conventional
7. Most perfect of its class	Metaphysics, esthetics, morals	Ideal

The first use of the word (Gaussian statistics) causes the biggest problem because it has little to do with the use of the word in any other sense. Gauss' law of errors applies to repeated measurements on the same object, *not* to a series of measurements on different objects. The law of errors implies that a plot of measurement errors made on the *same* object would fit a "normal" or Gaussian distribution. There is no known reason why an attribute of healthy or sick people should have a Gaussian distribution. The law, for example, applies to repeated measurements of one's own height, but not to the measurement of heights of different people.[2]

Furthermore, if we analyze data on blood levels for a nonphysiologic variable, such as lead, it is easier to see how we are mislead by the Procrustean bed of a Gaussian distribution. We need to define blood levels at which there is danger of morbidity and mortality. A statistical analysis of the distribution of lead values in a population and the subsequent definition of the "normal range" as those values that encompass 95% of the results tell us nothing about morbidity and mortality.

It may be more difficult to accept our argument for physiological variables, but it is just as valid. Let us consider cholesterol. In the United States the mean value for cholesterol for men between the ages of 40 and 60 is 225 mg/dl. However there are populations relatively free of atherosclerotic heart disease where the mean cholesterol level for the same age group is 150 mg/dl.[3] Therefore the mean value of 225 mg/dl is a normal value only in a statistical sense. With regard to morbidity and mortality, a value of 225 mg/dl may be quite "abnormal." In fact, according to Murphy, "normal" for cholesterol levels may have seven different meanings:

1. A bell-shaped probability distribution of cholesterol values.
2. The most representative cholesterol value as defined by a mean.
3. The most commonly encountered cholesterol values as defined by a range. This is the usual "laboratory normal range."
4. Cholesterol values most suited for reproduction and survival.
5. Cholesterol values unlikely to cause harm.
6. A committee's consensus, that is, "approved" cholesterol values.
7. The ideal cholesterol value.

The laboratory worker usually operates at level 3 in the above list. He defines the normal range by identifying the most commonly encountered values in various groups. The clinician, on the other hand, dealing with a single patient, does not care about Gaussian distributions or standard deviations, but wants to know whether the result is life threatening. He is interested in whether the result is optimum for survival, and he may have an interest in whether the result is common or even ideal.

An additional argument against the usefulness of a Gaussian approach to the definition of normality develops when we perform many tests on the same subject. If multiple tests are performed, and for each test normal is defined as those values that fall within ± 2 or 3 SD of the mean of a Gaussian or log-Gaussian distribution, the following *non sequitur* results—*the more tests performed on a healthy subject the more likely is the discovery of an abnormal result*. Table 2 shows the probability of obtaining such a result as the number of tests performed is increased. It is obvious that if this program were carried to its logical conclusion everyone would be classified as "abnormal" for one or more variables.

Table 2. Probability of obtaining an abnormal result

Number of independent tests	Percentage of times an abnormal result is found
1	5
2	10
4	19
6	26
10	40
20	64
50	92
90	99

THE USEFULNESS OF THE TEST

An additional problem is that many tests are not as useful as we think they are or would like them to be. Let us consider serum uric acid as an example. We can measure serum uric acid with a high degree of chemical specificity and accuracy. We can obtain superb statistics defining the usually encountered values by age and sex. But serum uric acid varies for a variety of nondisease reasons, such as race, intelligence, diet, physical activity, drugs, and genetic factors. Furthermore, it is often impossible to make the transition from test result to clinical syndrome or diagnosis. Gout, for example, does not have a high degree of correlation with serum uric acid levels. It is true that if the serum uric acid is above 9 mg/dl the diagnosis of gout is far more likely, but it is even truer that many cases of gout occur in subjects whose uric acid levels do not differ from those of the vast majority of the population.

Laboratory tests, if they are to be useful, cannot be interpreted simply in terms of "normal" or "abnormal." Dybkaer,[4] Grasbeck,[5] and Holland and Whitehead[6] propose the substitution of "reference values" for "normal values." This is a significant step forward. We, however, prefer the term referent value rather than reference value, because it emphasizes the *process of referring* to some bench mark rather than placing emphasis on the bench mark itself. We take up the subject of referent values in greater detail at the end of this chapter.

THE PREDICTIVE VALUE OF A TEST RESULT

Before we can expand on our concept of referent values, we must introduce the concept of predictive value.[7] The predictive value of a test answers the following questions: How accurately will a test predict the presence or absence of disease?; and, if you are given an abnormal result for a test, what are the chances that the abnormal result indicates disease? Again we find that a test result cannot be interpreted simply in terms of "normal" or "abnormal." Not only must we refer our result to a particular population, but we also require some estimate of the degree to which we can rely on that result in order to make a specific diagnosis. The predictive value of a test result gives us that estimate.

We discuss predictive value in greater detail in the next chapter, but a brief discussion is required at this point. The predictive value of a test is determined by the complex interaction of *three* variables: the incidence of false-negative results in patients with disease, the incidence of false-positive results in subjects without disease, and the prevalence of the disease itself in the group examined.

The prevalence of the disease is far more important than common sense would suggest. For example, if a test were so unbelievably good that there were never any false-negative results in patients with the disease and there was only 1 false-positive result per 10,000 subjects who were free of the disease—but the disease had a very low prevalence of between 5 and 10 per 100,000 (e.g., phenylketonuria)—then the predictive value of an abnormal result obtained with this unbelievably superb test would be only 50%! This means that half of the abnormal results would occur in subjects *who did not have true phenylketonuria* if the test were performed on *all* newborns—which is exactly what happened when legislators mandated routine PKU screening.

PERCENTILES

Clearly, the use of a normal range has limitations. What else can be substituted for the normal range? One way to avoid deciding what is normal, abnormal, or border-line is to report data in percentiles. This puts us into Murphy's third category in which "normal" means "commonly encountered in its class." By reporting percentile values we provide a linear measure of how unusual the result is in terms of a reference population. The clinician can decide for himself whether or not to consider a particular result abnormal.

However this approach still requires us to define a reference population, and, furthermore, *fails to indicate the likelihood of disease*. The physician is looking for answers in Murphy's category 5; that is, does the reported result carry any penalty, is it indicative of disease, and is it harmful?

Another problem with the percentile approach is the finite linearity of the scale. It is difficult to appreciate that a value in the 99.9999th percentile is 1000 times as rare as a value in the 99.9th percentile.

REFERENT VALUES

The usually encountered range of values (normal range) for a given measurement provides insufficient information to the physician. The usual "upper limit of normal" tells us nothing about disease, which is the main reason why concepts of normal, normal range, or percentile distribution have failed us. Such concepts have varying utility when applied to individual patients. The referent value concept, on the other hand, will make testing meaningful for diagnosis by indicating the predictive value of the test for particular diseases.

This can be illustrated by the measurement of serum uric acid. The usual range of values for uric acid in 95% of a particular population, based on age and sex, may be 3 to 6 mg/dl. But the usual range in a population tells us nothing about gout, renal disease, toxemia of pregnancy, or leukemia. The common solution is to refine our definition of the population by adding additional variables, such as race, geography, socioeconomic status, diet, activity, and medication. But such refinement would continue to mislead the clinician, because it would *fail to define a referent value for a specific disease.*

In order to obtain meaningful referent values for disease it is necessary to study and define meaningful reference populations, which should include:

1. Subjects who are free of any known disease.
2. Subjects who are free of the disease in question, *but who have other diseases.*
3. Subjects with the disease in question.

A major cause of trouble is that most data in the literature are based on studies of subjects in categories 1 and 3. Most tests (see Chapter 3) look very good when applied to subjects who are free of any known disease or to subjects having the disease in question. But these same tests fail in practice because most investigators do not study the results obtained when their test is applied to subjects *with other diseases.* It is usually not difficult for a physician to differentiate between good health and sickness. He has a problem, however, differentiating one disease from another disease with similar signs and symptoms, or defining the severity and the probable outcome of a disease process.

What the clinician requires, for example, is a table of referent values for uric acid for specific disease states, not a table of normal ranges. The particular referent value for a specific disease would be associated with a specific predictive value. Referent values vary by test, by population, by disease, *and by the predictive value desired.* We envision that future test reports may look something like Table 3. This report tells us that 21% of subjects in this population with a uric acid of 7 mg/dl or higher subsequently developed gout. This is more informative than simply noting that 7 mg/dl is outside the usual range. The report also tells us that 35% of subjects with a level of 8 mg/dl or higher and 82% of subjects with a level of 9 ml/dl or higher subsequently developed gout. These statistics were derived from the Framingham study.[8]

Table 3.   Future test report

Test: Serum uric acid
Population: To be characterized by age, sex, race,
geography, socioeconomics, etc.
Usual Range: 3 to 6 mg/dl

Referent Value	Diagnosis	Predictive Value, %
7.0	Gout	21
8.0	Gout	35
9.0	Gout	82

The ideal uric acid report would also include referent and predictive values for other diseases, such as leukemia, kidney disease, and toxemia of pregnancy. Unfortunately, we cannot give those values at this time, because most studies have not been designed with this purpose in mind. That, in fact, is the purpose of this book. Patients and physicians require referent and predictive values and this book shows how to obtain them.

REFERENCES

1. Murphy, Edmond A. The normal, and the perils of the sylleptic argument. *Perspect. Biol. Med.* **15:** 566–582, 1972.

2. Elveback, L. R., Guillier, C. L., and Keating, F. R., Jr., Health, normality, and the ghost of Gauss. *JAMA* **211:** 69–75, 1970.

3. McGill, Henry C., Jr. (Ed.). *The Geographic Pathology of Atherosclerosis.* Williams and Wilkins, Baltimore, 1968.

4. Dybkaer, R., Concepts and nomenclature in theory of reference values. *Scand. J. Clin. Lab. Invest.* **29,** Suppl. 126: 19.1, 1972.

5. Grasbeck, R., Types of reference groups. *Scand. J. Clin. Lab. Invest.* **29,** Suppl. 126: 19.2, 1972.

6. Holland, W. W. and Whitehead, T. P., Value of new laboratory tests in diagnosis and treatment. Lancet **ii:** 391–394, 1974.

7. Vecchio, Thomas J., Predictive value of a single diagnostic test in unselected populations. *N Engl. J. Med.* **274:** 1171–1173, 1966.

8. Hall, A. P., Farry, P. E., Dawber, R. R., and McNamara, P. M., Epidemiology of gout and hyperuricemia. *Am. J. Med.* **42:** 27–37, 1967.

CHAPTER 2

SENSITIVITY, SPECIFICITY, PREVALENCE, AND INCIDENCE

I N Chapter 1 we introduced the concept of predictive value and the three variables used in its determination: the incidence of true positive results in
patients with disease, the incidence of true negative results in subjects without
diseases, and the number of subjects with the disease in the group examined. The
academic terms for these variables are, respectively, sensitivity, specificity, and
prevalence or incidence.

What is the difference between sensitivity and specificity? What is the difference
between prevalence and incidence? The paired terms sound too much alike and are
too easily confused. Even the late Joseph Garland, the distinguished editor of the
New England Journal of Medicine from 1947 to 1967, was confused. When writing on "Clarity in Medical Writing" he stated:

> I confess that except among the biostatisticians and the more learned disciples of
> public health in its most esoteric form the differentiation of "incidence" and
> "prevalence" is difficult and even the biostatistical personality experiences at times
> a mild state of shock when accosted with the necessity of distinguishing the
> nuances of these common words.[1]

It is unfortunate that we are saddled with words that lack sharpness, but as
much as we'd like to dispose of these words they are so established in the special
literature of public health that we cannot eliminate them. On the other hand, we do
suggest some synonyms, and by example we hope to define more clearly what is
meant when these words are used and why we must distinguish between them.

SENSITIVITY OR POSITIVITY IN DISEASE

The term "the sensitivity of a test" is used to characterize the incidence of true-
positive results obtained when a test is applied to patients known to have the
disease. Let us illustrate this by example. If a pregnancy test were applied to 100
women who were *known* to be in the first trimester of pregnancy, and if the
sensitivity of the test were varied the results given in Table 1 would be obtained.

When a test has a sensitivity of 100% for a particular disease it gives positive
results in *all* patients with the disease. If the sensitivity is only 90%, then positive

Table 1.   **Results of pregnancy test given to 100 pregnant women**

Test sensitivity (%)	Number known to be pregnant	Number of true positives	Number of false negatives
100	100	100	0
99	100	99	1
95	100	95	5
90	100	90	10
85	100	85	15

results are obtained in only 90% of the subjects known to have the disease. Since sensitivity is equal to the percentage of positive results obtained in diseased subjects we prefer to replace the term sensitivity with "positivity in disease." If we remember the following we will never be confused: *A good test gives positive results in diseased subjects.*

SPECIFICITY OR NEGATIVITY IN HEALTH

Specificity is used to characterize the incidence of true-negative results obtained when a test is applied to subjects known to be *free* of the disease. If the same pregnancy test were applied to 100 subjects (men, women, and children) who were *not* pregnant and if the specificity of the test were varied, the results given in Table 2 would be obtained.

Table 2.   Results of pregnancy test given to 100 nonpregnant subjects

Test specificity (%)	Number known to be not pregnant	Number of true negatives	Number of false positives
100	100	100	0
99	100	99	1
95	100	95	5
90	100	90	10
85	100	85	15

When a test has a specificity of 100% for a particular disease it gives negative results in all subjects tested who are free of disease. If the specificity is only 90%, then negative results are obtained in only 90% of the subjects known to be free of the disease. Since specificity is equal to the percentage of negative results obtained in healthy subjects, we prefer to replace specificity with the term "negativity in health." If we remember the following we will never be confused: *A good test gives negative results in healthy subjects.*

PREVALENCE AND INCIDENCE

Prevalence derives from *prevail* and refers to that which is common, with less emphasis on time. The prevalence rate for a disease equals the number of patients per 100,000 population who have the disease at the time of the study.

Incidence derives from *incident* or *event* and refers to the frequency of occurrence of something, and is therefore always associated with a stated period of time.

The incidence rate for a disease is the number of patients per 100,000 population who develop the disease in a given year.

Let us illustrate this by example. If tuberculin tests are performed at the same time on everyone in a town of 100,000, and there are 10,000 positive tests, the *prevalence* of healed or active tuberculosis is 10% (10,000/100,000). If, on the other hand, the number of people who *change* from tuberculin negative to tuberculin positive each year are monitored and there are 1000 such cases in a 1-year period, then the *incidence* of tuberculosis is 1% (1000/100,000).

The incidence of a chronic disease can be low but its prevalence quite high. The incidence is low because a small percentage of the population may contract the disease each year, but the prevalence is high because the disease may last for a lifetime in each subject. On the other hand, the incidence of an acute disease may be high but its prevalence quite low. The incidence is high because the acute disease may occur in a large percentage of the population in the course of 1 year, but the prevalence is low because the disease has a very short duration and no long-term effects.

Pathologists commonly err in their use of prevalence and incidence because so many of their studies are based on autopsy findings. Disease statistics derived from autopsy diagnoses are misleading for many reasons, not the least of which is the inability of an autopsy study to define the true prevalence and incidence rates of disease states. The pathologist speaks glibly of the incidence of coronary artery disease, tumor, or trichinosis at autopsy, but such incidence figures are misleading. The population sampled at autopsy is not complete and is highly biased, and adequate historical data are usually lacking. Therefore true incidence and prevalence rates are not obtainable from a routine autopsy service. As a general rule:

$$\text{prevalence} = \text{incidence} \times \text{duration of disease}$$

PREDICTIVE VALUE

The predictive value of a positive test result is defined as the percentage of positive results that are true positives when the test is applied to a population containing both healthy and diseased subjects. Common sense would suggest that the predictive value of a test is dependent on the positivity of the test in disease and its negativity in health. Table 3 illustrates these relationships.

An ideal test would establish the presence or absence of disease in every individual screened. This ideal test would always give positive results in anyone with the disease and negative results in anyone without the disease. In other words, there would never be any false-positive or false-negative results. Unfortunately, there is no test that meets these ideal standards. Positivity in disease is coupled *inversely* to negativity in health. If there are more true-positive results in diseased subjects, then we are likely to find a smaller number of true-negative results in healthy subjects.

Even our tests for death never achieve 100% sensitivity and 100% specificity. For example, a flat electroencephalogram (EEG) is 100% sensitive for the occur-

Table 3.   Predictive value of test applied to healthy and diseased populations

	Model		
	Number with positive test result	Number with negative test result	Totals
Number with ⎯⎯⎯→ disease	TP	FN	TP + FN
Number without ⎯⎯⎯→ disease	FP	TN	FP + TN
Totals	TP + FP	TN + FN	TP + FP + TN + FN

TP = true positives, number of sick subjects correctly classified by the test.

FP = false positives, number of healthy subjects misclassified by the test.

TN = true negatives, number of healthy subjects correctly classified by the test.

FN = false negatives, number of sick subjects misclassified by the test.

$$\text{positivity in disease (sensitivity)} = \frac{TP}{TP + FN} \times 100$$

$$\text{negativity in health (specificity)} = \frac{TN}{TN + FP} \times 100$$

$$\text{predictive value of a positive result} = \frac{TP}{TP + FP} \times 100$$

rence of death because all dead people have a flat EEG; conversely, not all subjects who suddenly develop flat EEGs subsequently go on to die. Therefore, the EEG is *not* 100% specific. However, if death is diagnosed on the basis of rigor mortis and livor mortis 100% specificity will be achieved, because no one is ever found with rigor mortis and livor mortis who is not dead. On the other hand, 100% sensitivity will not be achieved because dead subjects can be found who have not yet developed rigor and livor.

When quantitative tests are used, it is possible to vary positivity and negativity by changing the level at which the test is considered positive. The positive screening level for anemia in women, for example, could be taken as either 11 or 12 grams of hemoglobin per 100 ml of whole blood. A cutoff of 12 grams will provide very high sensitivity for anemia but lower specificity since a larger proportion of healthy subjects will be classified as anemic. On the other hand, if the cutoff is 11 grams sensitivity will decrease but specificity will increase. The 11-gram cutoff will miss some borderline anemics, but the use of that level will avoid the misclassification of healthy subjects.

For certain qualitative tests (e.g., current pregnancy tests), sensitivity and specificity are inherent in the test system and cannot be varied by the laboratory; although different pregnancy tests have differing degrees of positivity and negativity.

Finally, which is better: very high sensitivity, or very high specificity? Remember we cannot have both. The decision must take into account certain epidemiological features of the population studied, as well as a judgement as to the number of false positives and the number of false negatives that would be tolerable. The decision should be based on the prevalence of the disease, the severity of the disease, the cost of the test, and the advantages and probability of early treatment. This subject is discussed further in Chapter 7.

REFERENCE

---

1. Garland, Joseph, *A Time for Remembering*. The Massachusetts Medical Society, Boston, 1972, pp. 128–129.

CHAPTER 3

MORE ON PREVALENCE AND PREDICTIVE VALUE, AND THEIR RELATIONSHIP TO MEDICAL PRACTICE

THE predictive value of a positive test (i.e., the percentage of all positive results that are true positives) varies with the prevalence of the disease. For example, during a raging influenza epidemic simply asking a patient how he feels would have high predictive value—those with influenza would feel miserable and almost everyone else would be free of the disease. If there is only *one* case of influenza in the entire community, however, this simple screening test (i.e., how do you feel?) would have nearly zero predictive value for influenza.

Prevalence is probably the most important—but least understood—factor affecting the usefulness of a test result. If we kept sensitivity and specificity constant at 95% each and changed prevalence, the predictive value of a test would vary widely, as shown in Table 1.

Table 1.   Effect of prevalence on predictive value when sensitivity and specificity equal 95%

Prevalence of disease (%)	Predictive value of a positive test (%)
0.1	1.9
1	16.1
2	27.9
5	50.0
50	95.0

Even if we have a test with superior characteristics; a test, for example, with a specificity of 99% and a sensitivity of 99%, prevalence still has a profound effect on predictive value (Table 2).

Tables 1 and 2 explain why so many reports of new tests look so good, but when those same tests are applied in the field failure is common. A typical research report is usually constructed as follows:

1.   An investigator collects 100 examples of subjects with a disease (e.g., rheumatoid arthritis) and shows that the new test is capable of detecting 99 of the 100 patients with the disease. Thus the sensitivity is 99%.

Table 2.   Effect of prevalence on predictive value when sensitivity and specificity equal 99%

Prevalance (%)	Predictive value of a positive test (%)
0.1	9.0
1.0	50.0
2.0	66.9
5.0	83.9
50.0	99.0

2. The investigator collects 100 subjects (laboratory workers, medical students, secretaries, etc.) who, he is fairly certain, are free of rheumatoid arthritis and shows that only 1 person out of 100 has a positive test result. Therefore the specificity is 99%.

3. The investigator publishes a paper extolling the virtues of the new test for the diagnosis of rheumatoid arthritis, believing it to be 99% correct.

4. Internists interested in rheumatoid arthritis insist that the hospital laboratory provide this excellent new test.

5. The laboratory obliges, and internists with interest in rheumatoid arthritis are delighted, because time after time the test is positive in patients with classic symptoms of the disease.

6. A conference is held and the laboratory director and the internists recommend that the test be used as a routine screen.

7. The laboratory director and other physicians then begin to find: positive results in patients coming in for elective gall bladder surgery but having no joint pains; positive results in patients on certain drugs; positive results in patients with acute hepatitis; positive results in adolescents during their acute growth spurt; and so on. What happened?

The original investigator, the internists, and the laboratory director *forgot that prevalence may be more important than sensitivity and specificity.* When the original investigator studied 100 subjects with the disease and 100 subjects without the disease, he had a disease prevalence of 50%! This is very high and would have a predictive value of 99%. When the internists studied patients with arthritis, they were examining patients in whom the prevalence of rheumatoid arthritis still was quite high—so again the predictive value of the test was excellent. However, when the hospital laboratory and the medical staff decided to use this "excellent" test on a routine basis, they forgot to consider the effect of prevalence. When applied to *all* admissions, the test did not change; only the prevalence of the disease changed. Instead of being 40 to 60%, prevalence dropped to less than 1%, because fewer than 1 out of every 100 admissions had occult or obvious rheumatoid arthritis. If the prevalence were 1%, the predictive value of the test would be 50%, which means that fully half of the positive results would be *false* positives. And if the prevalence were only 1 in a 1000, as is likely if the test were to be applied to all outpatients in a community, then the predictive value would be a low 9%, which means that 91 out of every 100 positive results would be *false*-positive results.

Our illustration is not exaggerated. In fact, we have purposely chosen a test with very high sensitivity and specificity. Most tests, however, do not have such high sensitivity and specificity, and the effects therefore would be worse.

APPLICATIONS OUTSIDE THE LABORATORY

The concepts of normality, referent value, predictive value, sensitivity, specificity, and prevalence are usually applied to the analysis of laboratory tests. But, in fact, these concepts are applicable to *all* areas of medicine, whether quantitative or not. It is easy to see how they would apply in radiology and in such areas as electrocardiography and electroencephalography, but the concepts also apply to physical diagnosis and history taking.

Physical diagnosis and laboratory diagnosis are identical. Physical diagnosis utilizes the science of gross anatomy to detect disease. The ability of a particular examination, such as auscultation, to predict the presence or absence of mitral stenosis also depends on sensitivity, specificity, and prevalence. The effect of prevalence in this setting is more complex—prevalence will alter sensitivity. In the examination of children with symptoms of acute rheumatic fever much more care is taken in the auscultation and therefore the sensitivity of the examination is automatically increased. In contrast, in the performance of routine screening physicals at an Army induction center, the sensitivity of the auscultation is decreased. One of the reasons automated laboratory tests are replacing physical diagnosis is that the sensitivity of an automated laboratory test usually is not affected by the index of suspicion of the physician or the skill of the technologist. Furthermore, laboratory tests broaden the scope of any examination and increase the certainty of the diagnosis. Laboratory tests are an extension of the physician's senses. Instead of limiting the physical examination to what can be seen, heard or felt, the laboratory examination permits the study of microscopic and molecular changes in structure and function, which otherwise would be undetectable. Indeed, the scope of such examinations has increased to such an extent that we now have many disease categories that are diagnosible *only* by laboratory examination. However, this should not blind us to the logical continuum that exists between the physical examination and the measurement of any laboratory variable.

It is easy to see how our principles apply to the physcial exam—but what about the taking of a history? Is medical history taking a pure art form unrelated to the mathematical principles outlined in prior chapters? We do not think so. True, good history taking requires much training and there are striking differences in skill among physicians, but the same variables of sensitivity, specificity, and prevalence apply if we wish to quantitate the predictive value of any particular question.

History taking probes the mind–body interaction. The question, How do you feel? has the same constraints as any objective laboratory test. The question is, in fact, a test of a patient's awareness of his overall function.

Furthermore, history taking can increase prevalence. In the diagnosis of hepatitis, for example, a history of a blood transfusion functions to segregate the population into two groups: those who received a transfusion, and therefore have a higher risk and a higher prevalence of type B hepatitis, and those who did not. Similarly, if not more strikingly, a history of sexual contact has 100% sensitivity for venereal disease. Without sexual contact, venereal disease is probably impossible. The history of contact increases the prevalence of the disease in the population to be tested.

A good physical examination and an excellent history are essential components of good medical practice, and they are equally essential for the effective use of laboratory tests. The experienced clinician has always known this and has been justifiably suspicious of routine laboratory screening procedures. Indiscriminate use of laboratory tests on subjects selected at random is doomed to failure if the prevalence of the disease is low. The history and the physical examination increase the prevalence of disease in the population selected for testing, and thereby increase the predictive value of any test procedure applied to this selected population.

We close with an example from the psychiatric literature. The powerful effect of prevalence on predictive value helps to explain the results of Rosenhan's controversial psychiatric study entitled, "On Being Sane in Insane Places."[1] In the Rosenhan study, 8 sane people had themselves admitted to 12 different psychiatric hospitals by feigning a *single* hallucinatory episode. Otherwise they told the truth, and they never had another "hallucination." Hospitalization lasted from 7 to 52 days, and they behaved while hospitalized in a totally sane manner and were fully cooperative. Many patients recognized the subjects as sane pseudopatients, *but not a single psychiatrist or hospital worker recognized the subjects as sane.* The psychiatric profession was shocked by the results of the study and much acrimonious debate ensued.

The results of the study should not be surprising, however, if we consider the effect of prevalence. Psychiatric tests are neither 100% sensitive nor 100% specific. When the prevalence of sanity is less than 0.1% (100/100,000), even the very best psychiatric tests fail. If we are relatively charitable and assume an average hospital psychiatrist can diagnose sanity with 95% sensitivity and 95% specificity, the predictive value of a positive result is only 2%. The psychiatrist will experience an extremely high failure rate in his attempt to discover sanity in an insane environment. A false-positive rate of 98% is so poor that any attempt to discover a very few sane among a massive number of insane will be dropped because it does not justify the extra effort. It was that revelation that stirred such emotional debate among psychiatrists. In addition, the Rosenhan study revealed serious shortcomings in the sensitivity and specificity of the tests used routinely by hospital psychiatrists. Indeed, the Rosenhan study should be interpreted as a call for psychiatrists, as well as other physicians, to define with greater care the sensitivity and specificity of all test procedures.

REFERENCE

---

1. Rosenhan, D. L., On being sane in insane places. *Science* **179:** 250–258, 1973.

CHAPTER 4

WHY DO DOCTORS ORDER LABORATORY TESTS?

THE LABORATORY AS FEEDBACK

I N his book *Management,* Peter Drucker stresses the importance of feedback information if one is to obtain reliable results. He recognizes the critical role played by the introduction of the routine autopsy in medical practice 150 years ago. The autopsy provided reliable and important feedback information to the physician, thereby improving his diagnostic and therapeutic skills. Drucker attributes the rise of modern medical practice to the introduction of the autopsy.[1]

Laboratory tests play the same important role as the autopsy, that of providing critical feedback information to the physician. It is difficult, if not impossible, to control and correct performance unless feedback is provided. The feedback information required, however, must be timely, relevant, and operational. The importance of timeliness is obvious both in theory and in practice. Every physician wants his laboratory results as soon as possible. The importance of relevance and of an operational effect is equally obvious in theory—but not so in practice.

This book provides a system for evaluating some aspects of the operational effect of a laboratory test. The sensitivity, specificity, and predictive value of a test define the operational characteristics of the test—characteristics that are not readily perceived unless quantitated.

THE LABORATORY AS AN EXTENSION OF PHYSICAL DIAGNOSIS

Laboratory tests are an extension of physical diagnosis. They "amplify" the physicians senses so that he can "see," "hear," or "feel" at cellular, molecular, and atomic levels. For example, a physician cannot smell, feel, or hear oxygen, but with a Po_2 electrode he can detect small changes in Po_2. As our understanding of disease mechanisms increases we begin to define a "disease" by a specific molecular or functional alteration that is measurable *only* by a laboratory test. Thus "disease" may be defined by a particular test and can only be diagnosed and monitored by that test.

If denied access to tests that define disease, or monitor the progress or therapy of disease, a physician will become extremely angry. It is as if he had been blindfolded, had plugs placed in his ears and heavy gloves placed on his hands—thus limiting the use of his senses in physical diagnosis. If he was then told that he could remove these impediments only when the laboratory was open, obviously the physician would prefer that the laboratory to be open and ready for tests at all times.

When we deny a physician a laboratory test, we are in effect cutting off his senses. If, for example, we deny a nephrologist ready access to creatinine measurements at any time of the day and night, we might just as well deny him physical access to his patients, because the only efficient way a nephrologist can detect deterioration of renal function in patients requiring dialysis or transplantation is to monitor creatinine clearance.

THE LABORATORY AS A FINITE RESOURCE

Granted that the physician is frustrated if he is blindfolded, but does that mean that any physician should be able to order any test he wants whenever he wants? The answer is no, since the laboratory is simply an extension of physical diagnosis. Can a physician examine any patient at any time and perform any physical diagnostic test he wishes? Of course not. Obviously, the patient would call a halt if he felt abused. He would also question the physician if the physical examination failed to cover areas of the body or organ systems producing his complaints. Finally, the physician realizes that he has finite resources. He has only so much time for each patient and can perform only a limited number of examinations. He therefore selects those questions and procedures that training and experience have taught him are most effective in resolving diagnostic and therapeutic problems.

However in the use of laboratory tests the physician does not sense any limitation. He considers the laboratory—like air, water, and telephones—to be an infinite resource. A simple, effortless, painless stroke of the pen is all that is required to command its use. It is not the physician's time that is used. It is not the physician's money that is consumed. It is not the physician's assistants who do the work.

THE NEED TO BE "ON TARGET"

A physician without blindfolds, however, may still not "see" correctly unless his vision is directed to the proper place. Similarly, a physician with total freedom to order any laboratory test may not order the correct test. In both examples "correct vision" comes from training, experience, and scientific experiment. It is also essential that the examination be directed to the problem under study. If, for example, a patient is being examined for genital lice, it will do no good to examine the head— no matter how accurate and precise an examination it is—because the head is not the target.

Being "off target" is the main reason why most laboratory tests lack sensitivity and specificity. It is essential to have a detailed understanding of the biochemical pathways in a particular disease *before* a chemical assay is established as a routine diagnostic test. Without such knowledge it is not possible to select the correct biochemical measurement. Most tests currently in use are *not* biochemically specific for the problem under study, and therefore they lack clinical sensitivity and specificity.

HOW CAN WE DEFINE A "GOOD" TEST OR A "BAD" TEST?

As an example, let us take a close look at the glucose tolerance test. This test is widely used, but it may be one of the most useless tests performed. Why? Because we do not know enough about diabetes. Diabetes is much more than glucose intolerance, but we fall back on the glucose tolerance test because we have no current way of measuring those other factors. The glucose tolerance test is way off target as far as the complications of diabetes are concerned.

The glucose tolerance test tells us nothing about whether a patient is prone to develop acute ketoacidosis, nonketotic diabetic coma, peripheral neuropathy, renal disease, cardiovascular disease, blindness, or impotence. In short, the test lacks specificity and sensitivity for the complications of diabetes. Therefore it has no predictive value for the major complications of diabetes. The only thing determined by the glucose tolerance test is glucose intolerance. But occult glucose intolerance does not predict clinical diabetes with a high degree of accuracy—and more significantly—it fails to predict the future occurrence of diabetic complications. For the patient it is the complications, not the glucose intolerance, that characterize the disease.

MULTIPLE FUNCTIONS OF LABORATORY TESTING

- Provide a correct diagnosis in a patient known to be sick.
- Provide a prognosis in a patient with a known disease.
- Provide an indication as to whether or not a disease is present in its early or subclinical stages in an otherwise "healthy" person.
- Provide data for monitoring the level of therapeutic drugs, or the effects of drugs, or both.
- Provide data that may indicate whether or not disease might develop at some future time, that is, delineation of risk factors.

Let us apply the multiple functions of laboratory tests to the measurement of glucose and see what effect they may have on required decision limits and accuracy limits.

Provide a Correct Diagnosis in a Patient Known to be Sick

When a patient is known to be urinating a great deal, and glucose and ketone bodies are found in the urine, a blood glucose serves to provide additional support for a diagnosis of diabetic ketoacidosis. It would not matter whether the glucose level were 250, 350, or 450 mg/dl. It would not matter if the "true" glucose were

300 mg/dl, but the laboratory reported 275 or 325 mg/dl. It would not matter whether the upper limit of normal for glucose were 90, 100, 110, or 120 mg/dl. The decision levels in a patient urinating a great deal and spilling sugar and ketone bodies into his urine might be:

>150 mg/dl = consistent with diabetes

>500 mg/dl = consistent with severe diabetes

>1000 mg/dl = consistent with hyperosmolar coma

An upper limit of normal derived from a healthy population has little or no value in the above circumstance. What are needed are referent values that provide information on the presence or absence of suspected disease states.

In the above example the referent values are well above the usual upper limit of normal and the ranges are broad. High accuracy is not required because anyone, with severe diabetes for example, has a very high blood sugar. The exact blood glucose level is not as important as the fact that the blood glucose is very elevated.

Provide a Prognosis in a Patient with a Known Disease

In diabetes the level of blood glucose is not as useful as commonly thought. It fails to provide information on the possible development of diabetic complications. The multiple complications of diabetes, such as neuopathy, retinitis, glomerulosclerosis, atherosclerosis, propensity to infection, and impotence, are not predictable from the glucose level *per se*.

The relative abnormality of the glucose tolerance test, for example, does not predict the future severity of any complication, nor when the complication might occur. Diabetes mellitus is more than hyperglycemia. The blood glucose level is too far removed from the fundamental pathogenesis of diabetes.

In this case, therefore, the definition of a referent value or the improvement of the accuracy of the measurement is relatively futile because *the measurement is not relevant.*

Indicate Whether or Not a Disease is Present in Its Early or Subclinical Stages in an Otherwise Healthy Person

---

Sometimes physicians order a glucose tolerance test to check for occult diabetes. A great deal of effort has been expended on determining what is "normal" or "abnormal" in glucose tolerance testing. However no one has demonstrated any practical value to be obtained from the discovery of occult diabetes, since we still do not know how to use the information. It does not require a glucose tolerance test to advise patients to remain lean, to remain active, and to maintain good mental health. The test has no *operational* function in this setting, since there is no action that should be taken on the basis of the test that would not be taken without the test.

Provide Data for Monitoring the Level of Therapeutic Drugs, the Effect of Drugs, or Both

The monitoring of drug action is one of the most persuasive reasons for ordering a laboratory test. Blood sugar levels provide one of the most direct measures of the effect of any given dose of insulin. The blood sugar level provides *direct feedback* to the therapist (patient or physician) on the functional effect of a specific drug regimen. Without this information, therapy might end in failure or even lead to injury.

When monitoring the effect of insulin precision is a prime requisite. It is highly desirable, but not essential, to have accuracy as well. Accuracy is not as essential as precision because the effect of insulin is studied by monitoring the *change* in blood glucose. The absolute level is not as important as the change in the level. Therefore it is essential that we be able to detect change, and for this high precision is required.

For many years the Folin-Wu blood glucose method provided adequate data for monitoring insulin therapy even though total reducing substances were measured and not true glucose. It is, of course, desirable to measure the absolute level of glucose itself, but the important point is that it is not essential as long as the *change* in glucose can be measured.

Glucose levels are not the only requirement. Insulin acts at several sites, and only one of its effects results in the lowering of blood sugar. As our knowledge of insulin action grows, we will probably require several new measurements to monitor its actions.

Provide Data that May Indicate Whether or Not Disease Might Develop at Some Future Time (Delineation of risk factors)

Does the measurement of blood glucose provide data that can be used to delineate risk factors? The answer is no. The future incidence of frank diabetes in subjects with abnormal glucose tolerance curves is nearly equal to that in subjects with normal glucose tolerance curves—if studied for at least 5 years. We have *no idea* why one patient, both of whose parents have frank diabetes, develops keto-acidosis at age 17, his brother or sister develops mild diabetes at age 55, and a third sibling never develops frank diabetes, but dies following a massive myocardial infarction. Until we understand what factors precipitate the development of frank diabetes mellitus we will lack the proper test(s). Glucose measurements are not useful in this context, and therefore their routine use is a relative waste of time and money.

The glucose tolerance test is *not relevant* to the problem posed by the question, Will this patient develop frank diabetes, and if so, when? Furthermore, the test has no *operational utility at this time*. Even if it did answer the question, the answer would fall into a therapeutic vacuum. At the present time we do not know what to do with the information.

SUMMARY

At the beginning of this chapter we suggested that laboratory tests play a critical role in providing essential feedback to the physician. The feedback information required, however, must be timely, must be relevant, and must be operational.

We have "dissected" the measurement of blood glucose and have shown that the relevant operational functions of blood glucose measurements are to monitor the effect of insulin and to provide confirmation of suspected frank diabetes mellitus. On the other hand, the use of blood glucose measurements to detect occult diabetes, or to predict the risk of developing diabetes, is neither relevant nor operational and is, therefore, essentially useless. Unfortunately, most of the blood sugar measurements performed in 1975 were ordered under the mistaken notion that they would provide useful predictive information as to the risk of developing diabetes *and its complications* in individual subjects.

REFERENCE

1. Drucker, Peter F., *Management*, Harper and Row, New York, 1974, pp. 268.

CHAPTER 5

HOW TO DETERMINE THE PREDICTIVE VALUE
AND EFFICIENCY OF A TEST
WHEN READING A SCIENTIFIC PAPER

I N this chapter we demonstrate, step by step, how to *apply* the general principles described in the preceding chapters.

1. First, the sensitivity of the test is calculated from the author's data. That is, what percent of sick patients tested had *positive test results?* Most scientific papers do not directly state the sensitivity of the test used. Furthermore, the sensitivity of the test may vary with the stage or duration of the disease, or with other population variables, such as sex, age, other diseases, and medications. The author usually provides data for calculating the best possible sensitivity. Let us also look for data indicating the sensitivity generally obtained under routine conditions in unselected cases. Such data is usually not provided by the developer of the test, but often can be found by examining subsequent papers by other authors.

2. Next, the specificity of the test is calculated from the author's data. That is, what percent of subjects without the disease under study had *negative test results?* Again, most scientific papers fail to define the specificity of the test. In addition, if specificity is defined, it is most often in terms of negative results in totally healthy or normal subjects. The use of healthy subjects provides data for an ideal specificity never seen in routine practice. An estimate of ideal specificity is made, but the real specificity is needed when the test is applied to patients with other or similar diseases. This data may be found in subsequent papers by other authors. As mentioned earlier, most physicians have little difficulty differentiating disease from perfect health—the problem is to differentiate one type of sickness from a variety of similar diseases.

3. An estimate is made of the prevalence of the disease in the population to be tested. Only a 'ball park" estimate is needed. Is the prevalence 10/100,000, 100/100,000, 1000/100,000 or 10,000/100,000? *When prevalence is 0/100,000 or 100,000/100,000 a test is not necessary.* In Appendix VIII we provide statistics on the prevalence of some diseases in our society.

4. The next step is to fill in the blanks of a worksheet table. On a worksheet make a blank table as shown in Table 1a.

5. In the lower right hand corner of the blank table 100,000 is entered as the grand total. The table now looks like Table 1b.

6. Now the estimate of *prevalence* is used to fill in the total number of sick and nonsick subjects. For example, if the estimated prevalence is 10,000/100,000 or 10%, then the total number of sick patients is 10% of 100,000, or 10,000; and the total number of nonsick subjects is 90,000. Thus, for a prevalence of 10% (10,000/100,000) the worksheet table looks like Table 1c.

Table 1a. Tabular format for calculating predictive value and efficiency

	Number with positive test	Number with negative test	Totals
Number sick			
Number not sick			
Totals			

Table 1b.   Total number of subjects equals 100,000

	Number with positive test	Number with negative test	Totals
Number sick			
Number not sick			
Totals			100,000

Table 1c.   The number of sick subjects equals 10,000 and the number of nonsick subjects equals 90,000

	Number with positive test	Number with negative test	Totals
Number sick			10,000
Number not sick			90,000
Totals			100,000

7. The next step requires the estimate of the *sensitivity* of the test. The sensitivity permits the calculation of the number of sick subjects who test positive and the number who test negative. For example, if the sensitivity of the test is 95%, then for every 10,000 sick subjects tested 9500 (95%) will test positive (true positives or TP) and 500 sick subjects will test negative (false negatives or FN). The table looks like Table 1d.

Table 1d.   The number of true positives equals 9500 and the number of false negatives equals 500

	Number with positive test	Number with negative test	Totals
Number sick	9500 (TP)	500 (FN)	10,000
Number not sick			90,000
Totals			100,000

8. Now the estimate of *specificity* is applied to determine the number of nonsick subjects who will test negative (true negatives or TN), and the number of nonsick subjects who will test positive (false positives or FP). If the specificity of the test is 95%, then 85,500 (95% of 90,000) healthy subjects will test negative, and 4500 healthy subjects will test positive. The table looks like Table 1e.

9. Next, the number of positive test results and the number of negative test results are summed. The grand sum, of course, equals 100,000. The completed table looks like Table 1f.

Table 1e.   The number of true negatives equals 85,500 and the number of false positives equals 4500

	Number with positive test	Number with negative test	Totals
Number sick	9500 (TP)	500 (FN)	10,000
Number not sick	4500 (FP)	85,500 (TN)	90,000
Totals			100,000

Table 1f.   The completed table

	Number with positive test	Number with negative test	Totals
Number sick	9500 (TP)	500 (FN)	10,000
Number not sick	4500 (FP)	85,500 (TN)	90,000
Totals	14,000	86,000	100,000

The completed table can now be used to determine the predictive value of a positive result, the predictive value of a negative result, and the overall efficiency of the test.

10. The *predictive value of a positive result* is represented by the percent of all positive results that are true positives; that is,

$$\text{predictive value of positives} = \frac{\text{true positives}}{\text{total positives}} \times 100$$

If we refer back to the completed table we find that there were 9500 true positives and 14,000 positives. (These numbers are shaded in Table 1g.)

Table 1g.   The shaded numbers are used to calculate the predictive value of a positive result

	Number with positive test	Number with negative test	Totals
Number sick	9500 (TP)	500 (FN)	10,000
Number not sick	4500 (FP)	85,500 (TN)	90,000
Totals	14,000	86,000	100,000

Therefore, the predictive value of a positive result is 9500 divided by 14,000 or 67.9%:

$$\text{predictive value of positives} = \frac{9500}{14,000} \times 100 = 67.9\%$$

11. The *predictive value of a negative result* is represented by the percent of all negative results that are true negatives; that is,

$$\text{predictive value of negatives} = \frac{\text{true negatives}}{\text{total negatives}} \times 100$$

If we refer back to the completed table we find that there were 85,500 true negatives and 86,000 total negatives. (These numbers are shaded in Table 1h.) Therefore the predictive value of a negative result is 85,500 divided by 86,000 or 99.4%:

$$\text{predictive value of negatives} = \frac{85,500}{86,000} \times 100 = 99.4\%$$

Table 1h. The shaded numbers are used to calculate the predictive value of a negative result

	Number with positive test	Number with negative test	Totals
Number sick	9500 (TP)	500 (FN)	10,000
Number not sick	4500 (FP)	85,500 (TN)	90,000
Totals	14,000	86,000	100,000

12. The *efficiency* of the test is represented by the percent of all results that are true results, whether positive or negative; that is,

$$\text{efficiency} = \frac{\text{true positives} + \text{true negatives}}{\text{grand total}} \times 100$$

If we refer back to the completed table we find that there were 9500 true positives and 85,500 true negatives for a total number of true results of 95,000. The grand total of all results was 100,000. (These numbers are shaded in Table 1i.) Therefore the efficiency of the test is 9500 plus 85,500 divided by 100,000, or 95.0%:

$$\text{efficiency} = \frac{9500 + 85,500}{100,000} \times 100 = 95.0\%$$

Table 1i. The shaded numbers are used to calculate efficiency

	Number with positive test	Number with negative test	Totals
Number sick	9500 (TP)	500 (FN)	10,000
Number not sick	4500 (FP)	85,500 (TN)	90,000
Totals	14,000	86,000	100,000

WHAT HAPPENS WHEN PREVALENCE IS CHANGED?

1. Utilizing the same worksheet, and the same sensitivity and specificity, let us see what happens when prevalence goes from 10 to 50%. We start with 100,000 subjects. The worksheet table looks like Table 2a.

Table 2a.   New blank table. Total number of subjects equals 100,000

	Number with positive test	Number with negative test	Totals
Number sick			
Number not sick			
Totals			100,000

2. Since *prevalence* is now 50,000/100,000 (50%), there are 50,000 sick subjects and 50,000 nonsick subjects. The worksheet table looks like Table 2b.

Table 2b.   The number of sick subjects equals 50,000 and the number of nonsick subjects equals 50,000

	Number with positive test	Number with negative test	Totals
Number sick			50,000
Number not sick			50,000
Totals			100,000

3. *Sensitivity* remains constant at 95%. Therefore 95% of the 50,000 sick subjects will test positive (true positives). The table looks like Table 2c.

Table 2c.   The number of true positives equals 47,500 and the number of false negatives equals 2500

	Number with positive test	Number with negative test	Totals
Number sick	47,500 (TP)	2500 (FN)	50,000
Number not sick			50,000
Totals			100,000

4. *Specificity* remains constant at 95%. Therefore 95% of the 50,000 nonsick subjects will test negative (true negatives). The completed table looks like Table 2d.

Table 2d. The completed table. The number of true negatives equals 47,500 and the number of false positives equals 2500

	Number with positive test	Number with negative test	Totals
Number sick	47,500 (TP)	2500 (FN)	50,000
Number not sick	2500 (FP)	47,500 (TN)	50,000
Totals	50,000	50,000	100,000

5. The *predictive value of a positive result* is obtained by dividing the number of true positives by the total number of positive results. Table 2d indicates that there were 47,500 true positives and 50,000 total positives. Therefore,

$$\text{predictive value of positives} = \frac{47,500}{50,000} \times 100 = 95.0\%$$

6. The *predictive value of a negative result* is obtained by dividing the number of true negatives by the total number of negative results. Table 2d indicates that there were 47,500 true negatives and 50,000 total negatives. Therefore,

$$\text{predictive value of negatives} = \frac{47,500}{50,000} \times 100 = 95.0\%$$

7. The *efficiency* of the test is obtained by adding the number of true positives to the number of true negatives and dividing by the total number of subjects tested. Table 2d indicates that there were 47,500 true positives, 47,500 true negatives, and a total of 100,000 subjects tested. Therefore,

$$\text{efficiency} = \frac{47,500 + 47,500}{100,000} \times 100 = 95.0\%$$

Let us now compare what happened to predictive values and efficiency when prevalence changed from 10 to 50%, but sensitivity and specificity remained constant at 95% each (Table 3).

Table 3. The effect of prevalence on predictive values and efficiency

Prevalence	Predictive value of a positive result (%)	Predictive value of a negative result (%)	Overall efficiency
10,000/100,000	67.9	99.4	95.0
50,000/100,000	95.0	95.0	95.0

In this particular example we see that as prevalence increased the predictive value of a positive result increased, whereas the predictive value of a negative result decreased. The exact effect in any particular case varies with sensitivity, specificity, and prevalence. Since there is no simple general rule, and since it is too time consuming to repeat the above calculations each time a predictive value is needed, we have appended a large number of computer-generated tables to this book. The tables make it possible to find positive and negative predictive values, and efficiency, for any combination of sensitivity, specificity, and prevalence.

The model that we have presented is easy to apply to published studies. The three examples detailed below include selected excerpts from recent journal articles and our critical analysis of the data based on the application of the predictive value model for interpreting laboratory data.

BRIEF EXAMPLES FROM THE MEDICAL LITERATURE

Alpha$_1$-Fetoprotein

Below is the published summary of a study by Kohn and Weaver on serum-alpha$_1$-fetoprotein in hepatocellular carcinoma.[1]

> Sera from 2225 patients, 107 with primary hepatocellular carcinoma and 2118 with other diseases, mainly hepatic disorders, were screened for alpha$_1$-fetoprotein (A.F.P.) in serum by a sensitive countercurrent immunoelectrophoretic technique. The screening test detects serum-A.F.P. at concentrations in the order of 200 ng. per ml.; 90 out of the 107 cases of hepatocellular carcinoma, including 5 cases of hepatoblastoma, were A.F.P. positive, and 4 cases which were negative on screening were shown by radioimmunoassay (R.I.A.) to have significantly raised serum-A.F.P. levels. R.I.A. does reveal a greater percentage of A.F.P.-positive cases, but it also poses serious problems of interpretation; however, R.I.A. is essential in monitoring progress and response to treatment, especially in hepatoblastoma and malignant teratoma. Raised A.F.P. levels after surgery or chemotherapy indicate failure of treatment, though the converse does not necessarily apply. In malignant testicular teratoma, the frequency of raised serum-A.F.P. was 32 out of 117 cases (27%). Significant amounts of A.F.P. were found in 9 cases of carcinoma other than hepatocellular. Raised A.F.P. levels, usually transient and in most cases small, were found in 16 cases of liver disease other than hepatocellular carcinoma, and in 14 cases in which a diagnosis was not available. *The frequency of false-positives was 1.8%. A. F. P. detection and assay correctly performed and interpreted is a valuable, sensitive, and specific serological marker of hepatocellular carcinoma.* The screening technique described here seems to be adequate for the detection of hepatocellular carcinoma in most cases.

The summary suggests that the false-positive rate for this test is only 1.8%. But this statistic is inaccurate, because the authors failed to calculate the predictive value of a positive result, and therefore they failed to appreciate that the false-positive rate is the percentage of all *positive* results that were false positives.

Let us arrange their data in our worksheet format (Table 4).

Table 4. Alpha$_1$-Fetoprotein data arranged in tabular format

	Number with positive test	Number with negative test	Totals
Cancer of liver	90	17	107
No cancer of liver	39	2079	2118
Totals	129	2096	2225

We can now derive the correct numbers:

$$\text{sensitivity} = 90/107 = 84.1\%$$

$$\text{specificity} = 2079/2118 = 98.2\%$$

$$\text{predictive value of positive result} = 90/129 = 69.8\%$$

$$\text{false-positive rate} = 100\% - 69.8\% = 30.2\%$$

The false-positive rate is *not* 1.8%, but rather 30.2%.[2]

Food Antibodies

Davies and associates reported on the association of food antibodies and myo-cardial infarction (MI), and they concluded that the possession of antibody to cow's milk protein and egg white seemed highly predictive of death. They published the following summary[3]:

> The presence and level of serum antibody to reconstituted heat-dried cow's milk, boiled egg white, and gluten, have been determined in 216 patients who had had a myocardial infarction (M.I.) and in 144 control hospital patients. A higher proportion of M.I. patients than controls had antibodies to dried milk and prob-ably to egg, but not to gluten. These differences in proportion were very striking in the M.I. patients who died within six months of infarction. The possession of antibody to cow's milk protein and egg white in blood-samples taken soon after infarction seems, therefore, to be highly predictive of death. Mortality was increased almost three fold if either antibody was present. It is considered that they are of considerable significance and have a causal relationship with myocardial infarction through an immunological mechanism. The results support an immunological hypothesis of coronary heart-disease and atheroma.[3]

Is the presence of antibody highly predictive of death? To answer this we arranged their data in our worksheet format. By consolidating the large array of data pre-sented in the author's tables we obtained Table 5.

Table 5.   Milk antibody data arranged in tabular format

Totals	Number with positive milk antibody	Number with negative milk antibody	Totals
MI—died	29	10	39
MI—alive	80	94	174
Totals	109	104	213

We can now derive the correct numbers:

$$\text{sensitivity} = 29/39 = 74.3\%$$

$$\text{specificity} = 94/174 = 54.0\%$$

$$\text{predictive value of a positive result} = 29/109 = 26.6\%$$

$$\text{efficiency} = (29 + 94)/213 = 57.7\%$$

This is an extremely poor test. The predictive value of a positive result is only 26.6%. The predictive value of the egg-antibody test is equally poor.[4]

Intravenous Pyelogram

Dr. Murray Katz described a probability graph that could be used to obtain the predictive value of a highly sensitive diagnostic test.[5] Unfortunately, the author's attempts to simplify the use of the predictive value concept resulted in the generation of misleading information. A quote from the penultimate paragraph of his paper follows:

> If a hypertensive patient is suspected of having a 10 percent chance of having renovascular hypertension, and one wished to know if a diagnostic test, such as an intravenous pyelogram, which, it is assumed has a 10 percent false-positive frequency, is worthwhile, what is the probability that the patient has the disease if the pyelogram is positive, assuming that the hypertensive intravenous pyelogram detects most of renovascular hypertension? From 0.10 on the abcissa, one draws a line to the 0.10 false positive frequency curve, and from this intersection, a horizontal line to the y-axis, which is intersected at about 53 percent. Hence, with a 10 percent chance that the patient had the disease before the test, and 10 percent false positivity, a positive test gives no more information than the flip of a coin, and is thus probably not worth doing.

Dr. Katz is confused. Let us examine his hypothetical example utilizing our worksheet and compare it to flipping a coin. In his hypothetical example the sensitivity of an intravenous pyelogram (IVP) equals 100%, the specificity of an IVP equals 90%, and the prevalence of renovascular hypertension is equal to 10% (10,000/100,000). If we put this into our worksheet format we obtain Table 6.

Table 6. Dr. Katz's hypothetical IVP data arranged in tabular format

	Number with positive IVP	Number with negative IVP	Totals
Renovascular hypertension	10,000	Zero	10,000
No renovascular hypertension	9000	81,000	90,000
Totals	19,000	81,000	100,000

Predictive value of a positive result = 10,000/19,000 = 52.6%.
Predictive value of a negative result = 81,000/81,000 = 100%.
Efficiency = (10,000 + 81,000)/100,000 = 91%.

Now let us examine the same situation, but this time we will substitute a coin-flip for the IVP (Table 7). A coin-flip has a sensitivity of 50% and a specificity of 50%. Prevalence remains at 10%.

Table 7. Coin flip data arranged in tabular format

	Number with positive coin flip	Number with negative coin flip	Totals
Renovascular hypertension	5000	5000	10,000
No renovascular hypertension	45,000	45,000	90,000
Totals	50,000	50,000	100,000

Predictive value of a positive result = 5000/50,000 = 10%.
Predictive value of a negative result = 45,000/50,000 = 90%.
Efficiency = (5000 + 45,000)/100,000 = 50%.

We can now compare the results obtained with the hypothetical IVP test to those obtained with the flip of a coin when prevalence equals 10% (Table 8).

Table 8. Comparison of hypothetical IVP data and coin flip

Test	Predictive value of a positive (%)	Predictive value of a negative (%)	Efficiency (%)
IVP	52.6	100	91.0
Coin flip	10.0	90.0	50.0

In every case the IVP test is better than a flip of the coin.[6]

REFERENCES

1. Kohn, J. and Weaver, P. C. Serum-alpha$_1$-fetoprotein in hepatocellular carcinoma. *Lancet* **ii:** 334–336, 1974.
2. Galen, Robert S. False-positives. *Lancet* **ii:** 1081, 1974.
3. Davies, D. F., Rees, B. W. G., Johnson, A. P., Elwood, P. C., and Abernethy, M. Food antibodies and myocardial infarction. *Lancet* **i:** 1012–1014, 1974.
4. Galen, Robert S. Food antibodies and myocardial infarction. *Lancet* **ii:** 832, 1974. 1974.
5. Katz, Murray A. A probability graph describing the predictive value of a highly sensitive diagnostic test. *N. Engl. J. Med.,* **291:** 1115–1116, 1974.
6. Galen, Robert S. Interpretation of laboratory tests. *N. Engl. J. Med.* **292:** 433–434, 1975.

CHAPTER 6

COMBINATION TESTING—MULTIPLE TESTING

SO far we have discussed the predictive value of a single test result. But in fact it is rare to use the result of a single test as the final arbiter of a medical decision. Therefore, let us explore some hypothetical and some actual examples of multiple test situations to illustrate what happens when we apply more than one test to a clinical problem.

Two independent tests in a screening or diagnostic situation, can be used in three different ways:

1. Test A is applied first and all those with a positive result are retested with test B. [Series approach: $(++) = +.$]
2. Test B is applied first and all those with a positive result are retested with test A. [Series approach: $(++) = +.$]
3. Tests A and B can be used together and all those with positive results for either or both tests are considered to be positives. [Parallel approach: $(+-) = +, (++) = +, (-+) = +.$]

Which approach or sequence is best? This depends on the testing situation and the sensitivity and specificity of the individual tests and their combinations. For the sake of this discussion, we examine the *hypothetical* data presented in Table 1.

Table 1.   Hypothetical data for two tests A and B

| | Test Results | | | | |
	A+B−	A−B+	A+B+	A−B−	Totals
Disease	190	40	760	10	1,000
Nondisease	9,800	4,850	100	84,250	99,000
Totals	9,990	4,890	860	84,260	100,000

The sensitivity of test A is $(190 + 760)/1000 = 95\%$. The sensitivity of test B is $(40 + 760)/1000 = 80\%$. The sensitivity of the series combination (A *and* B positive) $= 760/1000 = 76\%$, but the sensitivity of the parallel combination (A *or* B positive) is $(190 + 40 + 760)/1000 = 99\%$. With parallel testing, the combined sensitivity is greater than the individual sensitivities of the contributing tests.

Similarly, the specificity of test A is $(4850 + 84,250)/99,000 = 90\%$. The specificity of test B is $(9800 + 84,250)/99,000 = 95\%$. The specificity of the series combination is $(9800 + 4850 + 84,250)/99,000 = 99.9\%$, since A+B−, A−B+, and A−B− are all interpreted as negative results in series testing. The specificity of the parallel combination is $84,250/99,000 = 85.1\%$, since only A−B− is considered a negative response.

Parallel testing results in the highest sensitivity but the lowest specificity, whereas series testing results in the lowest sensitivity but highest specificity. Table 2 summarizes these findings.

The series approach can be taken as either A then B, or B then A. Let us use our hypothetical tests to see how test sequence affects the final outcome in screening for disease. We let disease prevalence be 1% in a population of 100,000. Test

Table 2.   Combination testing for hypothetical data

	Test(s)	Sensitivity (%)	Specificity (%)
Single	A	95.0	90.0
Single	B	80.0	95.0
Series	A and B	76.0	99.9
Parallel	A or B	99.0	85.1

A is applied first and all those with a positive result are retested with test B (Tables 3 and 4).

Table 3.   Series approach: A then B

	Test A positive	Test A negative	Totals
Disease	950	50	1,000 (sensitivity = 95%)
Nondisease	9,900	89,100	99,000 (specificity = 90%)
Totals	10,850	89,150	100,000

We see that on initial testing there are 10,850 positive test results using test A alone. These are, however, presumptive positives and will be retested with test B (Table 4).

Table 4.   Series approach: A then B

	Test B positive	Test B negative	Totals
Disease	760	190	950 (sensitivity = 80%)
Nondisease	495	9,405	9,900 (specificity = 95%)
Totals	1,255	9,595	10,850

The predictive value of a positive result is 60.6% (760/1255).

Now let us take the same tests and the same prevalence, but this time test B is applied first and all those with a positive result are retested with test A (Tables 5 and 6).

Table 5.   Series approach: B then A

	Test B positive	Test B negative	Totals
Disease	800	200	1,000 (sensitivity = 80%)
Nondisease	4,950	94,050	99,000 (specificity = 95%)
Totals	5,750	94,250	100,000

We see that on initial testing there are 5750 positive test results using test B alone. These are, however, presumptive positives and will be retested with test A (Table 6).

Table 6. Series approach: B then A

	Test A positive	Test A negative	Totals
Disease	760	40	800 (sensitivity = 95%)
Nondisease	495	4455	4950 (specificity = 90%)
Totals	1255	4495	5750

The predictive value of a positive result is 60.6% (760/1255).

The above analyses show the most effective way to use laboratory tests in series. The first sequence (A then B) resulted in the retesting of 10,850 patients. There were then 1255 patients diagnosed as positive with a predictive value of 60.6%. When the sequence was reversed to B then A, only 5750 patients needed retesting. There were 1255 positives with a predictive value of 60.6%. Both sequences, using the series approach, produced 1255 positives with 760 true positives in the group. However, the latter sequence (B then A) is considered more effective since fewer patients required retesting to get to the same end result. This analysis assumes that both tests cost about the same to perform in the laboratory. If two tests are going to be used in series, the optimal sequence can be determined using the predictive value model as described here.

What about parallel testing in this same situation? In this case tests A and B are applied simultaneously. If either A or B or both is positive, this is considered a positive test. A negative test requires A *and* B to be negative. (Table 7).

Table 7. Parallel approach: A or B positive = positive test

	A *or* B positive	A *and* B negative	Totals
Disease	990	10	1,000 (sensitivity = 99%)
Nondisease	14,750	84,250	99,000 (specificity = 85.1%)
Totals	15,740	84,260	100,000

The predictive value of a positive result is 6.3% (990/15,740).

For tests run in parallel (A and B determined simultaneously), but considered positive if *either* component is positive, and negative only if *both* are negative, the sensitivity is higher and the specificity is lower than in comparable series testing. The sensitivity is increased because some diseased patients are positive on one test, but not on the other. Similarly, there are more false-positive results in nondisease patients. The parallel approach outlined above has the highest sensitivity. It detects the greatest number of diseased patients in the population. However it also produces the greatest number of false positives. In this case the predictive value is so low (6.3%) that this test might be unacceptable for any disease. Of all the approaches, the parallel approach requires the most laboratory work since both tests are performed on all patients in the population.

We can now demonstrate these relationships with actual examples from laboratory studies. First we examine data obtained from our study of serum enzymes in myocardial infarction. [1,2] Utilizing the final clinical diagnosis as our reference point, we used a computer program to calculate the sensitivity and specificity of single and multiple enzyme assays. Positive results were defined as follows. CPK on day 1 $\geq$40 IU/l; SGOT on day 1 $\geq$40 IU/l; and LDH on day 3 $\geq$250 U/l. The results are summarized in Table 8.

Table 8. Sensitivity and specificity of single and combination enzyme tests in diagnosing myocardial infarction in the coronary care unit

TEST*	Sensitivity (%)	Specificity (%)
CPK	95.7	57.1
SGOT	91.4	73.5
LDH	87.2	90.5
SGOT and LDH	82.2	92.9
CPK and LDH	82.2	92.9
CPK and SGOT	87.2	83.7
CPK, SGOT, and LDH	77.7	95.2

* All combination results interpreted in series fashion as listed.

It can be seen that series testing always decreases sensitivity and increases specificity relative to single tests or smaller test combinations. It should be clear what effect this has on overall results, that is, more cases missed, but a higher predictive value for a positive result (fewer false positives).

What about parallel testing? As part of a multiple screening study conducted at the District of Columbia General Hospital, four commonly used screening tests for heart disease and hypertension were evaluated by Kurlander and co-workers.[3] A total of 858 persons underwent multiple screening and a complete diagnostic examination for cardiovascular disease. Only 690 of the 858 received all four screening tests, and the data that follow relate to this group (Table 9). Of these 690, only 233 were finally diagnosed as having heart disease, hypertension, or both.

Table 9. Sensitivity and specificity of individual screening tests and a complete battery of four tests in identifying heart disease and/or hypertension*

Test	Sensitivity (%)	Specificity (%)
Blood pressure	86.3	74.0
History	54.1	58.0
ECG	50.6	76.6
X-Ray	47.6	92.1
Total battery (parallel)	96.6	31.9

* Modified from Kurlander et al.[3]

We can see from Table 10 that there was a positive response in 96.6% (225/233) of patients diagnosed as having heart disease and/or hypertension when the four screening tests were administered in parallel (one or more positive tests equals a positive response). Unfortunately, parrallel testing has very low specificity and all four tests were negative in only 146 of the 457 patients without heart disease or hypertension (31.9% specificity).

Table 10.   Predictive value of four tests applied in parallel

	Any one of four tests positive	All four tests negative	Totals
Heart disease or hypertension	225	8	233 (sensitivity = 96.6%)
Nondisease	311	146	457 (specificity = 31.9%)
Totals	536	154	690

Prevalence is 33.8%. The predictive value of a positive test is 42.0% (225/536). Efficiency is 53.8%.

These results are startling because even with a prevalence of 33.8%, the predictive value is only 42%, and the efficiency, or number of patients properly classified by the test battery, is only 53.8%.

In an investigation of the value of different combinations of tests, Kurlander and co-workers interpreted their results in all cases in a parallel fashion (positive on any one test in the combination = positive screening test). Table 11 is from their study.[3]

Table 11.   Sensitivity and specificity of various test combinations for heart disease and hypertension*

Test	Sensitivity (%)	Specificity (%)
Blood pressure and history	93.1	43.5
Blood pressure and ECG	92.3	55.6
Blood pressure and X-ray	90.6	69.8
ECG and history	77.3	45.5
History and X-ray	72.5	52.7
ECG and X-ray	67.4	70.7
Blood pressure, ECG, and history	96.1	33.9
Blood pressure, ECG, and X-ray	94.4	52.7
Blood pressure, history, and X-ray	94.0	40.9
ECG, history, and X-ray	82.0	41.4

* Adapted from Kurlander et al.[3]

While it is clear that combining tests and interpreting them in parallel increases the sensitivity, the loss of specificity is equally striking. The effect of this approach is to increase the number of cases detected (high sensitivity) and to generate a very large number of false positives.

At this point a comment on statistically independent tests is in order. At the beginning of this chapter we discussed applying two independent tests and proceeded to illustrate our points with a hypothetical example. The application of sensitivity and specificity percentages in series testing can only be valid if the tests (A and B) are independent of each other. Otherwise the first test would serve to preselect the population for the second test. Therefore, if the tests are not independent, the sensitivity and specificity percentages are no longer valid in the selected subpopulation. If the tests are not independent, then it is not valid to use the available sensitivity and specificity to accurately predict the outcome. However, such an analysis would indicate the general effects to be derived from a series approach. Similarly, the performance of a repeat test and the use of the same sensitivity and specificity as applied to the unselected population will provide only an approximation of what would happen. An accurate analysis requires that the second sample (selected subpopulation) redistribute itself entirely to resemble the first population. This, of course, is unlikely. Therefore, the calculation of predictive values based on repeat testing with the same test, or a combination of tests in series, is fraught with statistical difficulties. It does however, demonstrate the general beneficial effects of repeat testing, but it does not result in a precise predictive value percent that can be affixed to the diagnostic process. The calculated predictive value is always higher than the actual predictive value of the testing situation. Furthermore, the degree of error depends on the degree to which the two tests are correlated.

We have heard from many of our colleagues that our predictive value model, while technically quite accurate, is nevertheless unrealistic. They claim it is unlikely that a single test would be used in isolation to arrive at a diagnosis and that the astute clinician or laboratorian utilizes several tests, trend analysis, and judgement to permit him to exceed the predictive value of a single test.

In an attempt to explore this point, we submitted laboratory test results on 96 subjects in our MI study (see Chapter 13) to five professors of clinical pathology at the 1974 Laboratory Medicine course held at Given Pathobiology Institute in Aspen, Colorado. For each case we gave the physician total CPK, LDH, and SGOT values on the day of admission and for 2 subsequent days. The clinical pathologists were assigned the task of placing each case into one of two categories, either myocardial infarction or no myocardial infarction. In addition, we processed the same data through a computer. The computer was programmed to report a positive result (MI) when all of the following results were obtained: CPK, >40 U/l on day 1, SGOT, >40 U/l on day 1, *and* LDH >250 U/l on day 3.

Table 12 provides a compact summary of the sensitivity, specificity, and so on for each individual and the computer. It is clear that most of the clinical pathologists, utilizing their judgement, favor specificity at the expense of sensitivity, and therefore they obtain a high predictive value. The computer, which was programmed by a clinical pathologist, gives similar results. The efficiency of most of the pathologists and of the computer is not too impressive, considering that the number of true MIs comprised 50% of the total. The results also suggest that a computer program is equal to, if not better than, the average professor of clinical

Table 12.   Summary of sensitivity, specificity, predictive value, and efficiency obtained by five pathologists and a computer program

Pathologist	Sensitivity (%)	Specificity (%)	Predictive value of a positive (%)	Efficiency (%)
A	71	96	94	83
B	73	96	95	84
C	75	94	92	84
D	77	98	97	88
E	92	90	90	91
Computer	80	95	95	86

pathology when it comes to analyzing a series of test results. It also appears that "judgement" may simply be a euphemism for "bias."

The predictive value format is a useful way of analyzing *any* diagnostic process, whether it be a single test, a series of tests, a panel of tests, a computer interpretation, a trend analysis, a multivariate analysis, or a clinical judgement. In each case the final product must be a positive or negative result, that is, a diagnosis. Therefore the predictive value format is a suitable method for evaluating the accuracy of any analytical process and the accompanying error rates.

REFERENCES

1. Galen, R. S., Reiffel, J. A., and Gambino, S. R. Diagnosis of acute myocardial infarction. *JAMA* **232:** 145–147, 1975.
2. Galen, R. S. and Gambino, S. R. Enzymes and isoenzymes. In *Pathology Annual*, Harry Ioachim (Ed.). Appleton, Century, and Crofts, New York, 1975.
3. Kurlander, A. B., Hill, E. H., and Enterline, P. E. An evaluation of some commonly used screening tests for heart disease and hypertension. *J. Chron. Dis.* **2:** 427–439, 1955.

CHAPTER 7

SENSITIVITY, SPECIFICITY, PREDICTIVE VALUE, OR EFFICIENCY

WHICH is preferable, a test with the highest sensitivity, the highest specificity, the highest predictive value for a positive result, *or* the highest efficiency? It is not possible to have all at the same time. The higher the sensitivity, the lower the specificity. As shown in Table 1 even tests for death are not 100% sensitive and 100% specific (see also Chapter 2).

Table 1.   Tests for death

Test	Sensitivity (%)	Specificity (%)
Flat EEG	100	<100
Rigor mortis and livor mortis	<100	100

The highest sensitivity (preferably 100%) is desired in the following situations:

- The disease is serious and should not be missed.
  AND
- The disease is treatable.
  AND
- False-positive results do not lead to serious psychologic or economic trauma to the patient.

Example   *Pheochromocytoma. This disease can be fatal if missed; but if diagnosed it is nearly 100% curable.*

Here we want the highest sensitivity possible. If we make a false-positive diagnosis we can repeat the test as well as perform a different test on urine before attempting surgery.

Other examples include phenylketonuria, venereal disease, and other treatable infectious diseases.

The highest specificity (preferably 100%) is desired in the following situations:

- The disease is serious but is *not* treatable or curable.
  AND
- The knowledge that the disease is absent has psychologic or public health value.
  AND
- False-positive results can lead to serious psychologic or economic trauma to the patient.

Example   *Multiple sclerosis. The disease is serious but not treatable or curable.*

We do not want *any* false-positive results; therefore, we must opt for the highest possible specificity and thereby sacrifice sensitivity. If a case of multiple sclerosis is missed, there is no need for concern because the patient will return. On the other hand, a false-positive diagnosis can cause serious psychologic harm.

Other examples include most occult cancers and any other serious but untreatable disease.

A high predictive value for a positive result is essential in the following situation:

- Treatment of a false positive might have serious consequences.

Example   *Occult cancer of the lung. A test for this disease should have a predictive value of a positive result of 100%, because the only treatment available at present is lobectomy or radiation.*

If a lobectomy is performed or radiation given to a patient without cancer, the consequences might be disastrous.

The highest efficiency is desired in the following situations:

- The disease is serious but treatable.
  AND
- False-positive results *and* false-negative results are essentially equally serious or damaging.

Example   *Myocardial infarction. The disease may be fatal but it is treatable.*

If a case is missed irreparable harm may result; but equal harm can be caused if the diagnosis is made when an infarct is not present. Therefore, the wise clinician has always opted for efficiency.

Other examples include lupus erythematosus, some forms of leukemia and lymphoma, and diabetes mellitus.

A full discussion of this subject, in relation to the diagnosis of myocardial infarction, can be found in Chapter 13.

CHAPTER 8

PKU—LOW INCIDENCE. A TEST OF THE MODEL

PHENYLKETONURIA (PKU), a disease with a very low incidence at birth, provides us with an opportunity to test our theoretical model against actual clinical data. Since screening for PKU is required in most states, there is abundant data available on incidence, sensitivity, specificity, and predictive value.

The biochemical defect in PKU is the absence in the liver of phenylalanine hydroxylase activity. This enzyme catalyzes the conversion of phenylalanine to tyrosine (Figure 1). The absence of phenylalanine hydroxylase results in the

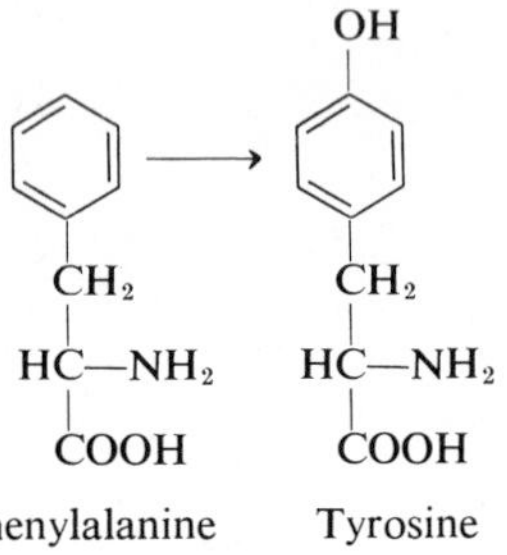

OH

CH_2 CH_2
HC—NH_2 HC—NH_2
COOH   COOH
Phenylalanine   Tyrosine

Figure 1. Conversion of phenylalanine to tyrosine.

accumulation of certain metabolites in the urine of these patients (Figure 2). If PKU is not treated, severe mental retardation will develop in the majority of children with this biochemical lesion. Most pediatricians agree that if an appropriate diet (low phenylalanine) is instituted before 3 months of age, normal intelligence will result. Children must follow the diet stringently until about the age of 5 or 6 years, at which time hyperphenylalaninemia seems to have no effect on growth and development. Given the above considerations it would seem obviously worthwhile to proceed to screen for PKU in all newborns.

Before proceeding with the obvious, however, additional essential information is needed. What, for example, is the incidence of PKU? The incidence at birth is estimated to be between 1/10,000 and 1/20,000, which is very low. Without knowing anymore about plans for a screening program, we can evaluate the ideal effectiveness of a screening program by referring to our tables of predictive values. Let us assume an ideal test—one with a sensitivity of 100% and a specificity of 99.99%. Such a test would never give a false-negative result, and there would be only 1 false-positive result in every 10,000 non-PKU children tested. Such a test does not exist, *but the predictive value of a positive PKU test under these ideal conditions should be only 50%.* Therefore we would be concerned about proceeding rapidly with widespread screening programs and legislation to regulate those activities.

Is the theoretical prediction of a high false-positive rate born out in practice? The answer is yes. MacCready and Hussey reported the results of the Massachusetts program after testing 135,000 newborns.[1] Fourteen cases of PKU were detected. Three of the cases had initial phenylalanine levels at the time of discharge of less than 20 mg/dl. All 14 cases, however, had levels above 6 mg/dl. In screening for a disease with such a low incidence, that may be amenable to treatment, we cannot afford to miss any cases. Therefore, a cutoff point of 6 mg/dl was instituted. When such a cutoff was used, however, the authors found that 1 in 2000 non-PKU infants had levels above 6 mg/dl.

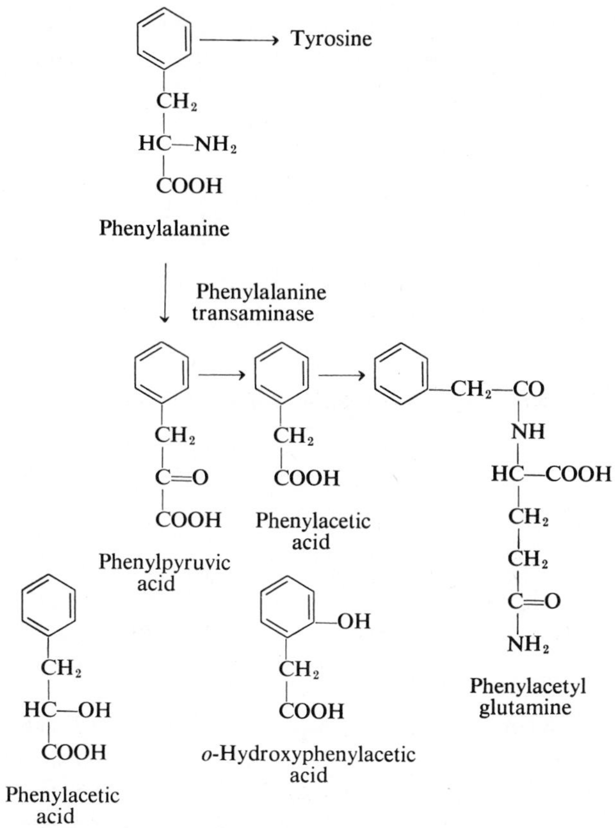

Figure 2. Metabolites of phenylalanine seen when conversion to tyrosine is blocked.

There are several reasons why newborns without PKU (or genetic variants of PKU, heterozygotes, etc.) may have this elevation in blood phenylalanine. Hyperphenylalaninemia may be found in premature infants with immature metabolic pathways. The most common example is the transient hyperphenylalaninemia associated with hypertyrosinemia. As many as 20% of low-birth-weight infants have delayed development of tyrosine transaminase and may exhibit increased phenylalanine on this basis. Hyperphenylalaninemia may also be found in liver disease, a variety of pathological conditions, and other metabolic diseases. These moderate and transient elevations cause "false positives" in screening for PKU, in that the hyperphenylalaninemia does not lead to mental retardation, and so forth. In the MacCready and Hussey report, only 3 babies and elevations about 20 mg% and did not have PKU. Two of them were premature.

A critical decision must be made. Should a cutoff of 6 mg/dl, which gives a sensitivity of 100% and a specificity of 99.95% be used or should a cutoff of 20 mg/dl, which gives a sensitivity of only 78.6% but a specificity greater than 99.99%, be used? The low cutoff gives 100% sensitivity and all cases of PKU will be found. However, a large number of false positives will be obtained that will require identification by retesting. On the other hand, the high cutoff of 20 mg/dl eliminates the false-positive problem and thereby minimizes the financial and emotional costs incurred with retesting. Retesting is expensive and requires family cooperation in excess of that required for the initial screening test performed at the time of discharge from the hospital. A cutoff point of 20 mg/dl, however, would actually miss 3 out of 14 or 21% of potentially affected children.

One might wonder why a baby with genuine PKU would not have a blood level above 20 mg/dl. The answer is really quite straightforward. Since discharge from the hospital is "as soon as possible," babies now often go home on day 3 of life, whereas at one time they stayed a week. By day 3, a PKU baby may not have had enough protein intake to challenge his or her defective enzyme pathway. Therefore, although the enzyme activity is absent, the level has not yet climbed to 20 mg/dl. Tables 1 and 2 detail the two screening alternatives. This data is taken

Table 1.   Screening with a 6 mg/dl blood level cutoff

	Number with positive test	Number with negative test	Totals
PKU	14	0	14
Non-PKU	67	134,919	134,986
Totals	81	134,919	135,000

from the screening of 135,000 Massachusetts newborns.[1] The incidence of 14/135,000 is approximately 1/10,000. The sensitivity is 100%. The specificity is 99.95% which is explained by the 1/2,000 non-PKU babies with elevations above 6 mg/dl. The predictive value is 14/81 or 17.3%, which means that when the above test is employed in screening newborns, 82.7% of the positive results will be in non-PKU babies and will be false-positive tests for PKU. Only 17.3% of the positive screenees will have PKU determined by further evaluation. This seems to be a poor approach, and yet *all* of the cases will be found. Let us examine the

Table 2.   Screening with a 20 mg/dl blood level cutoff

	Number with positive test	Number with negative test	Totals
PKU	11	3	14
Non-PKU	3	134,983	134,986
Totals	14	134,986	135,000

alternative approach (Table 2). With the higher cutoff point (20 mg/dl), the sensitivity is reduced to 11/14 or 78.6%. The specificity is raised, however, to 99.998%. The predictive value of this approach is 11/14 or 78.6%, meaning that over three-quarters of the positives on the screening test actually have the disease. With this approach, followup is required in fewer patients, with much less cost and emotional distress to parents of nondiseased children. This program also does not require the cooperation of patients to distinguish true positives from false positives. In terms of the entire population, 3 cases of the disease are missed. Because it may be possible to prevent the development of mental retardation in a child, this approach (screening with a cutoff point of 20 mg/dl) has been considered unacceptable. We have therefore proceeded to screen at the lower level.

According to the model, we see that a program using a level of 6 mg/dl to screen for PKU would have a predictive value of only 17%, which can be found simply by looking in the predictive value tables under a rate of 10/100,000. A test with a sensitivity of 100% and a specificity of 99.95% has a predictive value of 17%.

Have others verified the poor predictive value of screening for PKU? Dr. Neil Holtzman and co-workers at Johns Hopkins sent questionnaires to each state health department in the United States during 1970, as well as to the departments in the provinces of Ontario and Quebec. The authors verified and documented all of our theoretical expectations. They noted, "The infants in whom a diagnosis of PKU was confirmed constituted only 5.1% of all infants with presumptive positive screening tests." The predictive value of routine general screening appears to be only 5.1%, with a 94.9% false-positive rate. What is even more alarming is that, "More than 10% of infants with PKU are either not being screened or are not being detected by screening." In routine practice, even with the lower cutoff point, the sensitivity is not 100%.[2]

Holtzman and associates tried to identify factors associated with false-positive tests in their survey:

1. Low birth weight. Infants with birth weights of less than 2500 grams accounted for 44% of all elevated tests in infants screened at 9 days of age or older in regions in which screening was performed before nursery discharge.

2. Race. In the four southern states from which data were available, the estimated incidence of elevated tests was 2.7 times higher in nonwhite than white infants.

3. Elevated tyrosine. Among infants with elevated phenylalanine levels, 41% of those with birth weights of less than 2500 grams and 23.6% with birth weights of 2500 grams or more had elevated tyrosines. Since PKU involves a block in the conversion of phenylalanine to tyrosine, an elevation of tyrosine is unlikely in PKU. An elevation of tyrosine usually reflects a transient defect in tyrosine metabolism, often on the basis of prematurity.[3]

MORE PROBLEMS

We do not understand the biochemical basis for the mental defect in PKU. Furthermore, several assumptions underlying PKU screening have a profound effect on the decision to screen for this disease, and these assumptions need constant reevaluation.

Assumption 1   *All children with PKU will be retarded unless treated.*

This is not the case at all, and the discovery of persons with untreated PKU who have normal intelligence has been documented in the literature.[4,5] Therefore, how is it determined which babies with PKU really need treatment? What percentage of babies with PKU do not require treatment?

Assumption 2   *The treatment is harmless.*

This is not true. Complications and deficiency states in children placed on the low phenylalanine diet are on record. The incorrect diagnosis of PKU and subsequent treatment of children with mild forms of hyperphenylalaninemia have resulted in death from phenylalanine deficiency.[6] Furthermore, the diet requires strict co-operation on the part of parents and child.

Assumption 3   *The diet always works.*

This is not the case at all. Not all children with PKU who are started on the diet early in life achieve normal mental development. A possible explanation for this is *in utero* damage caused by hyperphenylalaninemia.

Assumption 4   *Treating children with PKU who would otherwise suffer mental retardation decreases the amount of mental retardation in society, and with it, the number of children requiring institutionalization for this problem.*

This may not be true at all. When phenylketonuric women become pregnant, their offspring may suffer from the *in utero* effects of hyperphenylyalaninemia unless the mother returns to a low phenylalanine diet during gestation. This is not a theoretical consideration. Three phenylketonuric mothers had among them *14 non-phenlyketonuric* but mentally retarded children.[7] Other similar cases have been reported, and there is now a demand for routine urine testing for PKU for all women at the first prenatal visit and at premarital examinations, so that dietary treatment can be instituted during their pregnancies.[5,8]

What are the alternatives? Most states now have laws requiring screening of all newborns for PKU, so the physician has very little choice. Presently, over 3 million neonates are screened for PKU each year in the United States at a cost of over $10 million.[9] This seems like a large sum of money to spend on the small group of children (300) who would be affected by PKU. A much simpler approach, which would cost a fraction of the amount, would be to perform an intensive examination of all newborns in PKU families who had already been identified. It is estimated that this would permit identification of approximately half of all new cases.[10] The massive and costly screening of all newborns would be required to find the other half. This index case approach seems to be a reasonable compromise. In fact, if the pursuit of index cases were carried out with the same emotional fervor as the institution of mandatory screening, the case-finding rate could be significantly higher and still remain less costly than mandatory routine screening.

REFERENCES

1. MacCready, R. A. and Hussey, M. G. Newborn phenylketonuria detection program in Massachusetts. *Am. J. Public Health.* **54:** 2075–2081, 1964

2. Holtzman, N. A., Meek, A. G., Mellits, E. D. Neonatal screening for phenylketonuria, I. Effectiveness. *JAMA* **229:** 667–670, 1974.

3. Holtzman, N. A., Meek, A. G., and Mellits, E. D. Neonatal screening for phenylketonuria, IV, Factors influencing the occurrence of false positives. *Am. J. Public Health* **64:** 775–779, 1974.

4. Perry, T. L., Hansen, S., Tischler, B., Bunting, R., and Diamond, S. Glutamine in phenyl-ketonuria: A possible cause of the mental defect. *N. Engl. J. Med.* **282:** 761–766, 1970.

5. Perry, T. L., Hansen, S., Tischler, B., Richards, F. M., and Sokol, M. Unrecognized adult phenylketonuria: Implications for obstetrics and psychiatry. *N. Engl. J. Med.* **289:** 395–398, 1973.

6. Buist, N. R. M., and Jhaveri, B. M. A guide to screening newborn infants for inborn errors of metabolism. *J. Pediatr.* **82:** 511–522, 1973.

7. Mabry, C. C., Dennison, J. C., Nelson, T. L., and Son, C. D. Maternal phenylketonuria: Cause of mental retardation in children without metabolic defect. *N. Engl. J. Med.* **269:** 1404–1408, 1963.

8. MacCready, R. A. and Levy, H. L. The problem of maternal phenylketonuria. *Am. J. Obstet. Gynecol.* **113:** 121–128, 1972.

9. Guthrie, R. Mass screening for genetic disease. *Hosp. Prac.* **7:** 93–100, June, 1972.

10. Knox, W. E. Phenylketonuria. In *The Metabolic Basis of Inherited Disease,* J. B. Stanbury, J. B. Wyngaarden, and D. S. Fredrickson (Eds.). McGraw-Hill, New York, 1972, 3rd ed. Chap. 11, pp. 266–295.

CHAPTER 9

METANEPHRINES AND VMA—
HIGH SENSITIVITY, HIGH SPECIFICITY

P HEOCHROMOCYTOMA is a good model for demonstrating the proper use of laboratory tests. In 1957 Armstrong and associates defined the major catabolic pathways of the catecholamines[1] (see Figure 1). They showed that less than 1% of normally synthesized norepinephrine is excreted unchanged in the urine. Thus measurement of epinephrine and norepinephrine is predictably insensitive. Their studies suggest that it would pay to measure vanillylmandelic acid (VMA), metanephrines, homovanillic acid, and 3-methoxy-4-hydroxypenylethyleneglycol (HMPG).

Without the detailed understanding of the metabolic pathways for catecholamines, which has been provided by Armstrong and associates, it would be difficult to select efficient tests. Where we lack such detailed understanding, as in diabetes for example, it is difficult, if not impossible, to find sensitive and specific tests capable of predicting the probable occurrence or absence of a particular diabetic complication.

Armed with the information provided by Armstrong and associates, Stanley Gitlow and his associates at Mt. Sinai Hospital in New York began a systematic study of laboratory screening procedures in 92 subjects with proved pheochromocytoma (pheo), and in 9500 subjects without pheochromocytoma, but with high blood pressure or with paroxysmal symptoms suggestive of pheochromocytoma.[2] The Gitlow study may be used as a model study for the following reasons:

1. Hypertensives and patients with symptoms similar to those seen in pheochromocytoma—not healthy individuals—were used as controls.

2. Ninety-two pateints with proven pheochromocytoma and 9500 controls were studied. Thus the prevalence of pheo in their study was 1%, which comes close the estimated true prevalence of 0.5% in a population of hypertensives.

3. Data were provided on the sensitivity and specificity of each of the tests studied.

Gitlow and associates do not directly state that an individual test has a specific sensitivity and specificity—but that is exactly what their tables provide.

Table 1. Rapid colorimetric screening for pheochromocytoma

Result (ratio o.d. 450 nm/550 nm)	Patients with phecohromocytoma (%)	Patients without pheochromocytoma (%)
>1.30	3.3	99.1
<1.30	96.7	0.9

A ratio of less than 1.30 has a sensitivity of 96.7% and a specificity of 99.1%.

Table 3 is the most interesting and important table because it illustrates what happens when the cutoff level for a positive result is changed. A urine metanephrine concentration of 2.2 μg/mg creatinine has a sensitivity of 100% and a specificity of 98%. If the cutoff point is raised to 4.5 μg/mg creatinine, then specificity rises to 100%, but sensitivity drops to 82%.

Table 2. Bidirectional paper chromatographic determination of vanillylmandelic acid

VMA Level	Pheochromocytoma (%)	Non-pheochromocytema (%)
>5 μg/mg creatine	96.4	0
<5 μg/mg creatinine	3.6	100

A urine VMA level of 5 μg/mg creatinine determined by bidirectional paper
chromatography has a sensitivity of 96.4% and a specificity of 100%.

Table 3. Column chromatographic determination of total metanephrines

Total metanephrines	Pheochromocytoma (%)	Nonpheochromocytoma (%)
>2.2 μg/mg creatinine	100	2
<2.2 μg/mg creatinine	0	98
>4.5 μg/mg creatinine	82	0
<4.5 μg/mg creatinine	18	100

In addition, Gitlow and co-workers provide data for a chromatoelectrophoretic
screening technique (Table 4). This qualitative test is designed to reveal border-
line elevations of VMA and metanephrine. From the table we can see that chromatoelectrophoresis has a sensitivity of 100% but a specificity of only 76% (many
false positives).

Table 4. Chromatoelectrophoretic screening

Result	Pheochromocytoma (%)	Nonpheochromocytoma (%)
Positive	100	24
Negative	0	76

Data on sensitivity, specificity, predictive value, and efficiency of five possible
screening tests are summarized in Table 5. These data make it possible to come to
a rational decision as to which tests are to be used and in which sequence.

SENSITIVITY, SPECIFICITY OR EFFICIENCY?

Of the five screening tests available, which is "best"? Should we choose the test
with the highest sensitivity, the highest specificity, or the highest efficiency? In the
case of pheochromocytoma we should look for the highest sensitivity. Pheochromocytoma is a serious disease that may be fatal if undiagnosed, but it is 100% cur-

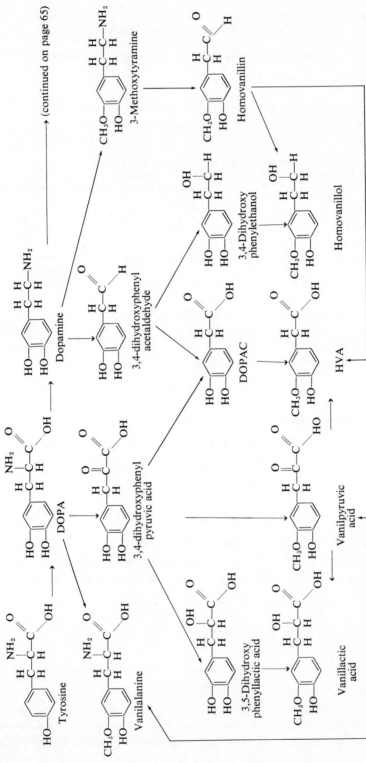

→ (continued on page 65)

Figure 1. The major metabolic pathways of the catecholamines. DOMA = dihydroxymandelic acid; DOPA = dihydroxyphenylalanine; DOPAC = dihydroxyphenylacetic acid; E = epinephrine; HMPG = 3 methoxy-4-hydroxyphenylethyleneglycol; HVA = homovanillic acid; M = metanephrine; N = norepinephrine; NM = normetanephrine; VMA = vanillylmandelic acid.

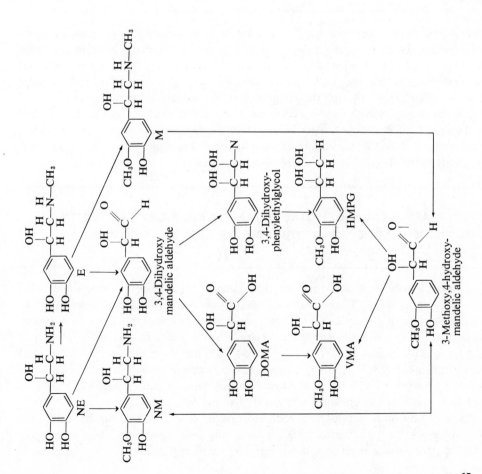

Table 5. Sensitivity, specificity, predictive value, and efficiency for five tests that can be used to screen for pheochromocytoma

Test	Sensitivity (%)	Specificity (%)	Pred. value of a positive result for prevalence of 500/100,000 (%)	Efficiency (%)
Colorimetric screening test for VMA	96.7	99.1	35	99.1
Qualitative chromatoelectrophoresis for metanephrine and VMA	100	76	2	76
Total metanephrine by column Chromatography; cutoff at 2.2 μg/mg creatinine	100	98	20	98
Same test but with cutoff at 4.5 μg/mg creatinine	82	100	100	99.91
Bidirectional paper chromatography for VMA	96.4	100	100	99.98

able if diagnosed. Therefore we do not want to miss a case. The problem of false-positive results and lower efficiency is not a major problem, because the false positives are easily handled, without harm to the patient, by repeating the test and by performing a different test. In each case we apply the repeat test and the new test to a population in which the prevalence of the disease is much higher.

Of the two tests with 100% sensitivity (i.e., chromatoelectrophoresis and total metanephrines) it is best to use the test with the highest efficiency. Thus Gitlow's data suggest that the measurement of total metanephrines by column chromatography is the single best test for pheochromocytoma.

PROPER APPLICATION OF TOTAL METANEPHRINE ASSAYS TO SCREEN FOR PHEOCHROMOCYTOMA. THE ROLE OF CLINICAL JUDGMENT

The test for total metanephrines is 100% sensitive for pheochromocytoma. This view is supported by Gitlow's data and also by those of Freier and associates.[3] In situations involving a serious but treatable disease, it is important not to miss any cases, so 100% sensitivity is most desirable. On the other hand, 100% sensitivity always results in less than 100% specificity. In this case the specificity of total metanephrines is 98%. If this test were applied *indiscriminately* to 1 million adults, all of the estimated 500 cases of pheochromocytoma in that population would be detected, but there would also be 20,000 false positive results!

How can the situation be improved? Most of the false positives can be eliminated by taking a history and performing a simple physical examination *before* ordering the test. If the test is used only in hypertensives and in patients with episodic symptoms, the prevalence of pheochromocytoma is increased by a factor of 10. False-positive results will then fall from 20,000 down to 1990, and all 500 pheochromocytomas will still be detected. The improved results are attributable to the application of clinical judgement, and not to any improvement in the test itself.

The laboratory is not a substitute for clinical judgement. Laboratory tests are an extension of physical diagnosis and form only part of the data base essential for the care of sick people. As Alvin Feinstein said, "Because contemporary clinicians have become preoccupied with the technology available for pathologic diagnosis, the 'science' produced by the technology has often obscured the difference between precise function in a machine and in a human mind."[4]

PROPER APPLICATION OF TOTAL METANEPHRINE ASSAYS TO SCREEN FOR PHEOCHROMOCYTOMA. THE ROLE OF REPEAT TESTING

The simplest way to decrease the number of false-positive results is to repeat the test on all subjects with positive results on the initial screen. Now it is very reasonable to wonder why reapplication of the same test should give anything but the same result. Theoretically, if a screening test and a repeat test are the same, then there should be no new information derived from the reapplication. Furthermore, the predictive value should not be increased by the repeat test. Yet it is common practice to repeat and "confirm" a positive laboratory finding. The clinical intent of this practice is to eliminate false positives. The reason why this works in practice (as opposed to theory) is that there are two inconstant factors responsible for false positives that may be operative on initial testing but inoperative on repeat testing with the same test: (1) physiological or pathophysiological conditions and (2) analytical errors.

A test result may be elevated, for example, by drugs, infection, or stress. The value of repeat testing lies in the observation that false positives caused by drugs, diet, other disease conditions, and so on, frequently revert to the "true-negative" status on a repeat test at some interval in the future, whereas true positives remain positive. A specific drug interference may be gone or an infection may have been treated, but the pheo will continue to grow and excrete more metanephrine with the passage of time. Similarly, an elevated false-positive metanephrine caused by analytical error or a statistical sampling error tends to revert to a true-negative status. A false-positive result in a healthy subject lies in the far-tail of the Gaussian distribution. A second measurement, however, has a higher probability of falling closer to the mean of the distribution for healthy subjects, and therefore we are more likely to obtain a negative result the second and third time around. This is referred to as "regression toward the mean."

In summary, the clinical practice of repeat testing decreases false positives, and this form of combination series testing results in an increase in the predictive value. Can we calculate this predictive value? Yes, but not with the simple methods we have been using up to now. It is not valid to apply the same sensitivity and specificity percentages to the repeat test population. This holds for repeat testing

Table 6. The overall effect when the *same test* is applied before and after performing a preliminary physical examination and when the same test is repeated

Conditions	Number tested	Prevalence (%)	Number of pheos expected	Number of pheos found	Number of false positives	Predictive value of a positive result (%)	Efficiency (%)
1. The metanephrine test is applied to 1 million adults selected at random	1,000,000	0.05	500	500	20,000	2.4	98
2. A physical examination is performed and the same test is applied to 10% of the population with hypertension	100,000	0.50	500	500	1,990	20.0	98
3. The test is repeated in the 2,490 hypertensives with positive results on initial screening	2,490	20.1	500	500	40	92.5	98.4

with the same test or repeat testing with any test (unless the tests are independent). If the tests are correlated, then the first preselects the population for the second. The calculated predictive value is always higher than the actual predictive value of the testing scheme. Therefore our calculation of the predictive value, based on repeat testing with the same test, is statistically inaccurate. It does demonstrate, however, the general beneficial effect of repeat testing, but it does not result in a precise predictive value that can be affixed to the diagnostic process. With this in mind, let us return to our discussion of repeat testing in the diagnosis of pheochromocytoma.

Table 6 shows our estimate of what happens with repeat testing. On repeat testing, the number of false-positive results may drop by a factor of 40. However, all, or nearly all, of the 500 pheos expected are detected, because our test has 100% sensitivity. Because it is performed on positives only, rather than on everyone, repeat testing in this case requires only about 3% more work in the laboratory.

PROPER APPLICATION OF TOTAL METANEPHRINE ASSAYS TO SCREEN FOR PHEOCHROMOCYTOMA. THE ROLE OF PERFORMING A DIFFERENT TEST

In the above example we discussed what happens when the same test is repeated, and we stressed that the results are best when the test has 100% sensitivity. But what happens if you combine a test having 100% sensitivity with a test having 100% specificity? This works well only for those tests that combine 100% sensitivity with very high specificity, and 100% specificity with very high sensitivity. The total metanephrine test for pheochromocytoma, which has a sensitivity of 100% and a specificity of 98%, and the paper chromatographic measurement of VMA which has a sensitivity of 96.4% and a specificity of 100% meet these requirements.

If both tests were applied to the 100,000 hypertensives, with an estimated prevalence of 0.5% for pheochromocytoma, we would obtain the results given in Table 7.

Table 7. Predictive value of combining two tests for pheochromotcytoma

Number of cases	Final diagnosis	Metanephrines	VMA	Predictive value (%)
482	482 pheos	Positive	Positive	100
2008	18 pheos 1990 nonpheos	Positive	Negative	1
97,510	97,510 nonpheos	Negative	Negative	100

The combination separates the 100,000 subjects into three groups, two of which have 100% certainty of having or not having pheochromocytoma. This clearcut separation on the first "cut" is most useful to the physician and the patient. A new indeterminate group is created comprising 2008 subjects with a positive metanephrine and a negative VMA test. There are 18 cases of pheochromocytoma among these 2008 subjects.

In summary, repeat testing utilizing a test with 100% sensitivity is the best way to screen for serious but treatable disease. Repeat testing of positive results has the effect of decreasing the total number of false positives without creating an excessive workload in the laboratory. On the other hand, when a test with 100% sensitivity is combined with a test having 100% specificity, it is possible to achieve a tripartite distribution in which subjects with either all-positive or all-negative results are classified as diseased or nondiseased with nearly 100% certainty.

REFERENCES

1. Armstrong, M. D., McMillan, A., and Shaw, K. N. F. 3-Methoxy-4-hydroxy-D-mandelic acid, a urinary metabolite of norepinephrine. *Biochem. Biophys. Acta.* **25:** 442–443, 1957.

2. Gitlow, Stanley E., Mendlowitz, Milton, and Bertain, Laura. The biochemical techniques for detecting and establishing the presence of a pheochromocytoma. *Am. J. Cardiol.* **26:** 270–279, 1970.

3. Freier, D. T. and Harrison, T. S. Rigorous biochemical criteria for the diagnosis of pheochromocytoma. *J. Surg. Res.* **14:** 177–180, 1973.

4. Feinstein, Alvan R. *Clinical Judgement,* Williams and Wilkins, Baltimore, 1967, p. 362.

CHAPTER 10

A VMA TEST STRIP FOR NEUROBLASTOMA—LOW PREVALENCE, LOW SENSITIVITY, HIGH SPECIFICITY

D RS. Rogers, Lyon and Porter (Department of Pediatrics of Duke University and the University of Texas) reported favorably on a spot test for vanillyl-mandelic acid and other guaiacols in the urine of patients with neuroblastoma.[1] They recommended routine use of the spot test, in association with other appropriate diagnostic measures, in all patients suspected of having neuroblastoma. Was their recommendation sound? Let us analyze their paper using our model. We begin with their abstract.

A spot test for vanillylmandelic acid and other guaiacol derivatives in the urine of patients with neuroblastoma is presented. The test is based on the reaction of these substances with 2,4-dinitrophenylhydrazine and sodium metaperiodate which, when alkalinized with sodium carbonate, form a bright blue color. Nine of 13 cases of clinically apparent neuroblastoma (69%) were detectable by this test. Urine from 255 control subjects on unrestricted diets produced only one false positive reaction. The test is simple to perform and utilizes random urine specimens.

Would we introduce this test in our laboratory? Should we introduce this test in our laboratory? Before we answer these questions let us determine the predictive value of a positive result from sensitivity, specificity, and prevalence.

Sensitivity

What is the sensitivity of this test? The authors give us the information—it is only 69%—but they do not call it sensitivity.

Specificity

What is the specificity of this test? The abstract tells us it is 99.6%, since there was only one false-positive in 255 controls.

Prevalence

The authors fail to provide data on prevalence. In their study they had 13 clinical cases of neuroblastoma and 255 controls, giving them a prevalence of 4850/100,000 (4.85%). In fact, however, the prevalence of neuroblastoma is extremely low, ranging between 2/100,000 and 3/100,000.

Predictive Value and Efficiency

Now that we have the sensitivity (69%), specificity (99.6%), and prevalence (3/100,000), we can calculate the predictive value of a positive result and a negative result, and the overall efficiency of this test (Table 1).

Table 1.   VMA spot test data arranged in tabular form

	Positive	Negative	Totals	
Sick	2	1	3	(sensitivity = 69%)
Not sick	400	99,597	99,997	(specificity = 99.6%)
Totals	402	99,598	100,000	

Predictive value of a positive result = 0.5%.
Predictive value of a negative result = 99.999%.
Overall efficiency = 99.6%.

Neuroblastoma is a serious but treatable disease. Therefore it is important not to miss any cases and a test with high sensitivity is preferable. The spot test has a low sensitivity and misses 1 out of every 3 cases.

The predictive value of a positive result is poor. For every true positive result there are 200 false-positive results. There will be an overwhelming number of false positives.

The predictive value of a negative result and the overall efficiency look good, but they do not compensate for the problems raised by the low sensitivity and the low predictive value of a positive result.

Leonard et al. have recommended that this spot test be performed during the first 7 years of life as a routine screening test for neuroblastoma.[2] Even the Pediatric Department of Massachusetts General Hospital recommended that, "The urine VMA screening dipstick should be done routinely on all infants, and annually on all children under four."[3] Were these recommendations justified? We do not think so, nor does George Hallet, Chief of Pediatrics at the Maine Medical Center,[3] who has analyzed the cost of carrying out the Leonard recommendations.

Leonard and associates recommended screening at birth and six additional times during the first year, three times during the second year, and twice a year thereafter until the child reaches 7 years of age. Since each test strip costs 14 cents, the total cost of 20 assays over the 7-year period would be $2.80. To find 2 out of 3 cases, 100,000 children would have to be tested at a cost of about $280,000! Since a good physical examination is probably capable of picking up at least half of the cases, the actual case-finding obtained with this test would be low.

If 1 million children were tested, 20 cases would be found and 10 would be missed. If a physical examination were performed on these 1 million children, most likely 15 cases would be found and 15 would be missed. The spot test would therefore "find" 5 additional cases in 1 million children at a cost of $2.8 million. The testing of 1 million children would also lead to 4000 false-positive results— with resultant anxiety, confusion, and additional cost. The basic problem with this test is the low sensitivity. A serious but treatable disease requires a test with 100% or nearly 100% sensitivity. When sensitivity drops below 95% a significant number of sick patients are missed. When sensitivity is as low as 69%, as in this VMA spot test, then it is probably better to do without the test.

REFERENCES

1. Rogers, L. E., Lyon, G. M., Jr., and Porter, F. Stanley. Spot test for vanillylmandelic acid and other guaiacols in urine of patients with neuroblastoma. *Am. J. Clin. Pathol.* **58:** 383–387, 1972.
2. Leonard, Arnold S., Roback, S. A., Nesbit, M. E., Jr., and Freier, Esther, The VMA test strip: A new tool for mass screening, diagnosis, and management of catecholamine-secreting tumors. *J. Pediatr. Surg.* **7:** 528–531 1972.
3. Hallett, George W., Letter to the Editor, *Pediatrics* **52:** 757, 1973.

CHAPTER 11

SERUM CEA—LOW SENSITIVITY, LOW SPECIFICITY

THE serum carcinoembryonic antigen (CEA) test is a good model for demonstrating when *not* to use a laboratory test, since the test has low sensitivity and low specificity. In 1974 Hansen and associates published the results of their extensive study of CEA, a laboratory adjunct in the diagnosis and management of cancer.[1] Their paper contains a wealth of data that can be used to derive the sensitivity, specificity, and predictive value of the CEA test in a variety of clinical situations. Their abstract follows:

A collaborative study evaluating the clinical usefulness of the carcinoembryonic antigen (CEA) assay by the Roche z-gel method has been performed on 35,000 plasma samples from more than 10,000 patients and healthy subjects from approximately 100 institutions. This study has shown the assay to be of value as an adjunct in the diagnosis and management of the cancer patient.

The highest percentage of elevated titers and the highest titer values were found in patients with colorectal, pulmonary, and pancreatic carcinoma. CEA values dropped following successful therapy and were a reliable indicator of the clinical status of the patient. A progressive increase in the CEA level as demonstrated by successive assays was of unfavorable prognostic significance.

Some elevated titers were also found in patients with noncarcinoma malignant disease and nonmalignant disease, primarily when the disease was in a clinically active state. Chronic, heavy cigarette smoking is a factor in titer elevations, but the significance of this is not fully understood. Ninety-seven percent of healthy nonsmoking subjects had CEA values in the normal range, 0 to 2.5 ng. per ml.

The abstract suggests that the serum CEA test may have great value in the clinical diagnosis and therapy of malignant disease, particularly colorectal, pulmonary, and pancreatic carcinoma. Fortunately, Roche scientists have provided us with complete data. This makes it possible to evaluate the sensitivity and specificity of the serum CEA test.

SENSITIVITY OF THE CEA ASSAY

Sensitivity is "positivity in disease." How positive is the serum CEA test in disease? A CEA level greater than 2.5 ng/ml was considered positive by Hansen and associates. Their Tables provide the percentage of subjects having CEA levels above and below 2.5 ng/ml for a large number of disease states. Roche scientists assayed more than 35,000 plasma samples from 10,000 patients and healthy subjects. They found positive results in a variety of disease conditions. Table 1 gives some major disease conditions and the percentage of subjects in each group with CEA values above 2.5 ng/ml.

These data indicate serious problems with the CEA test. Test sensitivity in biopsy-proven cases of colon carcinoma is only 72%, whereas cases of lung cancer and pancreatic cancer have a higher percentage of positive results. Furthermore, the 72% sensitivity for colon carcinoma includes all stages of carcinoma. When test results are correlated with Dukes' staging, there is far less sensitivity for early cancers as shown in Table 2. In addition to low sensitivity for colon cancer, the

Table 1. Percent positive CEA in major disease conditions

Disease	Percent Positive CEA	Disease	Percent Positive CEA
Colon cancer	72	Emphysema	57
Lung cancer	74	Alcoholics	65
Pancreatic cancer	91	Ulcerative colitis	31
Stomach cancer	61	Ileitis	40
Breast cancer	47	Transplants	56
Other cancers	49	Pneumonia	46
Hyperplasias	21	Pancreatitis	53

Table 2. Percent positive CEA and Dukes' staging

Dukes' Staging		Percent positive CEA[2]
Group A:	limited to wall of bowel	58
Group B:	extends into serosa	68
Group C:	metastases to local nodes	71
Group D:	distant metastases	81

CEA test is positive in a variety of noncancerous conditions. Depending on the condition, positive results are seen in 21 to 65% of subjects who are free of cancer. Thus the CEA test is relatively insensitive to colon carcinoma and too sensitive to other diseases. Alcoholics, for example, show nearly the same percentage of positive results as patients with colon carcinoma.

SPECIFICITY OF THE CEA ASSAY

Specificity is "negativity in health." How negative is the serum CEA test in patients who are free of cancer? Table 5 in the paper by Hansen and associates provides this information. The authors list, for a variety of noncancerous conditions, the percentage of subjects with CEA levels *below* 2.5 ng/ml. A selected sample of their list is shown in Table 3, along with the percentage of subjects with negative results (less than 2.5 ng/ml). The percent of noncancer subjects with negative results *is* the specificity of the test. It is obvious that the CEA test is in no way negative enough in patients who are free of cancer. The only way to achieve a specificity of 97%, which is the specificity assigned to the test in the author's abstract, is to find subjects who are *nonsmokers,* and who are free of any one or more of the conditions listed.

But the serum CEA test is not applied to such a healthy population. It is applied to patients suspected of having colon cancer, and most of these patients have one or more of the conditions in Table 3. In fact, there are few nonmalignant diseases or conditions in which negative CEA results are obtained in more than 80% of the subjects. In other words, most nonmalignant disease states, including smoking, lead to false positive CEA results in more than 20% of subjects.

Table 3.   Percent negative CEA in various disease states in subjects free of cancer

Condition	Percentage of negative CEA	Condition	Percentage of negative CEA
Emphysema	43	Hernia	77
Alcoholism (cirrhosis)	30	Diabetes	62
Alcoholism (no cirrhosis)	35	Heart disease	61
Ulcerative colitis	69	Hypertension	72
Gastric ulcer	55	Hepatitis, viral	70
Rectal polyps	81	Hemorrhoids	67
Diverticulitis	73	Cholelithiasis	82
Osteoarthritis	70	Pneumonia	54
Bronchitis	67	Miscellaneous conditions	67
Obesity	69	Smoking	81

EFFECT OF PREVALENCE

What is the effect of changes in prevalence on the predictive value and efficiency of the serum CEA test for colon carcinoma? We apply the average sensitivity of 72% and specificity of 80% to three different populations: one in which there are 1000 cases per 100,000 (1%), one with 10,000 cases per 100,000 (10%), and finally, one in which the prevalence of colon cancer is 50,000 cases per 100,000 (50%).

What happens when the CEA test is used in an unselected population with a colon cancer prevalence of 1%? By completing the worksheet, we obtain Table 4. There are only 720 true positive out of a total of 20,520 positive results; *therefore the predictive value of a positive result is only 3.5%*. There are a total of 79,920 true results; *therefore the efficiency is 79.9%*.

Table 4.   Worksheet tabular format for CEA test when prevalence equals 1%

	Number with positive test	Number with negative test	Totals
Colon cancer	720	280	1,000
No colon cancer	19,800	79,200	99,000
Totals	20,520	79,480	100,000

We now increase prevalence to 10,000/100,000 and the completed worksheet looks like Table 5. We now have 7200 true positives out of a total of 25,200 positive results; *therefore the predictive value of a positive result has been increased to 28.6%*. *Efficiency drops slightly to 79.2%*.

Table 5. Work sheet tabular format for CEA test when prevalence equals 10%

	Number with positive test	Number with negative test	Totals
Colon cancer	7,200	2,800	10,000
No colon cancer	18,000	72,000	90,000
Totals	25,200	74,800	100,000

Finally, let us see what happens when prevalence is equal to 50,000/100,000 (50%). The completed worksheet looks like Table 6. We now have 36,000 true positives out of a total of 46,000 positive results; *therefore the predictive value of a positive result has increased to 78.3%*. There were a total of 76,000 true results, so efficiency is now 76.0%.

Table 6. Worksheet tabular format for CEA test when prevalence equals 50%

	Number with positive test	Number with negative test	Totals
Colon cancer	36,000	14,000	50,000
No colon cancer	10,000	40,000	50,000
Totals	46,000	54,000	100,000

In summary, Table 7 shows what happens to the predictive value of a positive CEA test and to efficiency of the CEA test as we change prevalence.

Table 7. Effect of prevalence on the predictive value and efficiency of the CEA test

Prevalence of Colon cancer	Predictive value of positive CEA test (%)	Efficiency of CEA test (%)
1000/100,000	3.5	79.9
10,000/100,000	28.6	79.2
50,000/100,000	78.3	76.0

What do we want? High sensitivity, high specificity, high predictive value or high efficiency? No test can give us all four variables equal to 100%; therefore a choice must be made. When we deal with cancer of an internal organ, for which treatment is difficult and the outcome in doubt, it is essential that false-positive results be kept to a minimum. Cancer is a serious disease with a generally poor prognosis. Therefore it is important not to label someone as having cancer when he indeed does not have cancer.

A test for occult cancer should have very high specificity. Ideally a test for cancer should have a specificity of 100% which means that it should not give us any false-positive results.

The CEA test is a poor test for cancer because it has an average specificity of 80% when applied to sick patients who are free of cancer. When a physician is considering a diagnosis of cancer of the bowel he does not usually need a test to differentiate sickness from good health. Rather it is necessary for him to differentiate a variety of sicknesses, one from another.

A test for cancer should also have high sensitivity—ideally above 95%. Again the CEA test is a poor test, having an average sensitivity for colon carcinoma of only 72%.

It is apparent that the serum CEA test has little discriminatory capacity. It is not specific for colon cancer, and it is not sensitive to colon cancer.

But might not the test be useful for following patients who have known cancer and in whom surgery is performed?[2] The answer is yes and no. In fact, we can give a fairly good idea of how useful it can be. In such a group of patients the prevalence of recurrent colon carcinoma is quite high. If we permit a high recurrence rate, so that at any one time one-half of the subjects tested have had a recurrence, and we use the 2.5 ng/ml cutoff, we reproduce the worksheet table for a prevalence of 50%. The predictive value of a positive result is 78.3% and the efficiency is 76.0%.

Serial measurements should be more useful since each patient can be his own control. But again we are faced with the problem that the test can respond to noncancerous conditions or to other cancers. Furthermore, at present there are no supporting data to indicate the equality or superiority of the serum CEA test over a variety of other available tests for predicting the occurrence of metastatic disease. Therefore, the published reports on the usefulness of the serum CEA test for the detection of recurrent cancer are, *at present,* best classified as unconvincing.

REFERENCES

1. Hansen, H. J., Snyder, J. J., Miller, E., Vandevoorde, J. P., Miller, O. N., Hines, L. R., and Burns, J. J. Carcinoembryonic antigen (CEA) assay. *Human Pathol.* **5:** 139–147, 1974.
2. Mach, J. P., Jaeger, P. H., Bertholet, M. M., Ruegsegger, C. H., Loosli, R. M., and Pettavel, J. Detection of recurrence of large-bowel carcinoma by radioimmunoassay of circulating carcinoembryonic antigen (C.E.A.). *Lancet* **ii:** 535–540, 1974.

CHAPTER 12

SCREENING FOR GONORRHEA—
HOW THE MODEL DEFINES ESSENTIAL CRITERIA
FOR AN EFFICIENT SCREENING TEST

R EASONABLY accurate statistics are available on the incidence of gonorrhea in various populations. Therefore, we should be able to apply the predictive-value model to select, *a priori,* essential criteria for an efficient screening test. In the following discussion we demonstrate how the model can be used to define adequate and inadequate tests for gonorrhea.

The age-specific incidence of gonorrhea in the United States in 1972 is shown in Table 1[1]. It can be seen that the highest incidence is in the 20 to 24 year group, where the incidence is almost 2%, or 1813.5 cases per 100,000 population. These rates refer to the number of infections and not to the number of individual persons with infections. There are no reliable data available on the incidence of repeaters, that is, individuals with more than one infection a year.

Table 1.   Age-specific incidence of gonorrhea

Age group	Number of reported cases	Incidence (per 100,000)
0–9	2,191	6.1
10–14	7,777	37.4
15–19	204,635	1,035.4
20–24	311,051	1,813.5
25–29	135,220	921.6
30–39	79,789	347.2
40–49	19,897	84.6
50 +	6,655	12.9
Totals	767,215	371.6

Gonorrhea is highly infectious, has a short incubation period, and the infection does not result in immunity. In short, it is an epidemiologist's nightmare. In order to control a gonorrhea epidemic, contacts must be diagnosed and treated before they have the opportunity to spread the infection. This task is complicated by the occurrence of the "asymptomatic carrier." As many as 50 to 70% of female contacts have been shown to be culture positive (endocervical) while symptom free. Similarly, 10% of male contacts have positive urethral cultures while symptom free.[2]

Asymptomatic carriers, primarily women, create a reservoir of gonorrhea that practically defies detection. The current approach to the problem has been two pronged: physicians have been urged to perform endocervical cultures routinely during pelvic examination; and they have been urged to identify and treat female contacts of diagnosed men. The sensitivity of a culture in women is only 70 to 80%, which means that in 20 to 30% of infected women the diagnosis cannot be substantiated. Therefore, all women are treated following exposure to male gonorrhea. Unfortunately, much less attention is given to identifying male contacts of diagnosed females. Asymptomatic gonorrhea in men is also recognized as a significant public health problem.[3]

Here then lies the challenge for the laboratory—to provide an efficient, highly predictive screening test for gonorrhea. A screening test that is simple and that can be performed in the clinic or doctor's office would be ideal, since treatment could be instituted immediately. Such a simple screening test would eliminate the risk of further spread of infection while awaiting the result of a culture. Let us try to define the essential characteristics of this screening test in terms of sensitivity and specificity. Using an incidence of 2000/100,000, we can examine the predictive value table on page 175 and select target values that give a highly predictive test. Some of the data are shown in Table 2. We can see by scanning our table that a

Table 2. Predictive value of positives (%)
Incidence = 2000/100,000

Specificity (%)	Sensitivity					
	90%	92%	94%	96%	98%	100%
90.00	16	16	16	16	17	17
93.00	21	21	22	22	22	23
95.00	27	27	28	28	29	29
97.00	38	38	39	40	40	40
99.00	65	65	66	66	67	67
99.50	79	79	79	80	80	80
99.90	95	95	95	95	95	95
99.99	99	99	99	99	100	100
100.00	100	100	100	100	100	100

screening test for gonorrhea that is 100% sensitive and 95% specific would have a predictive value of only 29%. Therefore, 71% of all positives by this test would indeed be false-positive results. A predictive value of 29% is achieved only if the age group screened is between 20 and 24 years—the group with the highest morbidity rate. In other age groups, the test would perform with an even higher false-positive rate. A test to screen for gonorrhea in the *general* population would have to have a specificity of 99.00% before it could begin to be reasonably predictive. At 99.00% specificity, the predictive value would lie between 65 and 67% (if the sensitivity were between 90 and 100%).

Our discussion is *not* theoretical. A serological test for gonorrhea has been developed, but has yet to reach the marketplace. In 1973 Organon, Inc. organized a preview of their Gonosticon Dri-Dot serologic test for gonorrhea in several simultaneously held meetings across the country. An edited manuscript of the soundtrack of their videotape presentation was made available at the same time.[4] The discussion that follows is based largely on that presentation:

Gonosticon Dri-Dot is a qualitative, two-minute *in vitro,* latex agglutination test for the presence of gonococcal antibody in serum. The antigen is an extract of a strain of *Neisseria gonorrhoeae* having special antigenic properties, affixed to a polystyrene latex particle. A soluble fraction of the gonococcus is the antigen used to coat the latex, and absorbing antigen is provided to enhance specificity. The absorbing antigen is a mixture of guinea pig tissue extract and specially processed beef tissue. Serum antibody to the gonococcus will react with the antigen-coated latex, producing a visible agglutination of the latex.[4]

During the presentation, several investigators presented data from clinical trials. Dr. King K. Holmes, of the Department of Medicine at the University of Washington School of Medicine in Seattle, summed up his studies as follows:

It (the test) appears to be influenced by 3 things in addition to active gonococcal infection. One is a past history of gonococcal infection. Another is the presence of meningocci in the throat. A third is the duration of time that the patient has actively been infected. We feel that the percentage of patients who have infection who would also have a positive latex test goes up with increasing time after infection.[4]

In his concluding remarks, Dr. Holmes said,

I don't feel that it (Gonosticon) is useful by itself in the diagnosis of gonorrhea in an individual patient. I would not use the results of the test to treat a patient with gonorrhea without the results of a culture to substantiate the positive test, because of the problem of non-specificity. In addition, I think that the utility of the test, if it is to have any utility, will be in screening for gonorrhea among low-risk populations.[4]

Dr. Nicholas J. Fiumara, Director, Division of Communicable and Venereal Disease, Massachusetts Department of Public Health, concluded that the Gonosticon blood test had a sensitivity of 80% and a specificity of 95%, and recommended using it to screen for gonorrhea in asymptomatic females. In addition, he said,

This is a beautiful test for private practice. Just imagine all we need to do is draw some blood, send it to the laboratory, then while we are still examining the patient, two minutes later we get a call from the laboratory, a report from the laboratory— the test is positive or negative. That's a beautiful test to us—it's going to simplify our office procedures.[4]

Unfortunately, Dr. Fiumara overlooked the fact that the value of a laboratory test depends on the prevalence of the disease it is supposed to detect. In his concluding remarks, he stated,

A positive blood test for gonorrhea means either she has gonorrhea now, she had had it in the past or that 5% false positive rate (sic).[4]

Dr. Fiumara errs. The false-positive rate cannot be derived from the specificity alone (95%), as he suggested. It is a function of sensitivity, specificity, and incidence. In office practice, the incidence of asymptomatic gonorrhea *might* be as high as 3%. Let us look at the false-positive rate under those circumstances (Table 3). The predictive value of a positive result, that is, the number of positive results that are true positives is only 2400 out of 7200, or a lowly 33.3%. In other words, the false-positive rate is 66.6%—not the 5% indicated by Dr. Fiumara—if the test is used, as suggested, to screen asymptomatic women in private practice.

The Gonosticon test is not even useful in areas of high prevalence, because the test is unable to distinguish current infection, and its related need for immediate

Table 3. The Gonosticon slide test in office practice incidence rate $= 3\%$; sensitivity $= 80\%$; specificity $= 95\%$.

	Number with positive test	Number with negative test	Totals
Gonorrhea	2,400	600	3,000
No gonorrhea	4,800	92,200	97,000
Totals	7,200	92,800	100,000

treatment, from prior infections in the same patient requiring no treatment. In the unselected low-risk population (private practice), the test suffers from the same shortcomings, further compromised by the effect of low disease frequency, resulting in an intolerable false-positive rate. Finally, the sensitivity of the test is compromised by the variable and frequently low level of antibody production detected by Gonosticon during the first 2 weeks of infection. It is therefore greatly affected by the time interval between infection and testing.

The Gonosticon test was introduced as a possible replacement for bacteriologic culture studies. Unfortunately, cultures have significantly greater specificity, as shown in Table 4. The results obtained when each test is applied to a population with a gonorrhea incidence rate of 2% are shown in Table 5. The culture eliminates the serious problem of false positives. Each test, however, misses 20% of the true positives, since each test has a sensitivity of only 80%.

Table 4. A Comparison of Gonosticon with Culture

Test	Cost (dollars/test)	Time	Sensitivity (%)	Specificity (%)	Differentiate active from prior infection
Gonosticon	1.5	2 minutes	80	95	No
Culture	4	2 days	80	100	Yes

Table 5. The predictive value of a positive result and the false-positive rate in a population with 2% incidence rate for gonorrhea

Test	Predictive value of positive (%)	False positive rate (%)
Gonosticon	25	75
Culture	100	0

The results obtained when each test is applied to a population with a high incidence (30%) are shown in Table 6. When the test is used in a population with a high incidence rate, the false-positive rate drops significantly, but it remains at a high level of 20%.

Table 6.   The predictive value of a positive result and the false-positive rate in a population with 30% incidence rate for gonorrhea

Test	Predictive value of positive (%)	False positive rate (%)
Gonosticon	80	20
Culture	100	0

Our analysis reveals the characteristics required for an adequate screening test for gonorrhea. The minimum requirements include:

1. Sensitivity greater than 80%.
2. Specificity greater than 99%.
3. Ability to differentiate recent from old infection.

Until a screening test for gonorrhea meets the above requirements, it will not replace current culture techniques.

REFERENCES

1. U.S. Department of Health, Education, and Welfare. Public Health Service. Center for Disease Control. *Morbidity and Mortality*, Vol. 22, No. 53: July 15, 1974.
2. Pariser, H. Asymptomatic gonorrhea. *Med. Clin. North Am.* **56:** 1127–1132, 1972.
3. Handsfield, H. H., Lipman, T. O., Harnisch, J. P., Tronca, E., and Holmes, K. K. Asymptomatic gonorrhea in men: diagnosis natural course, prevalence and significance. *N. Engl. J. Med.* **290:** 117–123, 1974.
4. Organon, Inc. Report on a New Serologic Test for Gonorrhea. Edited transcript of the soundtrack of the videotape of the report, 1973.

CHAPTER 13

MYOCARDIAL INFARCTION—
EXPERIMENTAL APPLICATION OF THE MODEL

FROM 1972 through 1974 we carried out an extensive study of enzyme and isoenzyme tests in patients with myocardial infarction and a variety of similar diseases. The results of this study illustrate the importance of sensitivity, specificity, and prevalence, and their effect on predictive value and efficiency, in establishing a referent value useful in the diagnosis of disease.

CCU STUDY

We investigated 100 consecutive admissions to the Coronary Care Unit (CCU) of The Presbyterian Hospital in the City of New York.[1] Each patient was admitted with a clinical diagnosis of "rule out acute myocardial infarction." On discharge from the unit, the internist, Dr. James A. Reiffel, placed each patient into one of two classes: myocardial infarction (MI) or no myocardial infarction (non-MI). The division was made on the basis of clinical judgement and electrocardiographic changes (ECG), without knowledge of any enzyme result.

A blood sample was obtained at the time of admission to the CCU and at 8 AM for 10 consecutive days following admission. Each sample was assayed for total CPK, HBDH, LDH, and SGOT activity utilizing kinetic UV-coupled assays on the DuPont ACA. The measurements were made daily, including weekends, to avoid major storage problems. Serum from each sample, separated within 2 hours of collection, was stored at 4°C for no longer than 24 hours.

In addition, the isoenzymes of LDH and CPK were separated on agarose gel utilizing the Corning-ACI system. The enzyme activities of the separated LDH and CPK fractions were determined, after incubation with substrate, by fluorometric scanning. The CPK isoenzyme test was considered positive for CPK_2 (cardiac specific CPK or CPK-MB) when the CPK_2 fraction was 3% or more of the total. The CPK_2 fraction, when present in myocardial infarction, was invariably far in excess of 3% of the total; therefore the results of the test were not difficult to evaluate. The LDH isoenzyme test was considered positive when LDH_1 levels were higher than LDH_2 levels. We referred to this change as "flipped" LDH.

Of the 100 patients admitted to the study, 3 had to be eliminated because they were admitted more than 48 hours after the onset of their clinical episode, and 3 more were eliminated because they died within 48 hours of their clinical episode. This left 94 cases with adequate data for analysis.

A common method of presenting the results of enzyme studies is to graph the daily mean values in one clinical group (e.g., MI) along with the daily mean values in a second clinical group (e.g., non-MI). Our daily mean values are plotted for SGOT and CPK in Figures 1 and 2, respectively.

If we rank our enzyme tests solely on the basis of the largest separation between MI and non-MI, based on daily mean values over a period of 10 days, CPK would have the highest rank, followed by HBDH, LDH, and SGOT as shown in Table 1.

However, clinicians do not evaluate mean values in groups over a long period of time; instead they are required to pass judgement on individual values for a specific

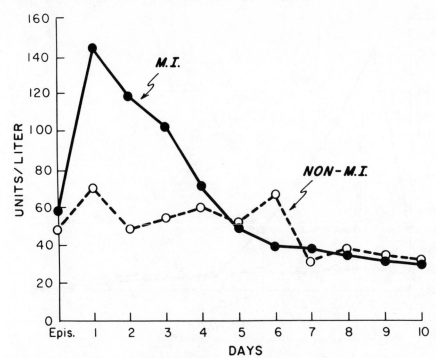

Figure 1. Daily mean values for SGOT in MI and non-MI.

Table 1. Rank order for discrimination based on mean values

Rank	Enzyme	Day of greatest discrimination	$\bar{X}$ MI Divided by $\bar{X}$ non-MI
1	Total CPK	1	11.9
2	Total HBDH	3	3.3
3	Total LDH	3	2.7
4	Total SGOT	1	2.0

patient on a specific day. Therefore a more appropriate way of looking at the data is to examine the frequency distribution of all values for all patients on a specific day. This was done on all days for all enzymes, and the results for SGOT and CPK at 24 hours are shown in Figures 3 and 4, respectively. Each figure shows that there is a significant overlap in enzyme values between the MI and the non-MI group.

If enzyme test results are ranked on the basis of the *least* amount of overlap between MI and non-MI, then the isoenzymes of CPK provide the greatest discrimination between the two groups, followed by the isoenzymes of LDH, total CPK, SGOT, total LDH, and finally, HBDH. This is shown in Table 2.

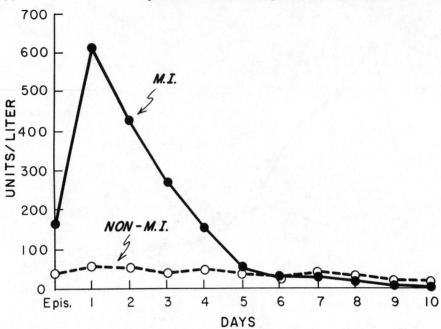

Figure 2. Daily mean values for CPK in MI and non-MI.

Table 2. Rank order for discrimination based on the size of the overlap, or "grey" zone, of the frequency distributions for MI and non-MI

Rank	Enzyme	Day of least overlap	Percentage of patients in "grey" zone
1	Isoenzymes of CPK	1	7
2	Isoenzymes of LDH	3	18
3	Total CPK	1	56
4	Total SGOT	1	70
5	Total LDH	3	82
6	Total HBDH	3	84

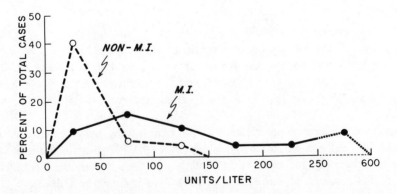

Figure 3. Frequency distribution of SGOT results at 24 hours in MI and non-MI.

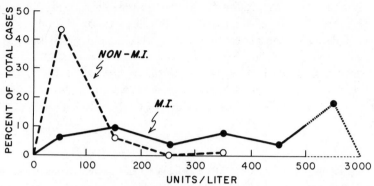

Figure 4. Frequency distribution of CPK results at 24 hours in MI and non-MI.

COMBINATION OF ISOENZYMES OF CPK AND LDH

The greatest discrimination between MI and non-MI patients is provided by the isoenzymes of CPK and LDH. As shown in Table 3, when CPK_2 was present and LDH was "flipped," all patients had a combined clinical and ECG diagnosis of MI. On the other hand, when CPK_2 was absent, all cases had a combined clinical and ECG diagnosis of non-MI.

Table 3. The predictive value of combined CPK-MB and flipped LDH for MI and non-MI in 94 patients

Lab Finding	Number of subjects	Combined clinical and ECG classification		Predictive value of the result (%)
		MI	Non-MI	
CPK-MB present LDH iso flipped	36	36	None	100
CPK-MB present LDH iso normal	17	10	7	60
CPK-MB absent	41	None	41	100

In both cases the combination of tests provided us with a predictive value of 100% when *both* were positive or *both* were negative. But when CPK_2 was positive and LDH isoenzymes were negative, a new type of overlap or grey zone resulted. In this new type of overlap zone we *know* we are in an indeterminate zone. There were 17 patients in this indeterminate zone, 10 of whom were classified as MI on the basis of combined clinical and ECG criteria. Although the remaining 7 were classified as non-MI, they most probably had some degree of myocardial ischemia.

Forty-six patients were classified as MI on the basis of combined clinical and ECG criteria. The presence of CPK_2 was 100% *sensitive* for MI when measured within the 48-hour period that followed the onset of the clinical episode. A test that is 100% sensitive is positive in all cases of the disease. On the other hand, the *specificity* of CPK_2 (as determined by the final clinical and ECG diagnosis) was only 85%, since only 41 of the 48 non-MI patients had an absent CPK_2.

The isoenzymes of LDH had an overall *sensitivity* for MI of 78%. This value varied with the type and extent of the infarct as shown in Table 4. Patients with classic infarcts associated with Q waves in the ECG showed a flipped LDH 85% of the time.

Table 4. Presence or absence of CPK-MB and flipped LDH in 46 patients classified as MI on the basis of combined clinical and ECG criteria

Number of cases	Clinical subclass for MI	Percentage with CPK-MB present	Percentage with flipped LDH
33	MI with typical Q wave changes	100	85
9	Nontransmural	100	67
4	MI with LBBB	100	50

WHICH IS BEST, LABORATORY TESTS OR CLINICAL DIAGNOSIS?

So far we have assumed, as most clinicians do, that the final clinical diagnosis is correct; and we have used the final clinical diagnosis for the determination of sensitivity and specificity. However, we must also consider that the final clinical diagnosis may not be as reliable as CPK_2. Since there is no absolute way to resolve this dilemma, we have developed the matrix shown in Table 5. The matrix utilizes four independent criteria for myocardial infarction: (1) positive new Q wave in the electrocardiogram, (2) classic clinical history, (3) presence of CPK_2, and (4) flipped LDH. Thus the matrix contains 16 possible combinations of positive and negative findings.

Since it is not possible to state *a priori* that any one of the four criteria is superior to the others, we suggest that a firm diagnosis of acute myocardial infarction can be made in a medical patient when three or four of the criteria are positive. On this basis we had 36 cases of acute myocardial infarction. Conversely, acute myocardial infarction can be ruled out if three or four of the criteria are negative. On this basis we had 48 cases that did not have an acute myocardial infarction.

A careful perusal of Table 5 suggests that CPK_2 has high specificity as well as high sensitivity. For example, there are no cases of myocardial infarction in cells 5, 9, 10, and 11. CPK_2 is absent in each of those cells, but two or more of the other criteria are present. Since there are no cases of myocardial infarction in those

Table 5. A four-fold matrix table indicating the presence or absence of four independent criteria for the diagnosis of acute myocardial infarction.

Cell	Number of cases	Final clinical diagnosis	Q Wave in ECG	Classic history	LDH flipped	CPK-MB present
1	24	MI	Yes	Yes	Yes	Yes
2	5	MI	No	Yes	Yes	Yes
3	4	MI	Yes	No	Yes	Yes
4	3	MI	Yes	Yes	No	Yes
5	None	—	Yes	Yes	Yes	No
6	3	MI	No	No	Yes	Yes
7	5	MI, 4; coronary insufficiency, 1	No	Yes	No	Yes
8	2	MI	Yes	No	No	Yes
9	None	—	Yes	No	Yes	No
10	None	—	Yes	Yes	No	No
11	None	—	No	Yes	Yes	No
12	None	—	Yes	No	No	No
13	7	Coronary insufficiency 4; angina, 2; chest pain, 1	No	Yes	No	No
14	1	Arrhythmia in patient with prosthetic valve, 1	No	No	Yes	No
15	7	MI, 1; angina, 3; heart failure, 1; pulmonary embolism, 1; coronary insufficiency, 1	No	No	No	Yes
16	33	Non-MI	No	No	No	No

cells, CPK_2 is probably highly specific for myocardial infarction. A test with high specificity is negative in the absence of a particular disease.

Cell 13 of the matrix contains 7 patients with a classic history for MI, but negative results for ECG, LDH_1, and CPK_2. Clinically these patients were finally judged *not* to have had an acute MI. In view of the high sensitivity of CPK_2 for MI, this final clinical judgement is probably correct.

The single patient in cell 14 is explained on the basis of hemolysis secondary to a valve replacement. Hemolysis always elevates LDH_1.

Cell 15 is the most controversial cell in our matrix. There were 7 patients in that cell and 1 of them was clinically diagnosed as MI. The other 6 were classified as non-MI. However, in each of those patients CPK_2 was present in serum. In view of the demonstrated high sensitivity of CPK_2 for myocardial ischemia, and the suggested high specificity of CPK_2 for acute myocardial infarction, each of the patients in cell 15 should probably have been classified as MI for purposes of treatment during the acute phase of the illness.

BEYOND NORMALITY—A REPRISE

Sensitivity versus Specificity versus Predictive Value versus Efficiency

Our study provides interesting data on the relative importance of sensitivity, specificity, predictive value, and efficiency. A change in the referent value (or the so-called upper limit of normal), alters sensitivity and specificity, and thereby the predictive value of a positive result and the efficiency. Table 6 gives the data derived from our MI study in which the prevalence of MI was approximately 50%.

Table 6.   SGOT
Prevalence = 50%

Referent value	Sensitivity (%)	Specificity (%)	Predictive value of positive (%)	Efficiency (%)
25	100	60	70	80
55	76	83	81	79.5
85	54	92	86	73
115	41	96	90	68.5
155	28	100	100	64

The highest sensitivity is obtained with a referent value of 25 U/l; the highest specificity with a referent value of 155 U/l; the highest predictive value of a positive result with a referent value of 155 U/l; and the highest efficiency with a referent value of 25 U/l.

These data clearly indicate why the problem of "limits" is far more complex than commonly thought. The naive physician believes there is a single well-defined upper limit, which can be agreed upon by all and which separates "normal" from "abnormal."[2] The more sophisticated approach, espoused by Holland and Whitehead,[3] is to define limits in terms of various population groups based on such variables as age, sex, nutrition, activity, and disease.

But, clearly, even this approach is not sufficiently sophisticated because, as our story indicates over and over again, it is essential to know the prevalence of the disease under investigation. It is equally essential to know whether you want the highest sensitivity, specificity, predictive value or efficiency. *There is no single upper limit, or referent value, that can be established immutably for any particular group.*

Efficiency is Best for MI

In a test for myocardial infarction we believe it is best to opt for the highest efficiency. To the patient and to the clinician it is equally bad to miss an infarct when one is present as it is to diagnose an infarct when one has not occurred. It is our impression, after working with cardiologists, that they have unconsciously recognized the need to seek the highest efficiency when evaluating test results in patients suspected of having a myocardial infarction.

We see from our Table 6 that a referent value of 25 U/1 provides the highest efficiency. The usual upper limit of normal for our SGOT method is published as 50 U/l. A very low referent value provides 100% sensitivity. That is, not a single case of myocardial infarction is missed; on the other hand, the false-positive rate is 30% (100 minus the predictive value). However, overall efficiency is highest with this low referent value. The highest efficiency is obtained when the largest number of correct diagnoses is made, whether positive or negative

Referent Value for Total CPK

The situation with regard to the proper referent value for total CPK is equally interesting. Again our study provides data that permits us to evaluate the effect of changing referent values in the setting of a coronary care unit in which the prevalence of MI is approximately 50%. Our data are shown in Table 7.

Table 7. Total CPK data derived from MI study
Prevalence = 50%

Referent Value (U/1)	Sensitivity (%)	Specificity (%)	Predictive value of positive (%)	Efficiency (%)
25	100	43	62	72
55	95	74	77	84.5
85	88	84	84	86
115	70	96	94	83
175	65	98	97	82

The highest sensitivity is obtained with a referent value of 25 U/l; the highest specificity with a referent value of 175 U/l; the highest predictive value of a positive result with a referent value of 175 U/l; and, the highest efficiency is obtained with a referent value of 85 U/l.

This time we have several possible limits (Table 8).

Table 8. Referent values for total CPK in the diagnosis of MI
Prevalence = 50%

Class	Referent value (U/1)
Usual upper limit	50
Highest sensitivity	25
Highest specificity	175
Highest predictive value of positive	175
Highest efficiency	85

Our analysis shows that a referent value of 85 U/l for our assay provides the highest efficiency for total CPK when prevalence is 50% and the clinical problem is "rule out MI."

No Single Upper Limit for Total CPK

If *all* conditions of the CPK assay were standardized across the nation, would it then be possible, as demanded by Gregory Duboff,[2] to provide an "official" cutoff point between health and disease. We think not. Creatine phosphokinase exemplifies, perhaps better than any other test, that a single cutoff point between health and disease, or between different diseases does not exist. Table 9, based on studies carried out in our laboratory, illustrates this point.[4] The data in the table show that there is no single upper limit that predicts the presence of disease or defines the risk of developing a disease.

Table 9. **What is normal for total CPK activity? The frequency distribution of total CPK activity 1 day after the clinical episode in four classes of patients**

CPK activity	Medical		Open heart surgery		Angiography	Hip surgery
(U /l)	Non-MI	MI	Non-MI	MI	Non-MI	Non-MI
0–49	32	2	—	—	9	—
50–99	10	4	—	—	2	1
100–149	5	6	1	—	3	—
150–199	1	3	2	—	2	—
200–299	—	3	6	—	7	2
300–399	1	8	8	—	5	2
400–499	—	4	6	1	—	5
500–599	—	—	4	—	1	—
600–699	—	4	5	—	2	2
700–799	—	1	1	—	—	—
800–899	—	2	—	—	—	—
900–999	—	3	1	—	—	1
1000–1999	—	6	3	3	—	—
2000–2999	—	—	—	1	—	—
3000–3999	—	1	—	—	—	—
Totals	49	47	37	5	31	13

Of the 96 medical patients suspected of having an acute myocardial infarction, 47 had a final combined clinical and ECG diagnosis of MI. Table 9 shows the frequency distribution of total CPK values 1 day after admission. The distributions for MI and non-MI show a considerable overlap as discussed previously. MI cannot be separated from non-MI on the basis of total CPK alone. A cutoff of 50 U/l, for example, had a sensitivity of 96%, but a specificity of only 65%. That is, 96% of the MI patients had a total CPK *above* 50 U/l, but only 65% of the non-MI patients in the CCU had a total CPK *below* 50 U/l.

Of the 42 patients who underwent heart surgery, 5 developed an MI during or immediately after surgery. The total CPK value 24 hours after surgery is shown in Table 9. There is no definable cutoff point for total CPK that permits separation of the 5 MI patients from the 37 non-MI patients following cardiac surgery. Elevation of total CPK following cardiac surgery has no diagnostic significance, since the total CPK level fails to predict disease or the risk of developing disease. All of the non-MI cases, even those with the highest levels of total CPK, made uneventful recoveries.

Of the 31 patients who underwent coronary angiography, none developed an MI. The distribution of total CPK values 1 day after angiography had little relationship to prognosis since the enzyme elevations were secondary to a variety of factors, such as intramuscular injections and cutdowns, and perhaps to transient myocardial ischemia during the procedure. Total CPK levels do not discriminate between myocardial and nonmyocardial origins of enzyme activity.

The last column in Table 9 shows data on 13 patients who underwent total hip replacement. There were no MI patients in this group, yet there were striking elevations of total CPK attributable to skeletal muscle trauma associated with the procedure.

It is *not* possible to define an absolute upper limit for total CPK that will be applicable to the majority of clinical situations. Following surgery, for example, a total CPK level of 1000 U/l may be "normal," in that it carries no clinical risk or predictive value for disease. It is far more important to ask, Where is the enzyme coming from?, than it is to ask, How much enzyme activity is present?

REFERENCES

---

1. Galen, R. S., Reiffel, J. A., and Gambino, S. R. Diagnosis of acute myocardial infarction: relative efficiency of serum enzyme and isoenzyme measurements. *JAMA* **232:** 145–147, 1975.
2. Duboff, G. S. Expressing results of enzyme assays. *Clin. Chem.* **20:** 402–403, 1974.
3. Holland, W. W. and Whitehead, T. P. Value of new laboratory tests in diagnosis and treatment. *Lancet* **ii:** 391–394, 1974.
4. Galen, R. S. and Gambino, S. R. What upper limit of creatine kinase activity defines disease? *Clin. Chem.* **21:** 272, 1975.

CHAPTER 14

THE ELECTROCARDIOGRAM—
APPLICATION OF THE MODEL TO A
NONLABORATORY TEST

IS THERE SUCH A THING AS A NORMAL ECG?

WHAT is a normal electrocardiogram (ECG)? Dr. Ernst Simonson, Professor of Physiological Hygiene at the University of Minnesota, has detailed the sources of normal variability in the ECG.[1] What is the diagnostic accuracy of the ECG? The answer varies with the respondent. The pathologist immediately conjures up those post-mortem cases of acute myocardial infarction that were "electrocardiographically silent." Post-mortem studies in the literature document the poor sensitivity of the ECG in the diagnosis of MI.[2] The cardiologist, on the other hand, can point to electrocardiographically diagnosed cases of MI that were "clinically silent." Studies in the literature document the problem of the "silent coronary," that is, cases with unequivocal ECG evidence of MI.[3] How good is ECG diagnosis? Simonson's answer is as follows:

> A precise evaluation of the diagnostic accuracy of any method can be made only by comparison of the frequency distribution in a sample of healthy population and in a sample of patients with known pathologic condition(sic). The distribution of ECG characteristics in well-defined groups of patients with proved cardiac disease is largely unknown. A fairly wide overlap of these values in healthy populations and in cardiac patients must be assumed, chiefly because the ECG may be normal in the presence of clinical heart disease.[1]

The situation is identical to that in clinical chemistry where the upper limit of normal, separating normal from abnormal, is determined by statistical analysis of data in normal individuals. The value of this cutoff point in diagnosis depends on the degree of overlap of the frequency distributions for normal and diseased populations. Depending on the diagnosis in question, there may be slight or significant overlap. Unfortunately, the cutoff point defining "normal" remains the same. Furthermore, the methods used to determine the limits of the normal range in electrocardiography are quite variable. In some cases, extreme limits encompassing 100% of the normal populations are used. In other cases, 95 or 98% limits are used. In those cases 5 or 2%, respectively, of healthy people are classified as abnormal for each variable. As expected, studies on the diagnostic value of ECG variables show a large degree of overlap between "health" and "disease." Weisbart and Simonson, in evaluating the presence of Q_3 in myocardial infarction, demonstrated a large degree of overlap because of a prominent Q_3 in the healthy population.[4] Simonson states that, "failure to take the frequency distribution into consideration may lead to erroneous conclusions regarding the diagnostic accuracy of the ECG."[1]

THE PRECISION OF THE ECG

Before considering several ECG studies, and evaluating the predictive value of the ECG, we think it worthwhile to comment on the precision of ECG interpretation. Several studies have documented both the intraobserver and interobserver variation in interpretation. Davies investigated 9 experienced physician readers who were required to interpret a series of 100 ECG tracings on two sparate occasions. The test tracings were selected so that half demonstrated myocardial infarction, a quarter showed other abnormalities, and a quarter were felt to be normal. "Complete agreement was reached in only one-third of the 100 tracings, majority agreement in half, but there was considerable dispute about one tracing in five. After the second reading, it was found that on average, the readers disagreed with one in eight of their original reports."[5] It should be noted that this variation was equally distributed among the normal, abnormal, and infarction categories. Summarizing his report, Davies commented, "From the standpoint of electrocardiographic diagnosis it is an illusion to believe there can be any arbitrary line between normal and abnormal tracings or between abnormal and infarction tracings. The ranges of each overlap and do so more widely than is generally realized."[5] Following Davies' study in the *British Heart Journal,* the following editorial comments appeared:

> If anyone thinks that a report on a single electrocardiogram can always decide whether it is normal or abnormal or whether there is or is not evidence of cardiac infarction, this valuable paper will show that he is wrong. No one, on reflection, does think this, but many write a routine report as if they did.[5]

Other studies further document the problems of intraobserver and interobserver variation in the interpretation of ECG tracings.[6,7]

THE SENSITIVITY OF THE ECG

In our myocardial infarction study, we analyzed data on 100 consecutive admissions to the coronary care unit. These patients had an admission diagnostic problem of "rule-out myocardial infarction." Our data have been presented in Chapter 13, and from the matrix in Table 6 (Chapter 13) we can determine the sensitivity and specificity of the development of a new and persistent Q wave in the ECG. From the matrix it can be seen that 33 out of 46 MI cases developed Q waves. Thus the sensitivity of the Q wave was 72%. In 48 non-MI cases there were no Q waves present. Thus the specificity of the Q wave in our study was 100%. In general, the appearance of a new Q wave is regarded as a highly specific, but not very sensitive test for myocardial infarction. In the coronary care unit setting, where the prevalence of myocardial infarction is extremely high (50%), the Q-wave criteria for MI has a predictive value of virtually 100%.[8] Unfortunately, an unacceptable number of MI cases (28)% would be missed if the sole criterion for diagnosis was the Q wave.

Autopsy studies further document the lack of sensitivity of the ECG in diagnosing acute myocardial infarction. Levine and Phillips analyzed 150 consecutive patients in whom at least one complete set of tracings had been taken during their terminal illness and who subsequently were autopsied. The authors found that "the electrocardiographic diagnosis of acute myocardial infarction was invariably correct (specificity = 100%). However, of all acute infarcts found at autopsy only 75% were detected electrocardiographically (Sensitivity = 75%). Only 20% of old infarcts found at autopsy were correctly diagnosed electrocardiographically."[2] After reviewing their findings, the authors concluded:

> However, since the electrocardiogram represents the composite effect of a number of factors operating simultaneously, the effect of certain changes may be obscured in the resulting tracing and thus may escape detection. Accordingly, restraint, caution, humility and sound judgment are still vital in its evaluation.[2]

In a more recent study by Garde and Rasmussen, of St. Josephs Hospital in Copenhagen, findings from 39 autopsies were compared with ECG localization of infarction.[9] Localization of infarction could not be determined in 8 patients because of widespread myocardial damage. In the remaining 31 patients, fairly good agreement was achieved; and 28 of the 31 infarcts localized by ECG were, in fact, found at post-mortem examination. The 3 cases in which the infarct could not be localized all had widespread infarction of the septum. In addition, there were 38 undiagnosed areas of infarction in these 31 patients. The lack of ECG sensitivity was demonstrated by the additional findings of 21 undiagnosed infarcts in the septum, 6 undiagnosed infarcts in the posterior wall, and 5 undiagnosed infarcts in the anterior wall. In 6 additional patients 2 infarcts were present in the same area.[9]

THE ECG AS A SCREENING TEST

Myocardial infarction is the most severe outcome in a spectrum of pathological conditions classified as variations of ischemic or coronary heart disease. Since myocardial infarction is the number one cause of death in this country, the possibility of screening for the presence of coronary heart disease is very attractive. The ECG has frequently been included as a screening tool in this regard. Unfortunately, the sensitivity is low. Data from the Framingham Study is enlightening relative to the ECG.[10] The Framingham report on the 6-year incidence of coronary heart disease (defined as angina pectoris, myocardial infarction, and sudden death) began with 2283 men free of coronary heart disease (CHD). There were 125 men who developed CHD in the subsequent 6-year period. The 6-year incidence in men, therefore, was 125/2283 = 5.5%; or about 1% per year. Table 1 is from the Framingham study. It can be seen that of 88 cases of myocardial infarction, 24 involved sudden death. Of these 24, 15 had no previous evidence of CHD, which included, therefore, negative ECG examinations. On the other hand, 7 men who suffered MI had clinically silent infarcts, and the diagnosis was made by ECG criteria alone. Table 1 shows that 73 of 88 cases of MI had prior positive ECG findings. Therefore the sensitivity of the ECG for predicting the development of CHD is 83%.

An earlier report from the Framingham Heart Disease Epidemiology Study discussed the value of an ECG in screening for heart disease. Multiple- and single-

Table 1.   Clinical manifestations of CHD developing in 6 years of followup[10]

Clinical manifestation	Men	
	Number	Percent
Total CHD	125	100
Angina pectoris	37	29.6
Myocardial infarction	88	70.4
Total myocardial infarction	88	100
By history and ECG	57	64.8
By ECG only	7	7.9
Sudden death	24	27.3
Total sudden death	24	100
With preexisting MI	3	12.5
With preexisting angina	6	25.0
Without preexisting CHD	15	62.5

lead ECG tracings were evaluated in 2000 individuals. Findings from the 12-lead ECG study are presented in Table 2. This table permits us to estimate the sensitivity and specificity of the ECG in screening for heart disease (coronary artery

Table 2.   Twelve-lead ECG versus final clinical impression: 2000 patients

Final clinical impression	Impression from 12-lead ECG			
	Normal	Doubtful	Abnormal	Total
No heart disease	1400	114	53	1567
	89.3	7.3	3.4	100.0%
Possible heart disease	100	32	24	156
	64.1	20.5	15.4	100.0%
Heart disease	147	51	79	277
	53.1	18.4	28.5	100.0%

disease, hypertensive cardiovascular disease, rheumatic heart disease, congenital heart disease, etc.) There was a normal ECG in 89.3% of patients with no heart disease. Therefore the specificity of the ECG was 89.3%. There was an abnormal or doubtful ECG in 46.9% (18.4 + 28.5) of patients with heart disease. Therefore the sensitivity of the ECG was 46.9%. Comparable figures for the single-lead ECG procedure reveal a specificity of 80.3% and a sensitivity of 49.3%[11] Dawber and co-workers concluded:

Either lead I alone or the 12-lead electrocardiogram will fail to classify correctly over half of the persons with clinically definite or possible cardiac disease. It is concluded that if the electrocardiogram is to be used for screening, the speed and ease of the technic and the slight loss of efficiency in the use of lead I alone compared with the 12-lead electrocardiogram would appear to make lead I the method of choice for the screening line.[11]

In another screening study, conducted at the District of Columbia General Hospital, four screening tests for heart disease and hypertension were evaluated in 690 persons. The ECG was included, and consisted of the standard lead I test. These investigators reported a sensitivity of 50.6% and a specificity of 76.6% for the ECG when applied to cases having *diagnosed* heart disease and/or hypertension.[12] This particular study is described in greater detail in Chapter 6.

Much of the present chapter has been devoted to the ECG diagnosis of myocardial infarction and ischemic heart disease; however ECG criteria have been used to evaluate other pathologic conditions. Dr. Roger W. Jeliffe, of the Cardiology Section at the University of Southern California School of Medicine, reviewed the effect of prevalence of left ventricular enlargement on errors in its ECG recognition. A cardiology service, a community hospital, and an outpatient population were evaluated. Dr. Jelliffe assigned the values of 25, 5, and 1%, respectively, to indicate the prevalence of left ventricular enlargement in the three groups. Several ECG criteria for the recognition of left ventricular enlargement have been reported, and Jelliffe constructed a table evaluating the effect of prevalence on the diagnostic accuracy of each. We have redrawn his table, converting data into sensitivity, specificity, and predictive value (Table 3).[13]

Jelliffe summarized his review by stating, "The results clearly show that (1) the electrocardiographic recognition of left ventricular enlargement is inaccurate at best, and (2) the influence of the incidence of the entity being sought for (left

Table 3.   Effect of prevalence of left ventricular enlargement upon errors in its electrocardiographic recognition*

Criteria	Sensitivity (%)	Specificity (%)	Predictive value of positives (%) Prevalence			False positive rate (%) Prevalence		
			25%	5%	1%	25%	5%	1%
Romhilt and Estes†								
(5 points)	58	97	87	50	16	13	50	84
Noth, Myers, and Klein	18	98	75	32	8	25	68	92
Schach, Rosenbaum,								
and Katz	12	98	67	24	6	33	76	94
Romhilt et al.	56	89	63	21	5	37	79	95
Allenstein	71	83	58	18	4	42	82	96
Gubner and Underleider	35	87	47	12	3	53	88	97
Goldberger	35	81	38	9	2	62	91	98
Sokolow and Lyon	88	44	34	8	2	66	92	98
Katz	41	73	34	7	2	66	93	98
Goulder and Kissane	12	92	33	7	1	67	93	99
Wilson et al.	94	23	29	6	1	71	94	99

*Modified from Jelliffe.
†Authors cited by Jelliffe.

ventricular enlargement in the population being tested) is profound." Jelliffe concludes his editorial with the admonition that "We must keep in mind not only the accuracy of the test itself, but also the incidence of what we expect to find in the population under study."[13]

Table 4 demonstrates the predictive value of one of the most accurate criteria, the point-score system of Romhilt and Estes, when the prevalence of left ventricular enlargement is 5% (community hospital setting).

Table 4. Predictive value of ECG diagnosis of left ventricular enlargement: community hospital setting

Prevalence = 5%

	ECG Positive	ECG Negative	Totals
Left ventricular hypertrophy	29	21	50 (sensitivity = 58%)
No left ventricular hypertrophy	28	922	950 (specificity = 97%)
Totals	57	943	1000

The predictive value of a positive result is 50%. The efficiency is 95.1%.

The ECG tracing is a set of diagnostic tests that are subject to the same theoretical considerations as the other diagnostic tests discussed in this book. As a panel of measurements of intervals, segments, and wave heights, it is really no different from a panel of biochemical measurements. If it is going to be used in a diagnostic fashion, criteria must be developed to separate positives from negatives, or "abnormals" from "normals." When this is done, the predictive value or diagnostic accuracy of the ECG depends on the sensitivity and specificity of the criteria and the prevalence of the disease. As with chemical tests, normal ranges can be altered to change sensitivity and specificity. Similarly, prevalence can be increased by careful patient selection.

The result of considering the ECG in light of the predictive value model will be the evolution of highly predictive or highly efficient criteria (depending on the clinical requirements). This will require evaluation of ECG changes in health and in a variety of disease states. It cannot be developed from the study of normal or healthy populations alone.

REFERENCES

1. Simonson, Ernst. Differentiation between normal and abnormal in electrocardiography. Mosby, St. Louis, 1961, pp. 328.
2. Levine, H. D. and Phillips, E. An appraisal of the newer electrocardiography: correlations in one hundred and fifty consecutive autopsied cases. *N. Engl. J. Med.* **245:** 833–842, 1951.

3. Stokes, J. and Dawber, T. R. *The "Silent Coronary":* the frequency and clinical charac-
    teristics of unrecognized myocardial infarction in the Framingham study. *Ann. Intern.
    Med.* **50:** 1359–1369, 1959.

4. Weisbart, Myron H. and Simonson, Ernst. The diagnostic accuracy of Q_3 and related
    electrocardiographic items for the detection of patients with posterior wall myocardial
    infarction. *Am. Heart J.* **50:** 62–81, 1955.

5. Davies, L. G. Observer variation in reports on electrocardiograms. *Br. Heart J.* **20:**
    153–161, 1958.

6. Kagen, Aubrey R. Interpretation of electrocardiograms. *Milbank Mem. Fund Q.* **43:**
    Part 2: 40–48, 1965.

7. Epstein, F. H., Doyle, J. T., Pollack, A. A., Pollack, H., Robb, G. B., and Simonson,
    E. Observer Interpretation of electrocardiograms. *JAMA* **175:** 847–850 1961.

8. Galen, R. S., Reiffel, J. A., and Gambino, S. R. Diagnosis of acute myocardial infarction:
    relative efficiency of serum enzyme and isoenzyme measurements. *JAMA* **232:** 145–147,
    1975.

9. Garde, A. Kjeld and Rasmussen, V. Elektrokardiografisk diagnosik af akut myokardiein-
    farkt sammenholtd med autopsifund. *Ugeskr Laeg* **135:** 4–7, 1973 (Translated by C.
    Nielsen and E. Sanden, Arhus, Denmark).

10. Kannel, W. B., Dawber, T. R., Kagan, A., Revotskie, N., and Stokes, J. Factors of
    risk in the development of coronary heart disease—six year follow-up experience. *Ann.
    Intern. Med.* **55:** 33–50, 1961.

11. Dawber, T. R., Kannel, W. B., Love, D. E., and Streeper, R. B. The electrocardiogram in
    heart disease detection: a comparison of the multiple and single lead procedure.
    Circulation **5:** 559–566, 1952.

12. Kurlander, A. B., Hill, E. H., and Enterline, P. E. An evaluation of some commonly
    used screening tests for heart disease and hypertension. *J. Chronic Dis.* **2:** 427–439, 1955.

13. Jelliffe, R. W. Quantitative aspects of clinical judgement. *Am. J. Med.* **55:** 431–433,
    1973.

CHAPTER 15

DIABETES—APPLICATION OF THE MODEL TO GLUCOSE MEASUREMENTS

I N Chapter 4 we explored glucose analysis in terms of some of the different ways the laboratory functions. A large percentage of the glucose analyses performed are related to the diagnosis and treatment of diabetes mellitus. Because the prevalence of diabetes is so high (2 to 6%), and the complications in terms of morbidity and mortality so significant, diabetes detection is the objective of many screening programs. In a recent review on screening, Professor J. M. Malins of the Diabetic Clinic of the General Hospital in Birmingham, England commented:

> Screening of whole populations with the object of case finding is not a rewarding exercise. In the Birmingham survey, self-testing by 18,532 subjects of urine passed after a meal revealed 119 known diabetics and only 55 new cases of definite diabetes. At the same time, there were many minor abnormalities of the glucose-tolerance test of doubtful significance. A follow-up of these doubtful tests after 10 years indicates that less than a quarter deteriorate to "clinical" diabetes during this time. Thus the problem of "borderline" diabetes is difficult to handle and one must hesitate before creating patients from volunteers who may have a trivial and harmless abnormality.[1]

Any discussion of diabetes and glucose should include (1) those levels at which to consider a test positive, (2) chemical methodology of the test used, (3) blood versus urine screening, and (4) reference criteria for diagnosing diabetes. A report by Remein and Wilkerson,[2] of the Public Health Service Study conducted at Boston City Hospital, provides comparative data on several blood and urine glucose tests. A total of 595 persons were studied and 72 were diagnosed as diabetics. The diagnostic criteria were established by a group of consultants and consisted entirely of the results of the 100-gram, 3-hour, oral glucose tolerance test. Relative to this classification, several blood and urine tests were evaluated to determine their individual sensitivity and specificity at different times. Tables 1 to 6 are from this study and are based on results for 70 persons diagnosed as diabetic from a sample of 580 patients. Tables 1 and 2 show the results obtained with two different chemical methods for measuring whole blood glucose.

It is interesting to explore the relationship between these two methods of glucose analysis. The Folin-Wu test measures total reducing substances and is clearly not a "specific" test for glucose. The Somogyi-Nelson, on the other hand, approximates a true glucose determination. Does a test that lacks chemical specificity also lack diagnostic specificity? From Tables 1 and 2, we see that at any given referent value, such as 120, 140, and 160 mg/dl, the specificity of the Somogyi-Nelson test is consistently higher than the specificity of the Folin-Wu test. Similarly, in order to achieve comparable diagnostic value and accuracy, a higher referent value is required for the Folin-Wu assay than for the Somogyi-Nelson test. The answer to our question, therefore, is yes, because chemical specificity is required to obtain diagnostic specificity.

Urine screening results for two tests are presented in Table 3. They are taken from the study by Remein and Wilkerson and are based on results for 61 patients diagnosed as diabetic from a sample of 515 patients. The sensitivity of urine testing is quite low.

We can compare the Somogyi-Nelson blood test with the Clinitest urine test at various prevalence rates of diabetes. The referent values have been selected to optimize the usefulness of each test. A referent value of 160 mg/dl has been

Table 1. Somogyi-Nelson blood test (venous). Sensitivity and specificity for diabetes at different referent values, by hours after test meal

Prevalence = 12.1%

Referent value (mg/dl)	Random hours after eating		One hour after test		Two hours after test		Three hours after test	
	Sensitivity (%)	Specificity (%)	Sensitivity (%)	Specificity (%)	Sensitivity (%)	Specificity (%)	Sensitivity (%)	Specificity (%)
80	91.4	36.3	97.1	22.4	97.1	25.5	91.4	34.7
90	82.9	65.7	97.1	39.0	94.3	47.6	82.9	67.5
100	65.7	84.7	95.7	57.3	88.6	69.8	70.0	86.5
110	54.3	92.7	92.9	70.6	85.7	84.1	60.0	95.3
120	50.0	96.7	88.6	83.3	71.4	92.5	51.4	98.2
130	44.3	99.0	78.6	90.6	64.3	96.9	48.6	99.8
140	37.1	99.6	68.6	95.1	57.1	99.4	41.4	100.0
150	30.0	99.8	57.1	97.8	50.0	99.6	32.9	100.0
160	25.7	99.8	52.9	99.4	47.1	99.8	28.6	100.0
170	25.7	99.8	47.1	99.6	42.9	100.0	28.6	100.0
180	22.9	99.8	40.0	99.8	38.6	100.0	28.6	100.0
190	21.4	100.0	34.3	100.0	34.3	100.0	24.3	100.0

selected for the blood test at 1 hour after the test meal, giving a sensitivity of 52.9% and a specificity of 99.4%. A referent value of 1+ has been selected for the Clinitest urine test at 2 hours after the test meal, giving a sensitivity of 44.3% and a specificity of 96.5%. Table 4 lists the predictive value, false-positive rate, and efficiency for these tests at three prevalence rates. It is reasonable to look at varying prevalence rates, because, by selecting high-risk groups for screening, we can increase the prevalence. High-risk groups can be defined by age (over 45), family history of diabetes, and obstetrical history.

Table 4 shows that the number of cases found would not be high for either test because of the low sensitivity of both tests; but the blood test would result in substantially fewer false positives and is more efficient because it is more specific than the urine test.

In addition, we see that at comparable specificities, the Somogyi-Nelson test has greater sensitivity than the urine tests. The differences can be further illustrated with the following hypothetical example:

Example *A population of 10,000 adults with a prevalence of diabetes of 5% is to be screened.*

Patients can be tested 2 hours postprandially. Because of limited retesting facilities and resources, and the desire to keep false-positive results to a reasonable level, we compare the outcome using a blood test and urine test that have approximately the same specificity. This will result in similar predictive values for both approaches. The 2 hour Clinitest (1+) has a sensitivity of 44.3% and a specificity of 96.5%. A Somogyi-Nelson blood sugar with a referent value of 130 mg/dl at 2 hours has a sensitivity of 64.3% and a specificity of 96.9%. Table 5 compares these two approaches.

Table 2. Folin-Wu blood test (venous). Sensitivity and specificity for diabetes at different values by hours after test meal

Prevalence = 12.1%

Referent value (mg/dl)	Random hours after eating		One hour after test		Two hours after test		Three hours after test	
	Sensitivity (%)	Specificity (%)	Sensitivity (%)	Specificity (%)	Sensitivity (%)	Specificity (%)	Sensitivity (%)	Specificity (%)
80	100.0	1.6	—	1.6	100.0	1.2	100.0	1.0
90	95.7	8.2	100.0	8.8	98.6	7.3	97.1	6.1
100	85.7	33.9	98.6	21.4	97.1	25.3	92.9	34.5
110	81.4	67.1	98.6	38.4	92.9	48.4	81.4	67.8
120	67.1	82.2	97.1	55.9	88.6	68.2	68.6	86.5
130	55.7	92.7	92.9	70.2	81.4	82.4	60.0	94.3
140	50.0	96.3	85.7	81.4	74.3	91.2	57.1	98.2
150	44.3	98.8	80.0	90.4	64.3	96.1	48.6	99.6
160	35.7	99.6	74.3	94.3	55.7	98.6	42.9	100.0
170	34.3	99.8	61.4	97.8	52.9	99.6	35.7	100.0
180	27.1	99.8	52.9	99.0	50.0	99.8	28.6	100.0
190	24.3	99.8	44.3	99.8	44.3	99.8	28.6	100.0

Table 3. Sensitivity and specificity of two urine tests for diabetes at different referent values by hours after test meal

Prevalence = 11.8%

Referent value	Random hours after eating		One hour after test		Two hours after test		Three hours after test	
	Sensitivity (%)	Specificity (%)	Sensitivity (%)	Specificity (%)	Sensitivity (%)	Specificity (%)	Sensitivity (%)	Specificity (%)
Clinitest*								
trace	34.4	88.3	37.7	83.5	54.1	80.6	45.9	86.6
1+	29.5	98.7	31.1	96.9	44.3	96.5	36.1	98.5
2+	23.0	100.0	27.9	98.9	37.7	98.7	34.4	99.3
3+	19.7	100.0	24.6	99.3	31.1	99.1	29.5	100.0
4+	9.8	100.0	21.3	99.8	24.6	99.3	2.2	100.0
Benedict's								
trace	42.6	73.6	68.9	54.4	88.5	34.6	80.3	51.1
1+	32.8	92.1	49.2	84.6	59.0	79.3	49.2	86.3
2+	21.3	99.8	34.4	97.4	41.0	97.4	34.4	99.3
3+	19.7	100.0	24.6	99.3	34.4	99.8	29.5	99.8
4+	4.9	100.0	11.5	100.0	13.1	100.0	9.8	100.0

*Clinitest, a copper sulfate reagent table for urine sugar determinations, is manufactured by the Ames Company, Inc., Elkhart, Indiana.

Table 4. Blood versus urine. Comparison of screening tests for diabetes

Prevalence (%	Test	Sensitivity	Specificity	Predictive value	False positive rate	Efficiency
1	Blood	52.9	99.4	47.1	52.9	98.9
1	Urine	44.3	96.5	11.3	88.7	96.0
3	Blood	52.9	99.4	73.2	26.8	98.0
3	Urine	44.3	96.5	28.1	71.9	94.9
5	Blood	52.9	99.4	82.3	17.7	97.1
5	Urine	44.3	96.5	40.0	60.0	93.9

Table 5. Blood versus urine. Comparison of screening tests at 2 hours after test meal

Tests have similar specificities

	Blood test				Urine test		
	Diabetes	Other	Total		Diabetes	Other	Total
Test				Test			
+	322	294	616	+	222	332	554
−	178	9,206	9,384	−	278	9,168	9,446
Total	500	9,500	10,000	Total	500	9,500	10,000

Prevalence	= 5.0%	Prevalence	= 5.0%
Sensitivity	= 64.3%	Sensitivity	= 44.3%
Specificity	= 96.9%	Specificity	= 96.5%
Predictive value	= 52.0%	Predictive value	= 40.0%
False positive	= 48.0%	False positive	= 60.0%
Efficiency	= 95.3%	Efficiency	= 93.9%

The blood test detects 322/222 = 1.5 times as many cases as the urine test with equal specificity.

At 2 hours postprandially, a 1+ Clinitest has a sensitivity of 44.3% and a specificity of 96.5%. Therefore 44.3% of the diabetics in the population tested will test positive. A Somogyi-Nelson blood glucose, 2 hours postprandially, at a referent value of 170 mg/dl has a similar detection rate with a sensitivity of 42.9% and a specificity of 100.0%. Let us compare these two approaches in our same hypothetical population (Table 6).

Each test detects about 220 true cases of diabetes. The blood test results in no false positives, whereas the urine test results in 554 positives, 60% of which are false positives. With equal sensitivity, the blood test is more predictive because it leads to fewer false positives than the urine test.

It should be noted that Remein and Wilkerson caution against generalizing their findings to other populations. The general relationships, however, can be expected to remain true; for example, the inferior value of the urine test versus the blood test. The relationship between blood and urinary glucose levels has been further investigated by Service and co-workers at the Mayo Clinic.[3]

Table 6. Blood versus urine. Comparison of screening tests at 2 hours after test meal

Tests have similar sensitivities

	Blood test				Urine test		
	Diabetes	Other	Total		Diabetes	Other	Total
Test				Test			
+	215	0	215	+	222	332	554
−	285	9,500	9,785	−	278	9,168	9,446
Total	500	9,500	10,000	Total	500	9,500	10,000

Prevalence	=	5.0%	Prevalence	=	5.0%
Sensitivity	=	42.9%	Sensitivity	=	44.3%
Specificity	=	100.0%	Specificity	=	96.5%
Predictive value	=	100.0%	Predictive value	=	40.0%
False Positive	=	0	False Positive	=	60.0%
Efficiency	=	97.2%	Efficiency	=	93.9%

The data presented, although not meant to be absolute or directly applicable to more commonly used glucose tests, such as glucose oxidase, hexokinase, and *ortho*-toluidine, do indicate several fundamental guidelines that probably hold true regardless of the glucose method employed. These include (1) blood tests are more accurate than urine tests in screening for diabetes, that is, results are more highly predictive (fewer false positives) and more efficient; and (2) blood tests taken following a glucose load are more accurate than either random or fasting samples. It should be noted that since mean postprandial blood sugar levels increase with age, and this is probably not abnormal, age-specific referent values should be applied when screening for diabetes.

DIAGNOSTIC CRITERIA

At present the reference test for establishing the diagnosis of diabetes mellitus is the oral glucose tolerance test. The test measures fasting, 1-, 2-, and 3-hour blood glucose levels following an oral glucose load of 40 grams per square meter of body surface. There is lack of agreement as to the optimum criteria to be used for making an interpretation, but the Committee on Statistics of the American Diabetes Association has recommended several comparable point systems. Their first choice is the Wilkerson point method shown in Table 7.[4]

In comparing the oral and intravenous glucose tolerance tests, Olefsky and co-workers at Stanford University School of Medicine note that, "depending upon the criteria used, the number of individuals with diabetes in a given population can vary from 0.5 to 24 percent."[5] The authors continue to probe the problem as follows:

Furthermore, it has been shown that a large proportion of patients in whom diabetes mellitus has been diagnosed by an abnormal tolerance test can have

Table 7. The Wilkerson point method for interpreting the oral glucose tolerance test

Time (hours)	Referent value (plasma or serum)	Point value
Fasting	130 or more	1
1	195 or more	$\frac{1}{2}$
2	140 or more	$\frac{1}{2}$
3	130 or more	1

Two points or more are required for the test to be considered positive for diabetes.

subsequent normal tests, and that many patients with a "diabetic" glucose tolerance test do not demonstrate significant decompensation of their glucose tolerance with time. Thus, the significance of designating asymptomatic individuals with fasting euglycemia as being diabetic on the basis of a glucose tolerance test is not clear.[5]

To investigate whether the oral and intravenous glucose tolerance tests provide similar information about carbohydrate tolerance, these investigators performed both tests in 45 patients. In addition they studied the pancreatic suppression test in these patients as a reference procedure. Their results indicated that the two tests were not providing the same information and that diagnostic classification of a patient as normal or diabetic would depend on whether the oral or intravenous test was used. The comparison between these two tests is seen in (Table 8).

Table 8. Comparison between oral glucose tolerance test and intravenous glucose tolerance test performed in 45 patients

OGTT result	IVGTT		
	Normal	Abnormal	Total
Normal	18*	12†	40
Abnormal	6†	9*	15
Total	24	21	45

* Total agreement 60%.
† Total disagreement 40%.

Further data presented from the pancreatic suppression test, which is based on measurement of the plasma glucose response to a continuous infusion of exogenous insulin, glucose, epinephrine, and propranolol, validated the reliability of the OGTT. The authors caution against interpreting their study as a defense of the OGTT.

The reproducibility of this test leaves a good deal to be desired, factors such as age, diet, activity, and various medications can profoundly affect the results; whether a patient is classified as diabetic or normal often depends upon which of several sets of criteria are used; and the meaning of an abnormal test in the subsequent development of the diabetic syndrome is certainly debatable.[5]

There is clearly a problem relating to uniform diagnostic criteria for diabetes and it is sheer folly to think that standardizing glucose analysis will help resolve the dilemma. A better glucose method or a more precise glucose assay is not the answer to the problem.

REFERENCES

1. Malins, J. M. Diabetes. *Lancet* **ii:** 1367–1368, 1974.
2. Remein, Q. R. and Wilkerson, H. L. C.: The efficiency of screening tests for diabetes. *J. Chronic Dis.* **13:** 6–21, 1961.
3. Service, F. J., Molnar, G. D., and Taylor, W. F. Urine glucose analyses during continuous blood glucose monitoring. *JAMA* **222:** 294–298, 1972.
4. Report of the Committee on Statistics of the American Diabetes Association. Standardization of the oral glucose tolerance test. *Diabetes* **18:** 299–310, 1969.
5. Olefsky, J. M., Farquhar, J. W., and Reaven, G. M. Do the oral and intravenous glucose tolerance tests provide similar diagnostic information in patients with chemical diabetes mellitus? *Diabetes* **22:** 202–209, 1973.

GLOSSARY

TRUE POSITIVES (TP).   Number of sick subjects who are correctly classified by the test.

FALSE POSITIVES (FP).   Number of subjects free of the disease who are misclassified by the test.

TRUE NEGATIVES (TN).   Number of subjects free of the disease who are correctly classified by the test.

FALSE NEGATIVES (FN).   Number of sick subjects who are misclassified by the test.

SENSITIVITY.   Percent positivity in disease:

$$\text{sensitivity} = \frac{\text{true positives}}{\text{all sick subjects}} \times 100$$

$$\text{sensitivity} = \frac{TP}{TP + FN} \times 100$$

SPECIFICITY.   Percent negativity in the absence of the disease:

$$\text{specificity} = \frac{\text{true negatives}}{\text{all subjects free of the disease}} \times 100$$

$$\text{specificity} = \frac{TN}{TN + FP} \times 100$$

PREVALENCE.   Number of subjects with the disease per 100,000 population.

INCIDENCE.   Number of *new* cases per year per 100,000 population.

PREDICTIVE VALUE OF A POSITIVE RESULT.   Percent of positive results that are true positives.

$$\text{Predictive value of } (+) = \frac{TP}{TP + FP} \times 100$$

PREDICTIVE VALUE OF A NEGATIVE RESULT.   Percent of negative results that are true negatives.

$$\text{Predictive value of } (-) = \frac{TN}{FN + TN} \times 100$$

EFFICIENCY. $\text{Efficiency} = \dfrac{TP + TN}{TP + FP + FN + TN} \times 100$

The interrelationships of true and false results is best appreciated by arranging the data according to Table 1.

Table 1. Interrelationships of true and false results

Clinical cases	Test result		Totals
	Positive	Negative	
Sick	TP	FN	TP + FN
Not sick	FP	TN	FP + TN
Totals	TP + FP	FN + TN	TP + FP + FN + TN

SELECTED READING

NORMALITY

Barnett, R. N. Medical significance of laboratory results. *Am. J. Clin. Pathol.* **50:** 671–676, 1968.

Childs, Barton. Sir Archibald Garrod's conception of chemical individuality: a modern appreciation. *N. Engl. J. Med.* **282:** 71–77, 1970.

Elveback, L. R., Guillier, C. L., and Keating, F. R., Jr., Health, normality, and the ghost of Gauss. *JAMA* **211:** 69–75, 1970.

Mainland, Donald. Remarks on clinical "norms." *Clin. Chem.* **17:** 267–274., 1971.

Martin, Horace F., Gudzinowicy, Benjamin J., and Fanger, Herbert. *Normal Values in Clinical Chemistry—A Guide to Statistical Analysis of Laboratory Data.* Marcel Dekker, Inc., New York, 1975.

Murphy, Edmond A. One cause? Many causes? The argument from the bimodal distribution. *J. Chronic Dis.* **17:** 301–324, 1964.

Murphy, Edmond A., A scientific viewpoint on normalcy. *Perspect. Biol. Med.* **9:** 333–348, Spring 1966.

Murphy, Edmond A. The normal, and the perils of the sylleptic argument. *Perspect. Biol. Med.* **15:** 566–582, Summer 1972.

Murphy, Edmond A. and Abbey, H. The normal range—a common misuse. *J. Chronic Dis.* **20:** 79–88, 1967.

Schoen, Irwin and Brooks, S. H. Judgement based on 95% confidence limits: a statistical dilemma involving multitest screening and proficiency testing of multiple specimens. *Am. J. Clin. Pathol.* **53:** 190–195, 1970.

Hoffman, Robert G. *Establishing Quality Control and Normal Ranges in the Clinical Laboratory*, 1st ed. (Exposition Press, New York) 1971.

PREDICTIVE VALUE

Blumberg, Mark S. Evaluating health screening procedures. *Oper. Res.* **5:** 351–360, 1957.

Chiang, C. L., Hodges, J. L., Jr., and Yerushalmy, J. Statistical problems in medical diagnosis. In *Berkeley Symposium on Mathematical Statistics and Probability (III)*. Berkeley, University of California Press, 1956, pp. 121–133.

Henry, R. J. and Reed, A. H. Normal values. In *Clinical Chemistry: Principles and Techniques,* 2nd ed., R. J. Henry, D. C. Cannon, and J. W. Winkelman (Eds.). Harper and Row, Hagerstown, Md. 1974, pp. 343–371.

Holland, W. W. and Whitehead, T. P. Value of new laboratory tests in diagnosis and treatment. *Lancet* **ii:** 391–394, 1974.

Jelliffe, Roger W. Quantitative aspects of clinical judgement, *Am. J. Med.* (editorial) **55:** 431–433, 1973.

Katz, Murray A. A probability graph describing the predictive value of a highly sensitive diagnostic test. *N. Engl. J. Med.* **291:** 1115–1116, 1974.

Krieg, A. F., Gambino, S. R., and Galen, R. S., Why are clinical laboratory tests performed? When are they valid? *J.A.M.A.* **233:** 76–78, 1975.

Sunderman, F. W., Jr. Conceptual problems in the interpretation of multitest surveys. In *Clinical Oriented Interpretation of Laboratory Data.* E. R. Gabrieli (Ed.). Academic Press, New York, 1972, 39–68.

Sunderman, F. W., Jr., and Van Soestbergen, A. A. Laboratory suggestions: probability computations for clinical interpretation of screening tests. *Am. J. Clin. Pathol.* **55:** 105–111, 1971.

Thorner, R. M., and Remein, Q. R. Principles and procedures in the evaluation of screening for disease. United States Public Health Service, Division of Chronic Diseases, Government Printing Office, Washington, D.C., 1961. Monograph No. 67.

Vecchio, Thomas J. Predictive value of a single diagnostic test in unselected populations. *N. Engl. J. Med.* **274:** 1171–1173, 1966.

Werner, M., Brooks, S. H., and Wette, R. Strategy for cost-effective laboratory testing. *Human Pathol.* **4:** 17–30, 1973.

Youden, W. J. Index for rating diagnostic tests. *Cancer* **3:** 32–35, 1950.

SCREENING

Bradwell, A. R., Carmalt, M. H. B., and Whitehead, T. P. Explaining the unexpected abnormal results of biochemical profile investigation. *Lancet* **ii:** 1071–1074, November 2, 1974.

Cochrane, A. L. and Holland, W. W. Validation of screening procedures. *Br. Med. J.* **27:** 3–8, 1971.

Galen, R. S. Multiphasic screening and biochemical profiles, state of the art. *Progr. Clin. Pathol.* **6:** 1975, in press.

Grant, John A. Qualitative evaluation of a screening program. *Am. J. Public Health* **64:** 66–71, 1974.

Hartz, Stuart C. A statistical model for assessing the need for medical care in a health screening program. *Clin. Chem.* **19:** 113–116, 1973.

Raine, D. N. Inherited metabolic disease. *Lancet,* **ii:** 996–998, October 26, 1974.

Sackett, David L. The usefulness of laboratory tests in health screening programs. *Clin. Chem.* **19:** 366–372, 1973.

Wilson, J. M. G. Current trends and problems in health screening. *J. Clin. Pathol.* **26:** 555–563, 1973.

Wilson, J. M. G., and Jungner, G. Principles and practice of screening for disease. Public Health Papers No. 34. World Health Organization, Geneva, 1968.

Wilson, J. M. G., and Hilleboe, H. E. Mass health examinations. Public Health Papers No. 45. World Health Organization, Geneva, 1971.

Cohen, Lord, Williams, E. T., and McLachlan, G. (Eds.) *Screening in Medical Care.* A Collection of Essays. Oxford University Press, London, 1968.

DECISION THEORY

Gorry, G. A., Kassirer, J. P., Essig, A., and Schwartz, W. B. Decision analysis as the basis for computer-aided management of acute renal failure. *Am. J. Med.* **55:** 473–484, 1973.

Ingelfinger, F. J. Decision in medicine. *N. Engl. J. Med.* **293:** 254–255, 1975.

Lusted, Lee B. Decision-making studies in patient management. *N. Engl. J. Med.* **284:** 416–424, 1971.

McNeil, B. J., Keeler, E., and Adelstein, S. J. Primer on certain elements of medical decision making. *N. Engl. J. Med.* **293:** 211–215, 1975.

Schwartz, W. B., Gorry, G. A., Kassirer, J. P., and Essig, A. Decision analysis and clinical judgement. *Am. J. Med.* **55:** 459–472, 1973.

Raiffa, Howard. *Decision Analysis: Introductory Lectures on Choices under Uncertainty.* Addison-Wesley, Reading, Mass., 1970.

APPENDICES

APPENDIX I FORMULA FOR THE EQUATION:
BAYES' THEOREM

Although predictive value theory has only recently been seen in the literature of clinical pathology, the formula and concept are not at all new. The formula for calculating predictive value is frequently referred to as Bayes' formula or Bayes' theorem and was published posthumously in 1763.[1] His formula allows us to calculate $p(\Theta_1/R)$ from the quantities $p(\Theta_1)$, $p(\Theta_2)$, $p(R/\Theta_1)$, and $p(R/\Theta_2)$.

$p(\Theta_1)$ is the *a priori* probability of a disease in a population. It is an estimate of the prevalence of a disease, Θ_1 (Θ_1 is read as "theta sub one").

$p(\Theta_2)$ is the *a priori* probability of nondisease or other disease states in a population. It is an estimate of the prevalence of nondisease or other disease states (excluding Θ_1) in a population. Θ_1 and Θ_2 are mutually exclusive of each other. $p(\Theta_1) + p(\Theta_2) = 1$.

$p(R/\Theta_1)$ is the probability of a positive test result R given that the patient has disease Θ_1. It represents the test sensitivity.

$p(R/\Theta_2)$ is the probability of a positive test result R given that the patient has other diseases or no disease Θ_2. It is equal to 1 minus test specificity.

$p(\Theta_1/R)$ is the *a posteriori* probability of disease Θ_1 given a positive test result R. It is the predictive value of a positive test result.

$$p(\Theta_1/R) = \frac{p(\Theta_1)\, p(R/\Theta_1)}{p(\Theta_1)\, p(R/\Theta_1) + p(\Theta_2)\, p(R/\Theta_2)}$$

We can place these symbols into their appropriate cells in our predictive value table and illustrate how this equation represents what we have been discussing throughout this book (Table 1).

Table 1. Predictive value table

	Number with positive test result	Number with negative test result	Totals
No. with disease	$p(\Theta_1)p(R/\Theta_1)$	$p(\Theta_1)[1 - p(R/\Theta_1)]$	$p(\Theta_1)$
No. without disease	$p(\Theta_2)p(R/\Theta_2)$	$p(\Theta_2)[1 - p(R/\Theta_2)]$	$p(\Theta_2)$
Totals	$p(\Theta_1)\, p(R/\Theta_1)$ $+ p(\Theta_2)\, p(R/\Theta_2)$	$p(\Theta_2)[1 - p(R/\Theta_1)]$ $+ p(\Theta_2)[1 - p(R/\Theta_2)]$	$p(\Theta_1) + p(\Theta_2) = 1$

Table 2 represents the more familiar presentation of this approach. We see that

$$\text{predictive value of a positive test} = \frac{\text{TP}}{\text{TP} + \text{FP}} \times 100$$

Similarly from Table 1, we see that

$$\text{predictive value of a positive test} = p(\Theta_1/R) = \frac{p(\Theta_1)p(R/\Theta_1)}{p(\Theta_1)p(R/\Theta_1) + p(\Theta_2)p(R/\Theta_2)}$$

Table 2.   Predictive value table

	Number with positive test result	Number with negative test result	Totals
Number with disease	TP	FN	TP + FN
Number without disease	FP	TN	FP + TN
Totals	TP + FP	FN + TN	TP + FP + TN + FN

TP = true positives; the number of sick subjects correctly classified by the test.

FP = false positives; the number of subjects free of the disease who are misclassified by the test.

TN = true negatives; the number of subjects free of the disease who are correctly classified by the test.

FN = false negatives; the number of sick subjects misclassified by the test.

Prevalence = percent of total subjects examined who are diseased

$$\text{Sensitivity} = \text{positivity in disease} = \frac{TP}{TP + FN} \times 100$$

$$\text{Specificity} = \text{negativity in health} = \frac{TN}{TN + FP} \times 100$$

$$\text{Predictive value of a positive test} = \frac{TP}{TP + FP} \times 100$$

It is clear from the current medical literature that Bayes' theorem is becoming increasingly popular. The formula may be presented in several variations and it is important that these be recognized as the same equation presented here. For example, if p were the prevalence of disease, then $(1 - p)$ would be the prevalence of non-disease or other disease. We could let a = sensitivity and b = specificity. The result would be Table 3.

Table 3.   Predictive value table

	Number with positive test result	Number with negative test result	Totals
Number with disease	pa	$p(1 - a)$	p
Number without disease	$(1 - p)(1 - b)$	$(1 - p)b$	$(1 - p)$
Totals	$pa + (1 - p)(1 - b)$	$p(1 - a) + (1 - p)b$	1

Sensitivity = a.

Specificity = b.

$$\text{Predictive value of positive} = \frac{pa}{[pa + (1 - p)(1 - b)]}$$

If we convert back to our starting terminology,

$$\text{predictive value} = \frac{(\text{prevalance})(\text{sensitivity})}{(\text{prevalence})(\text{sensitivity}) + (1 - \text{prevalence})(1 - \text{specificity})}$$

In the initial definitions presented here, we referred to prior and posterior probabilities. The difference in meaning between these probabilities is explained as follows. Before we examine the test result for a given patient, we know he belongs to Θ_1, with an *a priori* probability $p(\Theta_1)$, the disease prevalence; after we examine his test results, we know he belongs to Θ_1, with an *a posteriori* probability of $p(\Theta_1/R)$, the predictive value of the positive test result.

How do the equations presented above compare to the tables in this book? The predictive value and efficiency tables were generated by a computer program using these same equations. Solving the equation or using the tables should always result in the same answer:

$$\text{predictive value} = \frac{(\text{prevalence})(\text{sensitivity})}{(\text{prevalence})(\text{sensitivity}) + (1 - \text{prevalence})(1 - \text{specificity})}$$

Let us use this equation to calculate the predictive value of a test that has a sensitivity of 90% and a specificity of 80% when the disease prevalence is 10%.

$$\text{Predictive value} = \frac{(.10)(.90)}{(.10)(.90) + (1 - .10)(1 - .80)}$$

$$= \frac{(.10)(.90)}{(.10)(.90) + (.90)(.20)}$$

$$= \frac{.09}{.09 + .18}$$

$$= \frac{.09}{.27} = .33 = 33\%$$

This value can be found in the Predictive Value Tables. Remember, a disease prevalence of 10% is listed in the tables as 10,000/100,000.

REFERENCE

---

1. Bayes, Reverend Thomas. An essay toward solving a problem in the doctrine of chance. *Philo. Trans. Roy. Soc.* **53**: 370–418, 1763.

APPENDIX II   ALPHA AND BETA ERRORS

We frequently hear decision makers, including clinicians, discussing alpha and beta errors, Type I and Type II errors, errors of omission and commission, and false negatives and false positives. What do they mean? There are basically two errors that can be made in trying to classify a patient as diseased or nondiseased. They are shown in Table 1 as they relate to our fourfold table.

Table 1.   Two types of errors in making a diagnosis

	Number with positive test result	Number with negative test result
No. with disease	Correct decision Probability $= 1 - \alpha$	Type I error Probability $= \alpha$ False negative
No. without disease	Type II error Probability $= \beta$ False positive	Correct decision Probability $= 1 - \beta$

$1 - \alpha =$ test sensitivity; $1 - \beta =$ test specificity.

Alternate terminology has arisen over the years in an attempt to clarify the problem of errors in decision making (Table 2). It is unfortunate that all of the terms have survived and that we must suffer with their constant misuse.

Table 2.   Two types of errors in making a diagnosis: terminology

False positives	False negatives
Type II error	Type I error
Beta error	Alpha error
Error of commission	Error of omission
Proportion of well patients diagnosed as sick	Proportion of sick patients diagnosed as well

APPENDIX III   STANDARD ERROR OF A PERCENTAGE

Since values for sensitivity and specificity are unknown, and are only approximated from sample studies in the population, they are subject to error. It is much more accurate, in a statistical sense, to present sensitivity and specificity data with their ± 2 standard errors as 95% confidence limits than it is to simply state the percent sensitivity or specificity.

We can calculate the standard error of the sensitivity or specificity as follows:

$$SE_p = \sqrt{\frac{pq}{n}}$$

where SE_p is the standard error of the percent sensitivity or specificity, p is the percent sensitivity or specificity, and q equals $1 - p$. The sample size is n. Based on the normal curve, we can say that 95% of the time the true value for sensitivity or specificity is between $p + 2 SE$ and $p - 2SE$. With a small sample (less than 30), confidence limits should be derived from a t table.

Let us assume that we are studing a new immunological slide test for pregnancy. The test is positive in 90 out of 100 pregnant women. What are the confidence limits for this sensitivity? The sensitivity is 90%. The sample size is 100.

$$SE_p = \sqrt{\frac{pq}{n}}$$

$$SE_p = \sqrt{\frac{(.90)(.10)}{100}}$$

$$SE_p = \sqrt{\frac{.09}{100}}$$

$$SE_p = \sqrt{.0009}$$

$$SE_p = .03$$

The 95% confidence limits are calculated as the percent ± 2 SE.

$$.90 \pm 2(.03) = .90 \pm .06 = 84 \text{ to } 96\%$$

Therefore 95% of the time the sensitivity value lies between 84 and 96%, for this test, in this population.

APPENDIX IV EVALUATION OF LABORATORY TESTS: COMPARING SENSITIVITY AND SPECIFICITY DATA

Two situations are found in the clinical pathology literature that involve test comparisons and that require additional statistical methods.

1. Two different tests are evaluated in the same patient population (correlated data).

2. Two different tests are evaluated in two different patient populations (independent data).

The same question is asked in both situations. Which test is better? To obtain an answer, we must be certain that any difference in sensitivity and specificity noted between the two tests is real. We want to be certain that the difference is statistically significant, and that it is not caused by chance alone (sampling error).

The statistical methods presented in this appendix allow us to make this comparison.[1] We evaluate two types of tests in this way: qualitative and quantitative. For qualitative tests we merely compare different test sensitivity and specificity values. For quantitative tests, it is necessary to compare test sensitivities at equal specificities and test specificities at equal sensitivities. It is then possible to determine which test is more sensitive and/or specific.

CORRELATED DATA

In this situation two different tests are evaluated in the same patient population. The sensitivity and specificity data are formatted as shown in Table 1 and 2 respectively.

Table 1. Comparing sensitivity

Test 1 results for diseased patients	Test 2 results for diseased patients		
	Positive	Negative	Total
Positive	A	B	$A + B$
Negative	C	D	$C + D$
Total	$A + C$	$B + D$	$A + B + C + D = n$

$$\text{Test 1: sensitivity} = \frac{A + B}{A + B + C + D}$$

$$\text{Test 2: sensitivity} = \frac{A + C}{A + B + C + D}$$

The discrepancy cells are cells B and C. If there were no difference between these sensitivities, we would expect no cases in cells B and C. In reality, however, there would be some random discrepancies and these should fall equally into cells B and C. If either cell has more than 50% of the discrepancies (that cannot be attributed to sampling error), then the difference in sensitivities is statistically significant. This hypothesis is tested with a t test.

$$t = \frac{(B/n) - (C/n)}{\sqrt{(B + C)/n^2}}$$

If the numerator is negative, the sign is ignored. With small samples a t table is used to interpret the result; otherwise, a value of 2 or more represents the 95% confidence interval. If $B + C$ equals 20 or less, it is necessary to subtract $1/n$ from the numerator to correct for continuity (continuous normal curve distribution has been used as an approximation of discrete binomial distribution).

Table 2.   Comparing specificity

Test 1 results for nondiseased patients	Test 2 results for nondiseased patients		
	Positive	Negative	Total
Positive	A	B	$A + B$
Negative	C	D	$C + D$
Total	$A + C$	$B + D$	$A + B + C + D = n$

$$\text{Test 1:} \quad \text{specificity} = \frac{C + D}{A + B + C + D}$$

$$\text{Test 2:} \quad \text{specificity} = \frac{B + D}{A + B + C + D}$$

The discrepancy cells are still $B + C$, and we proceed in the same way as for sensitivity.

An example serves to clarify this approach. In Chapter 13 we described our myocardial infarction study. CPK and LDH isoenzyme studies were performed in the same patients (correlated data). Is there a statistically significant difference between these correlated specificities? From the matrix (Table 5, Chapter 13), we can derive the data in Tables 3 to 5.

Table 3.   Test 1—LDH flip

	Positive	Negative	Total
MI	36	10	46
Non-MI	1	47	48
Total	37	57	94

Specificity = 47/48 = 97.9%.

Table 4. Test 2—CPK-MB

	Positive	Negative	Total
MI	46	0	46
Non-MI	7	41	48
Total	53	41	94

Specificity = 41/48 = 85.4%

Table 5. Comparing specificity

LDH-flip results for Non-MI patients	CPK-MB results for Non-MI patients		
	Positive	Negative	Total
Positive	0	1	1
Negative	7	40	47
Total	7	41	48

Using the t test described above, we substitute in the formula:

$$t = \frac{|(B/n) - (C/n)| - (1/n)}{\sqrt{(B + C)/n^2}}$$

$$= \frac{|(1/48) - (7/48)| - (1/48)}{\sqrt{(1 + 7)/(48^2)}}$$

$$= \frac{|.021 - .146| - .021}{\sqrt{8/2304}}$$

$$= \frac{.104}{\sqrt{.0035}} = \frac{.104}{.059}$$

$$= 1.76$$

The t value does not exceed 2 (theoretically we should use 1.96 as the critical value). Therefore, the difference between the specificity of CPK-MB and LDH isoenzymes in the diagnosis of acute myocardial infarction in our study is due to chance or sampling variation and is not statistically significant.

Instead of using a t test to test the above hypothesis, we could use a chi-square test, which is similarly based on the expected equal distribution of discrepancy cases in cells $B + C$. The organization of the data is the same as for the t test. The formula for chi-square is as follows:

$$\chi^2 = \frac{[|B - C| - 1]^2}{B + C}$$

When $B - C$ is negative, the sign is ignored. When $B + C$ equals 20 or less, it is necessary to subtract 1 from the numerator as shown in the formula above as a correction for continuity. A value of 3.84 represents the 95% confidence interval, and when exceeded, indicates a statistically significant difference. Returning to our example, we substitute in the χ^2 formula as follows:

$$\chi^2 = \frac{[|B - C| - 1]^2}{B + C}$$

$$= \frac{[|1 - 7| - 1]^2}{1 + 7}$$

$$= \frac{(5)^2}{8}$$

$$= \frac{25}{8}$$

$$= 3.125$$

Since the value for χ^2 does not exceed 3.84, the difference in specificities between CPK-MB and LDH isoenzymes can be explained by chance, and LDH isoenzymes are not more specific than CPK isoenzymes in the diagnosis of myocardial infarction. It is interesting to note that $\sqrt{\chi^2} = t$ when the chi-square test has one degree of freedom:

$$\sqrt{3.125} = 1.76$$

INDEPENDENT DATA

In this situation two different tests are evaluated in two different patient populations. If there is no difference in their sensitivity and specificity, at a given sensitivity, their specificities are equal, and vice versa. If there are differences, we can test for their statistical significance by either a t test or a chi-square test. The approach is the same for sensitivity or specificity. We present the formula and an example comparing sensitivities.

In performing the t test, we need to calculate the "pooled sensitivity." When dealing with a quantitative test, sensitivities are compared at a constant specificity. The pooled sensitivity is given by:

$$\frac{TP_1 + TP_2}{(TP + FN)_1 + (TP + FN)_2} = \frac{\Sigma\ TP}{\Sigma\ \text{Diseased}}$$

We then calculate the standard error for the distribution of differences.

$$SE_{\text{diff}} = \sqrt{\frac{pq}{n_1} + \frac{pq}{n_2}}$$

Where p = pooled sensitivity

$q = 1 - p$

n_1 = total diseased, sample 1

n_2 = total diseased, sample 2

We then calculate t.

$$t = \frac{p_1 - p_2}{SE_{diff}}$$

Where p_1 = sensitivity, test 1

p_2 = sensitivity, test 2

When $p_1 - p_2$ is negative, the sign is ignored. With small samples a t table is used to interpret the result: otherwise, a value of 2 or more represents the 95% confidence interval. When using a t table, note that degrees of freedom equal $n_1 + n_2 - 2$. Furthermore, with small samples (20 or less), it is necessary to subtract $.5 [(1/n_1) + (1/n_2)]$ from $|p_1 - p_2|$.

We illustrate the use of this formula with a hypothetical example. Suppose that Galen collects 200 admissions to the CCU and studies the frequency distribution of HBD in MI and non-MI patients (diagnosis determined by ECG and clinical findings) on the third day following the episode. The prevalence of MI is 50%. His data are presented in Table 6. He considers the possibility that HBD is more accurate in this setting (CCU) than LDH; and discusses the data with Gambino, who produces Table 7. This represents the frequency distribution of LDH in MI and non-MI patients (diagnosis determined by ECG and clinical findings) on the third day following the episode, for 400 admissions to the CCU, collected several years earlier. The prevalence of MI was 50%. Is HBD more sensitive than LDH?

Table 6. Galen's study: HBD, day 3, 200 cases

Prevalence of MI = 50%

RV (U/l)	Sensitivity (%)	Specificity (%)	PV (%)
70	100.0	21.4	54.4
150	88.9	90.5	89.8
250	66.7	95.2	92.9
450	28.9	97.6	91.9
670	13.3	100.0	100.0

Table 7. Gambino's study: LDH, day 3, 400 cases

Prevalence of MI = 50%

RV (U/l)	Sensitivity (%)	Specificity (%)	Predictive value (%)
130	100.0	16.7	53.0
250	84.1	90.5	89.3
550	34.1	95.2	87.0
750	13.6	95.2	72.7
930	11.4	100.0	100.0

To compare two independent tests that have variable referent values (quantitative determinations), we compare sensitivity at a fixed specificity. From Tables 6 and 7, we see that at a specificity of 100%, HBD has a sensitivity of 13.3% and LDH has a sensitivity of 11.4%. Galen's series had 100 MI cases, whereas Gambino's had 200 MI cases. Let us return to our calculations:

$$\text{pooled sensitivity} = \frac{13.3 + 22.8}{100 + 200}$$

$$= \frac{36.1}{300}$$

$$= 12.0\%$$

We can now calculate t:

$$t = \frac{p_1 - p_2}{\sqrt{(pq/n_1) + (pq/n_2)}}$$

$$= \frac{.133 - .114}{\sqrt{(.12)(.88)/100 + (.12)(.88)/200}}$$

$$= \frac{.019}{\sqrt{.106/100 + .106/200}}$$

$$= \frac{.019}{\sqrt{.001 + .001}}$$

$$= \frac{.019}{\sqrt{.002}}$$

$$= \frac{.019}{.045}$$

$$= 0.42$$

The t value does not exceed 2 (theoretically we should use 1.96 as the critical value). Therefore, the difference between the sensitivity of HBD and LDH in the diagnosis of acute myocardial infarction, in these studies, is due to chance or sampling variation and is not statistically significant.

A chi-square test could be used instead of a t test in which case the data should be formatted as shown in Table 8.

Table 8.   Comparing independent test sensitivity

| | Results for diseased patients | | | | |
| | Positive test | | Negative test | | Total diseased |
Test	Observed	Expected	Observed	Expected	patients
Test 1	A	a	B	b	$A + B$
Test 2	C	c	D	d	$C + D$
Total	$A + C$	$a + c$	$B + D$	$b + d$	$A + B + C + D$

The total expected sensitivity is given by the pooled sensitivity:

$$a + c = \frac{A + C}{A + B + C + D}$$

This is multiplied by the total number of diseased patients $(A + B)$ to get the expected sensitivity for test 1 (a), and by the total number of diseased patients $(C + D)$ to get the expected sensitivity for test 2 (c). The expected negatives are derived by subtraction.

Chi-square is calculated as follows:

$$\chi^2 = \sum \frac{(O - E)^2}{E}$$

$$= \frac{(A - a)^2}{a} + \frac{(B - b)^2}{b} + \frac{(C - c)^2}{c} + \frac{(D - d)^2}{d}$$

Where O = observed value

E = expected value

If an expected value is less than 10, a correction for continuity should be made, as follows:

$$\frac{(|A - a| - .5)^2}{a}$$

Let us return to our hypothetical example (Table 9).

Table 9. Comparing HBD and LDH sensitivity

| | Results for MI patients | | | | |
| | Positive test | | Negative test | | |
Test	Observed	Expected	Observed	Expected	Total MI patients
HBD	13.3	12	86.7	88	100
LDH	22.8	24	177.2	176	200
Total	36.1	36	263.9	264	300

The total expected sensitivity is given by the pooled sensitivity:

$$36.1/300 = 12\%.$$

The expected positives for HBD are calculated by $(.12)(100) = 12$ and for LDH by $(.12)(200) = 24$. The expected negatives are calculated by subtraction:

$$\text{chi-square} = \sum \frac{(O - E)^2}{E}$$

$$= \frac{(13.3 - 12)^2}{12} + \frac{(86.7 - 88)^2}{88} + \frac{(22.8 - 24)^2}{24} + \frac{(177.2 - 176)^2}{176}$$

$$= \frac{(1.3)^2}{12} + \frac{(-1.3)^2}{88} + \frac{(-1.2)^2}{24} + \frac{(1.2)^2}{176}$$

$$= \frac{1.69}{12} + \frac{1.69}{88} + \frac{1.44}{24} + \frac{1.44}{176}$$

$$= 0.14 + 0.02 + 0.06 + 0.01$$

$$= 0.23$$

Since the value of χ^2 does not exceed 3.84, the difference in sensitivity between HBD and LDH can be explained by chance and HBD is not more sensitive than LDH in the diagnosis of acute myocardial infarction.

The next question follows logically: Is HBD more specific than LDH? To compare two independent tests that have variable referent values, we compare specificity at a fixed sensitivity. From Tables 6 and 7, we see that at a sensitivity of 100%, HBD has a specificity of 21.4% and LDH has a specificity of 16.7%. These independent test specificities may then be compared by either a t test or a chi-square analysis, both of which would indicate no statistically significant difference for test specificity. In conclusion, according to this study, HBD offers no advantage over LDH in the diagnosis of acute myocardial infraction. The format for comparing independent test specificity by the chi-square approach is shown in Table 10.

Table 10.   Comparing independent test specificity

	Results for nondiseased patients				
	Positive test		Negative test		Total nondiseased patients
Test	Observed	Expected	Observed	Expected	
Test 1	A	a	B	b	$A + B$
Test 2	C	c	D	d	$C + D$
Total	$A + C$	$a + c$	$B + D$	$b + d$	$A + B + C + D$

The total expected specificity is given by the pooled specificity:

$$b + d = \frac{B + D}{A + B + C + D}$$

This is multiplied by the total nondiseased patients $(A + B)$ to get the expected specificity for test 1 (b), and by the total nondiseased patients $(C + D)$ to get the expected specificity for test 2 (d). The expected positives are derived by subtraction. Chi-square is calculated as in the example above for comparing independent test sensitivity.

REFERENCE

1. Thorner, R. M. and Remein, Q. R. Principles and procedures in the evaluation of screening for disease. U.S. Public Health Service, Division of Chronic Diseases. Monograph No. 67. Government Printing Office, Washington, D.C., 1961.

APPENDIX V IS A LABORATORY TEST BETTER THAN CHANCE?

Clinicians frequently compare the predictive value of laboratory tests to flipping a coin. This analogy is not as straightforward as it might appear. The most common error made is to equate a 50% predictive value with flipping a coin. It is possible to achieve a 50% predictive value with a coin, but only if disease prevalence equals 50%. Flipping a coin has a sensitivity of 50% and a specificity of 50%. The predictive value, therefore, depends entirely on disease prevalence. This situation is discussed in detail in Chapter 5 and in a letter to the editor of the *New England Journal of Medicine*.[1]

If a test is equal to chance, will the sensitivity and specificity always be equal to 50%? To answer this question, we need to return to our fourfold table (Table 1).

Table 1. Predictive value table

	Number with positive test result	Number with negative test result	Totals
Number with disease	pa	$p(1 - a)$	p
Number without disease	$(1 - p)(1 - b)$	$(1 - p)b$	$1 - p$
Totals	$pa + (1 - p)(1 - b)$	$p(1 - a) + (1 - p)b$	1

a = sensitivity.
b = specificity.
p = disease prevalence.

$$\text{Predictive value} = \frac{pa}{[pa + (1 - p)(1 - b)]}$$

If the percentage of patients with a positive test result in the diseased group (pa/p) equals the percentage of patients with a positive test result in the nondiseased group $(1 - p)(1 - b)/(1 - p)$, a random selection is suspected. Since $(pa/p) = a$, the test sensitivity, and $(1 - p)(1 - b)/(1 - p)$ is equal to $1 - b$, $(1 - \text{specificity})$, we see that if the sum of sensitivity and specificity is 100%, we have a random test. Furthermore, the sensitivity (a) is equal to the total percent positive $[pa + (1 - p)(1 - b)]$. In addition, the predictive value is equal to the prevalence.

Let us look at the hypothetical example (Table 2) of a test that has a sensitivity of 30% and a specificity of 70%. We let the disease prevalence equal 100/100,000.

In this case we see that the sum of sensitivity and specificity is 100% (30% + 70%). Sensitivity (30%) is equal to 1 minus specificity or 100% minus 70%. The sensitivity (30%) is equal to the total precent positive (30,000/100,000) = 30%. We are not looking at a laboratory test, but rather at a random selection process. The predic-

Table 2.   Hypothetical example

	Number with positive test result	Number with negative test result	Totals
Number with disease	30	70	100
Number without disease	29,970	69,930	99,900
Totals	30,000	70,000	100,000

Sensitivity = 30%.
Specificity = 70%.
Prevalence = 100/100,000.
Sensitivity + specificity = 100%.

tive value of a positive result is (30/30,000) or 0.1%. The predictive value of a negative result is (69,930/70,000) or 99.9%. The efficiency of this "test" is (69,960/
100,000) or 70%. Note that the predictive value (30/30,000) equals the prevalence
(100/100,000). Therefore, the *a posteriori* probability of disease, given a test result,
equals the *a priori* probability of disease without any test result. Obviously, this is not
a test! Using a statistical approach presented in Appendix IV, we can compare
test results to those of chance, and determine if the test is significantly better than
or equal to chance. The dangers of developing laboratory tests and only reporting
clinical trials in diseased patients is obvious. When such a report describes a test with
90% sensitivity, there is no way of knowing whether the specificity is better than
10%.

REFERENCE

1. Galen, R. S. Interpretation of laboratory tests. *N. Engl. J. Med.*, **292:** 433–434, 1975.

APPENDIX VI MINIMIZING ERROR:
THOUGHTS ON OVERLAPPING DISTRIBUTIONS

Much attention has already been given to the problem created by overlapping frequency distributions between healthy and diseased patients and between various groups of diseased patients. One question that *predictive-value-users* frequently ask is, "How do I select the best cut-off point for a particular test?" Let us create a hypothetical data base and attempt to answer this question. Suppose we study a serum enzyme test in 2000 admissions to the CCU and divide the population into MI and non-MI, based on ECG and clinical criteria. We might expect to find the data distribution shown in Table 1.

Table 1. Raw data: hypothetical enzyme study

Enzyme activity (U/l)	Non-MI		MI	
	Number of cases	Percent of total	Number of cases	Percent of total
0– 20	600	30.0	—	—
21– 40	150	7.5	50	2.5
41– 60	100	5.0	100	5.0
61– 80	100	5.0	150	7.5
81–100	50	2.5	200	10.0
101–120	—	—	300	15.0
121–140	—	—	100	5.0
141–160	—	—	50	2.5
161–180	—	—	50	2.5
Totals	1000	50.0	1000	50.0

Although the mean level of enzyme activity for MI patients is 97 U/l and the mean level for non-MI patients is 27 U/l, the classical problem of overlapping distributions still exists. Figure 1, which is a graph of the above data, demonstrates the problem. Table 2 lists six possible referent values (cutoff points, upper limits) for this test.

By now sensitivity, specificity, predictive value, and efficiency are familiar terms and should not pose a problem in interpreting the data in Table 2. There are, however, some new terms that require definition.

- "Presumptive positive" is the percent of the total tested that have positive test results: (TP + FP)/total tested.

Table 2. Ten different ways of evaluating a laboratory test

Referent value	Sensitivity (%)	Specificity (%)	Predictive value of a positive test (%)	Predictive value of a negative test (%)	Efficiency (%)	Presumptive positive (%)	Detection rate (%)	Youden index	Error ratio (%)	Combined error (%)
20	100.0	60.0	71.4	100.0	80.0	70.0	50.0	.60	40.0	20.0
40	95.0	75.0	79.2	93.8	85.0	60.0	47.5	.70	31.6	15.0
50	90.0	80.0	82.8	88.9	85.0	55.0	45.0	.70	33.3	15.0
60	85.0	85.0	85.0	85.0	85.0	50.0	42.5	.70	35.3	15.0
80	70.0	95.0	93.3	76.0	82.5	37.5	35.0	.65	50.0	17.5
100	50.0	100.0	100.0	66.7	75.0	25.0	25.0	.50	100.0	25.0
Chance test*	50.0	50.0	50.0	50.0	50.0	50.0	25.0	0	200.0	50.0
Perfect test*	100.0	100.0	100.0	100.0	100.0	50.0	50.0	1.00	0	0

Disease prevalence = 50%.
*Hypothetical situation.

142

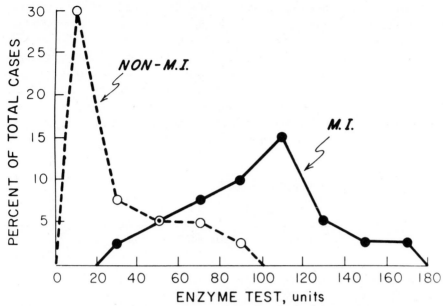

Figure 1.   Frequency distribution of enzyme activity in MI and non-MI.

- "Detection rate" is the percent of the total tested that are true positives: TP/total tested.

- "Youden index" is equal to [(sensitivity + specificity) − 1] and therefore can range from 0 to 1. A Youden index score of zero means that the test is no better than chance, since sensitivity + specificity = 1. This has been discussed in Appendix V. A perfect test scores 1, since sensitivity plus specificity can never exceed 2. The Youden index completely ignores the effect of prevalence on the testing situation.[1]

- The "error ratio" is the ratio of the total number of false diagnoses to the number of true-positive diagnoses: (FP + FN)/TP. The best discriminating referent value in terms of this parameter has the smallest error ratio.[2]

- The "combined error" is the percent of the total tested that are either false positives of false negatives: (FP + FN)/total tested.

We have presented 10 rates that can be calculated from the basic predictive value table and additional ratios can be created. Which one is best in selecting a referent value? The answer is, unfortunately, none! All of these parameters assume that alpha and beta errors (false negatives and false positives) are equally costly in the decision-making process. Since this is seldom the case in clinical practice, several of these should be considered in the light of the complexities of the clinical setting before a referent value is selected. But what if alpha and beta errors were equally costly, which referent value would be best? Murphy and Abbey propose that the smallest error is then made, on the average, if a referent value at the intersection of the two distribution curves is selected.[3] In our example, this would be at 50 U/l. At this point, several of our calculated parameters are optimized. For example, efficiency is at its highest, and the combined error is at its lowest. Since this example is an enzyme test for myocardial inferction, and the risk of alpha and of beta errors is very similar in this setting, 50 U/l would be a reasonable referent value to select.

How are these 10 rates affected by disease prevalence? To determine this we return to our original hypothetical data base (Table 1) and change the prevalence from 50 to 25%. The new distribution for the data is shown in Table 3.

Table 3. Raw data: Hypothetical enzyme study

Enzyme activity (U/l)	Non-MI		MI	
	Number of cases	Percent of total	Number of cases	Percent of total
0– 20	900	45.00	—	—
21– 40	225	11.25	25	1.25
41– 60	150	7.50	50	2.50
61– 80	150	7.50	75	3.75
81–100	75	3.75	100	5.00
101–120	—	—	150	7.50
121–140	—	—	50	2.50
141–160	—	—	25	1.25
161–180	—	—	25	1.25
Totals	1500	75.00	500	25.00

By comparing Tables 2 and 4, we can determine which rates are affected by disease prevalence and which are not. As expected, only sensitivity, specificity, and the Youden index are independent of prevalence.

If we assume that these hypothetical data represent an enzyme test for myocardial infarction and that the risk of alpha and beta errors are very similar, which referent value would be best? By evaluating the rates in Table 4, we would select a referent value of 80. At this level we achieve the highest efficiency and the lowest error ratio. Furthermore, the test has relatively high positive and negative predictive values, which are comparable to the predictive values achieved with a referent value of 50, when the disease prevalence is 50% (see Table 2). Tables 2 and 4 show the importance of selecting a referent value with an appreciation of the effect of disease prevalence.

When alpha and beta errors carry different risks, it is necessary to consider the relative cost of each type of error. The total cost of errors then can be minimized in selecting a referent value. Following the same principle, Murphy and Abbey suggest factoring disease prevalence to reflect the relative risk of alpha and beta errors.[3]

Tab.e 4. The effect of prevalence on selection of referent value

Referent value	Sensitivity (%)	Specificity (%)	Predictive value of a positive test (%)	Predictive value of a negative test (%)	Efficiency (%)	Presumptive positive (%)	Detection rate (%)	Youden index	Error ratio (%)	Combined error (%)
20	100.0	60.0	45.5	100.0	70.0	55.0	25.0	.60	120.0	30.0
40	95.0	75.0	55.9	97.8	80.0	42.5	23.8	.70	84.2	20.0
50	90.0	80.0	60.0	96.0	82.5	37.5	22.5	.70	77.8	17.5
60	85.0	85.0	65.4	94.4	85.0	32.5	21.3	.70	70.6	15.0
80	70.0	95.0	82.4	90.5	88.8	21.3	17.5	.65	64.3	11.2
100	50.0	100.0	100.0	85.7	87.5	12.5	12.5	.50	100.0	12.5
Chance test*	50.0	50.0	25.0	75.0	50.0	50.0	12.5	0	400.0	50.0
Perfect test*	100.0	100.0	100.0	100.0	100.0	25.0	25.0	1.00	0	0

Disease prevalence = 25%.
*Hypothetical situation.

145

REFERENCES

1. Youden, W. J. Index for rating diagnostic tests. *Cancer* **3:** 32–35, 1950.
2. Simonson, Ernst. *Differentiation between Normal and Abnormal in Electrocardiography.* Mosby, St. Louis, Mo., 1961.
3. Murphy, Edmond A., and Abbey, Helen. The normal range—A common misuse. *J. Chronic Dis.* **20:** 79–88, 1967.

APPENDIX VII   THE INTERPRETATION OF LABORATORY DATA IN THE FUTURE

If the appropriate research were conducted and predictive value information were available for the most common tests there would exist a compilation of upper limits of normal that would defy the memory of even the most astute medical student. What are the alternatives?

One alternative is a computer-based system that would calculate the predictive value of a test or test panel for a particular disease. Unfortunately, this approach is still in the planning stage.

Another alternative is to have tables that present predictive value data for test combinations. These are available in a usable format for coronary heart disease.[1] The tables give, for each sex and age group, the probability of developing coronary heart disease in 6 years. In addition to sex and age, the tables take into account cigarette smoking, left ventricular hypertrophy, glucose intolerance, and the combined risk of serum cholesterol values and systolic blood pressure.

The data for a 40-year-old man are given in Table 1. Rather than just indicating that a serum cholesterol of 310 mg/dl is abnormal, the table permits us to determine that a patient had a 26.6% chance of developing coronary heart disease in 6 years. This is the predictive value of a serum cholesterol of 310 mg/dl in a 40-year-old man who smokes cigarettes, has ECG evidence of LVH, demonstrates glucose intolerance, and has a systolic blood pressure of 180. This interpretation conveys much more information than the comment "abnormal cholesterol."

The value of compiling such tables for other diseases is clear. The task is enormous, but it would certainly put an end to the question, Is this laboratory result normal?

The tabular approach reviewed here is very interesting for the following reasons:

1. It combines multiple test data and presents a predictive value (actually a prognostic value) of developing a disease within a 6-year period.
2. It considers test results at their quantitatively determined level and not as positive or negative relative to a predetermined referent value.

Throughout this book, in our predictive value tables, we refer to tests as positive or negative. With qualitative tests there is no other alternative. However, with quantitative tests, there are varying degrees of positivity and negativity relative to any preselected referent value. Should this affect the predictive value? Can the predictive value be calculated for the individual quantitative test result? The answer to both of these questions is yes.

Doctor F. William Sunderman, Jr., Director of the Department of Laboratory Medicine at the University of Connecticut School of Medicine, has adapted the basic predictive value formula to quantitative test results.[2] His approach is detailed below (where In equals incidence).

147

Table 1. Probability (per 100) of developing coronary heart disease in 6 years according to specified characteristics

Does not smoke cigarettes and LVH-ECG negative

	Systolic blood pressure:	105	120	135	150	165	180	195
	Cholesterol							
Glucose	185	0.7	0.9	1.1	1.3	1.5	1.9	2.2
intolerance	210	1.0	1.2	1.4	1.7	2.1	2.5	3.0
absent	235	1.3	1.6	1.9	2.3	2.8	3.3	4.0
	260	1.8	2.2	2.6	3.1	3.7	4.4	5.3
	285	2.4	2.9	3.5	4.1	4.9	5.9	7.0
	310	3.2	3.8	4.6	5.5	6.5	7.8	9.2
	335	4.3	5.1	6.1	7.3	8.6	10.2	12.1
Glucose	185	1.0	1.2	1.4	1.7	2.0	2.4	2.9
intolerance	210	1.3	1.6	1.9	2.2	2.7	3.2	3.9
present	235	1.7	2.1	2.5	3.0	3.6	4.3	5.1
	260	2.3	2.8	3.3	4.0	4.8	5.7	6.8
	285	3.1	3.7	4.5	5.3	6.3	7.6	9.0
	310	4.2	5.0	5.9	7.0	8.4	9.9	11.7
	335	5.5	6.6	7.8	9.3	11.0	12.9	15.2

Does not smoke cigarettes and LVH-ECG positive

		105	120	135	150	165	180	195
Glucose	185	1.5	1.9	2.2	2.7	3.2	3.8	4.6
intolerance	210	2.1	2.5	3.0	3.6	4.3	5.1	6.1
absent	235	2.8	3.3	4.0	4.8	5.7	6.8	8.0
	260	3.7	4.4	5.3	6.3	7.5	8.9	10.5
	285	4.9	5.9	7.0	8.3	9.9	11.6	13.7
	310	6.5	7.8	9.2	10.9	12.8	15.1	17.6
	335	8.6	10.2	12.0	14.2	16.6	19.3	22.4
Glucose	185	2.0	2.4	2.9	3.5	4.1	4.9	5.9
intolerance	210	2.7	3.2	3.8	4.6	5.5	6.5	7.8
present	235	3.6	4.3	5.1	6.1	7.3	8.6	10.2
	260	4.8	5.7	6.8	8.1	9.6	11.3	13.3
	285	6.3	7.5	8.9	10.6	12.5	14.7	17.1
	310	8.3	9.9	11.7	13.7	16.1	18.8	21.8
	335	10.9	12.9	15.1	17.7	20.6	23.8	27.3

We let

probability of result R in presence of Y disease $= p(R/Y)$

probability of result R in absence of Y disease $= p(R/\overline{Y})$

Then, given any result R,

$$\text{probability of } Y \text{ disease} = \frac{\text{In} \cdot p(R/Y)}{(1 - \text{In}) \cdot p(R/\overline{Y}) + \text{In} \cdot p(R/Y)}$$

For example, let us suppose that a fasting serum glucose concentration of 150 mg/dl represents the 99th percentile of values in the healthy population and the 50th percentile of values

Smokes cigarettes and LVH-ECG negative

Systolic blood pressure:		105	120	135	150	165	180	195
	Cholesterol							
Glucose	185	1.2	1.4	1.7	2.0	2.4	2.9	3.5
intolerance	210	1.5	1.9	2.2	2.7	3.2	3.8	4.6
absent	235	2.1	2.5	3.0	3.6	4.3	5.1	6.1
	260	2.8	3.3	4.0	4.8	5.7	6.8	8.1
	285	3.7	4.4	5.3	6.3	7.5	8.9	10.6
	310	4.9	5.9	7.0	8.3	9.9	11.7	13.7
	335	6.5	7.8	9.2	10.9	12.9	15.1	17.7
Glucose	185	1.5	1.8	2.2	2.6	3.1	3.7	4.5
intolerance	210	2.0	2.4	2.9	3.5	4.1	5.0	5.9
present	235	2.7	3.2	3.9	4.6	5.5	6.6	7.8
	260	3.6	4.3	5.1	6.1	7.3	8.7	10.3
	285	4.8	5.7	6.8	8.1	9.6	11.3	13.3
	310	6.3	7.5	9.0	10.6	12.5	14.7	17.2
	335	8.4	9.9	11.7	13.8	16.2	18.9	21.9

Smokes cigarettes and LVH-ECG positive

Glucose	185	2.4	2.9	3.4	4.1	4.9	5.9	7.0
intolerance	210	3.2	3.8	4.6	5.5	6.5	7.8	9.2
absent	235	4.3	5.1	6.1	7.2	8.6	10.2	12.0
	260	5.7	6.8	8.0	9.5	11.3	13.3	15.6
	285	7.5	8.9	10.5	12.4	14.6	17.1	19.9
	310	9.9	11.6	13.7	16.1	18.7	21.7	25.1
	335	12.8	15.1	17.6	20.5	23.7	27.3	31.1
Glucose	185	3.1	3.7	4.4	5.3	6.3	7.5	8.9
intolerance	210	4.1	4.9	5.9	7.0	8.3	9.9	11.7
present	235	5.5	6.5	7.8	9.2	10.9	12.9	15.1
	260	7.3	8.6	10.2	12.1	14.2	16.6	19.4
	285	9.6	11.3	13.3	15.6	18.2	21.2	24.5
	310	12.5	14.7	17.1	20.0	23.1	26.6	30.4
	335	16.1	18.8	21.8	25.2	28.8	32.8	37.1

in patients with untreated diabetes mellitus, and that the approximate incidence of diabetes in the population is 5%. Then the probability that a fasting glucose concentration of 150 mg/dl is indicative of the presence of diabetes is .72.[2]

Using this data in the above equation, the probability of diabetes given the result 150 mg/dl is

$$\frac{(.05)(.5)}{(.95)(.01) + (.05)(.5)} = .725 = 72.5\%$$

Doctor Sunderman's approach is very interesting and, with computer-based data files, would permit the reporting of the laboratory test result together with its predictive value for the disease under investigation. Several difficulties with this approach, however, make it less reliable than it would seem. These include the analytical error of a single laboratory determination, the time trend found in most disease states, and the effect of treatment on levels of biochemical constituents. For these reasons, we prefer the referent value approach as described in this book. Consideration of analytical error in the Bayesian model has been reported by Krause and co-workers.[3]

REFERENCES

1. Insull, William, Jr., Committee Chairman. *Coronary Risk Handbook*. American Heart Association, New York, 1973.
2. Sunderman, F. William, Jr., and Van Soestbergen, A. A. Probability computations for clinical interpretations of screening tests. *Am. J. Clin. Pathol.* **55:** 105–111, 1971.
3. Krause, R. D., Anand, V. D., Gruemer, H. D., and Willke, T. A. The impact of laboratory error on the normal range: A Bayesian Model. *Clin. Chem.* **21:** 321–324, 1975.

APPENDIX VIII   EPIDEMIOLOGICAL COMMENTS

The predictive value and efficiency tables in this book use prevalence as the rate of disease frequency. Is disease incidence ever important? Will the tables still apply? How are incidence and prevalence related to each other? These are all reasonable questions and are readily answered in the epidemiology literature. One of the most lucid explanations of these measures of disease frequency is to be found in *Epidemiology: Principles and Methods* by MacMahon and Pugh.[1]

Incidence: The incidence of a disease is the number of cases of the disease which come into being during a specified period of time. The incidence rate is this number per specified unit of population. Prevalence: Point prevalence of a disease is a census type of measure. It is the frequency of the disease at a designated point in time. Expressed for a specified population at a specified time, point prevalence rate is the proportion of that population which exhibits the disease at that particular time. The numerator includes all persons having the disease at the given moment, irrespective of the length of time which has elapsed from the beginning of the illness to the time when the point prevalence is measured. The denominator is the total population (affected and unaffected) within which the disease is ascertained. In contrast to incidence rates, which measure events, point prevalence rates are measures of what prevails or exists.

Tables 1 and 2 are taken from MacMahon and Pugh[1] and consist of data on patients with leukemia in Brooklyn, New York, between 1948 and 1952. The total population base is estimated to be 2,525,000.

The prevalence rate for any year is simply the number of patients alive at the beginning of the year with leukemia per 100,000 population. For example, the prevalence rate of acute leukemia in Brooklyn in 1952 is calculated as follows:

$$\frac{(21)(100,000)}{2,525,000} = 0.83 \text{ cases}/100,000$$

Table 1.   Data on patients with acute leukemia, Brooklyn, New York, whites, 1948–1952

Year	Prevalence Patients alive at beginning of year	Incidence New cases diagnosed in year	Mortality Deaths in year
1948	7	69	54
1949	15	91	86
1950	17	83	73
1951	24	99	101
1952	21	68	81
Total	84	410	395

Table 2.   Data on patients with chronic leukemia, Brooklyn, New York, whites 1948–1952

Year	Prevalence — Patients alive at beginning of year	Incidence — New cases diagnosed in year	Mortality — Deaths in year
1948	129	79	50
1949	150	83	71
2950	157	90	90
1951	151	61	84
1952	121	53	89
Total	708	366	384

The incidence, on the other hand, consists of the number of new cases diagnosed in that year. Therefore, the incidence rate of acute leukemia in Brooklyn in 1952 is calculated as follows:

$$\frac{(68)(100,000)}{2,525,000} = 2.69 \text{ new cases}/100,000/\text{year}$$

The mortality is the number of persons dying of the disease during a stated period, per population. For acute leukemia in Brooklyn in 1952, the mortality rate is calculated as follows:

$$\frac{(81)(100,000)}{2,525,000} = 3.2 \text{ deaths}/100,000/\text{year}$$

How are incidence and prevalence rates related? The relationship in theory is:

$$P = (I)(D)$$

where P = prevalence

I = incidence

D = duration of disease from onset (diagnosis) to termination

Using this formula and the data in Tables 1 and 2 we can answer questions such as, What is the difference in duration of disease between acute and chronic leukemia?

$$D = \frac{P}{I}$$

Let us calculate D for 1952.

Acute leukemia

$$D = \frac{0.83}{2.69} = 0.31 \text{ years} = 3.7 \text{ months}$$

Chronic leukemia

$$D = \frac{4.79}{2.09} = 2.29 \text{ years} = 27.5 \text{ months}$$

Note that duration and incidence must be in the same units.

For a particular disease, will the prevalence be higher than the incidence? This depends on duration and explains why $P > I$ for chronic disease and $I > P$ for acute disease. Can $P = I$? Obviously, this can happen only when the average duration of a disease is 1 year.

Should prevalence or incidence data be sought when calculating the predictive value of a laboratory test? Since both incidence and prevalence are rates of disease frequency the answer depends on the circumstances of testing and the nature of the disease. For example, we could determine both the incidence and prevalence of a disease such as PKU. From a public health perspective, the diagnosis of the new case is of utmost concern, therefore the incidence is critical. Cases that would contribute to the prevalence are unimportant since they are either beyond hope of treatment or under treatment. Therefore, we want to work with incidence, the number of new cases per year. For PKU, this is believed to be 10 to 15 per 100,000 births. Although the tables in this book list prevalence, incidence is equally appropriate. Our tables are set up to take *disease frequency* into account in the calculation of predictive value or efficiency. We could just as easily have labeled the prevalence column "disease frequency" or "probability of disease." Most of the time, we are dealing with prevalence data. However, any appropriate disease frequency rate could be applied to these tables.

Where can incidence and prevalence data for a particular population or geographical area be found? The library is a good place to start. Tables 3 to 10 contain examples of the type of material that can be found in the epidemiology literature.

Table 3 is taken from *Morbidity and Mortality* and illustrates the type of reportable conditions dealt with by this publication.[2] This reference contains tables for these diseases by geographical division, by months of the year, and by patient age groups. *Morbidity and Mortality* is a good place to search for frequency data for evaluating a laboratory test for any of these diseases.

The Office of Information, National Center for Health Statistics, publishes a series of reports that provide frequency data on a number of disease conditons. Tables 4 to 10 are from these reports. Tables 4 and 5 are from *Current Estimates from the Health Interview Survey;*[3] Tables 6 to 9 are from *Prevalence of Chronic Circulatory Conditions*[4] and Table 10 is from *Limitation of Activity Due to Chronic Conditions.*[5]

Various agencies may also provide data on disease frequency, such as the American Cancer Society. Table 11 is taken from their literature.[6]

Other useful sources of data include the State Department of Health which maintains a registry on certain diseases. The list of reportable diseases in New York State is shown in Table 12.

Finally, if a disease frequency rate cannot be obtained in a reliable reference, an estimate may be used quite successfully in the model. An idea of the frequency might be obtained in disease-specific literature and then generalized to another area. If the laboratory test looks promising with this approach, then it might be

Table 3. Reported cases of specified notifiable diseases per 100,000 population: United States, 1964–1973

DISEASE	1973	1972	1971	1970	1969	1968	1967	1966	1965	1964
Amebiasis	1.07	1.06	1.33	1.42	1.44	1.50	1.60	1.49	1.43	1.73
Anthrax	0.00	0.00	0.00	0.00	0.00	0.00	0.00	0.00	0.00	0.00
Aseptic meningitis	2.33	2.23	2.51	3.18	1.82	2.25	1.56	1.56	1.20	1.14
Botulism	0.02	0.01	0.01	0.01	0.01	0.00	0.00	0.00	0.01	0.01
Brucellosis (undulant fever)	0.10	0.09	0.09	0.10	0.12	0.11	0.13	0.13	0.14	0.21
Chickenpox	97.68	87.34	. . . . . Not previously reportable nationally							
Diphtheria	0.11	0.07	0.10	0.21	0.12	0.13	0.11	0.11	0.08	0.15
Encephalitis, primary	—	0.51	0.74	0.78	0.80	0.89	0.75	1.08	0.89	1.05
Encephalitis, post infectious	—	0.12	0.21	0.18	0.15	0.25	0.54	0.49	0.51	0.83
Hepatitis A	24.18	25.97	28.90	27.87	23.98	22.96	19.67	16.77}	17.47	19.72
Hepatitis B	4.03	4.52	4.74	4.08	3.02	2.49	1.28	0.79}		
Leprosy	0.07	0.06	0.03	0.06	0.05	0.06	0.04	0.06	0.04	0.05
Leptospirosis	0.03	0.02	0.03	0.02	0.04	0.03	0.03	0.04	0.04	0.07
Malaria	0.11	0.36	1.15	1.50	1.54	1.16	1.02	0.29	0.08	0.05
Measles (rubeola)	12.72	15.50	36.50	23.23	12.79	11.12	31.69	105.41	136.73	242.20
Meningococcal infections	0.66	0.64	1.10	1.23	1.46	1.31	1.09	1.73	1.57	1.48
Mumps	36.23	38.42	65.33	55.55	48.65	87.87	. . . . Not previously reportable nationally			
Pertussis (whooping cough)	0.84	1.58	1.47	2.08	1.63	2.41	4.91	3.98	3.55	6.80
Poliomyelitis, total	0.00	0.01	0.01	0.02	0.01	0.03	0.02	0.06	0.04	0.06
Paralytic	0.00	0.01	0.01	0.02	0.01	0.03	0.02	0.05	0.03	0.06
Psittacosis	0.02	0.02	0.02	0.02	0.03	0.02	0.02	0.03	0.03	0.03
Rabies in man	0.00	0.00	0.00	0.00	0.00	0.00	0.00	0.00	0.00	0.00
Rheumatic fever, acute	1.92	2.01	2.16	2.45	2.48	2.67	3.12	3.63	4.25	5.93
Rubella (German measles)	13.25	12.25	21.86	27.75	28.91	25.67	25.74	24.57		
Rubella congenital syndrome	0.02	0.02	0.03	0.04	0.02	0.01	0.01	0.01		
Salmonellosis, excluding typhoid fever	11.35	10.64	10.63	10.84	9.12	8.26	9.16	8.60	8.86	8.96
Shigellosis	10.79	9.70	7.83	6.79	5.92	6.09	6.81	6.07	5.69	6.78
Tetanus	0.05	0.06	0.06	0.07	0.09	0.09	0.13	0.12	0.15	0.15
Trichinosis	0.05	0.04	0.05	0.05	0.11	0.04	0.03	0.06	0.10	0.10
Tuberculosis (newly reported active cases)	14.78	15.79	17.07	18.22	19.37	21.33	23.07	24.38	25.29	26.58
Tularemia	0.08	0.07	0.09	0.08	0.07	0.09	0.11	0.11	0.14	0.18
Typhoid fever	0.32	0.19	0.20	0.17	0.18	0.20	0.20	0.19	0.23	0.26
Typhus fever — flea-borne (murine)	0.02	0.01	0.01	0.01	0.02	0.02	0.03	0.02	0.02	0.02
Typhus fever — tick-borne (Rocky Mountain spotted)	0.32	0.25	0.21	0.19	0.25	0.15	0.15	0.14	0.14	0.14
Venereal diseases (newly reported civilian cases)										
Syphilis	42.03	44.15	47.00	45.30	46.28	48.84	52.53	54.37	58.89	60.44
Gonorrhea	404.92	371.61	328.16	297.47	268.58	235.67	207.33	181.85	169.58	158.96
Other specified venereal diseases:										
Chancroid, granuloma inguinale, and lymphogranuloma venerum	0.79	1.09	1.03	1.07	0.89	0.75	0.67	0.67	1.05	1.12

Total resident population used to calculate all rates except venereal diseases for which civilian resident population was used.

Table 4. Incidence of acute conditions, percent distribution, and number of acute conditions per 100 persons per year, by condition group, according to sex. United States, 1973 (Data are based on household interviews of the civilian, noninstitutionalized population)

CONDITION GROUP	BOTH SEXES	MALE	FEMALE	BOTH SEXES	MALE	FEMALE	BOTH SEXES	MALE	FEMALE
	INCIDENCE OF ACUTE CONDITIONS IN THOUSANDS			PERCENT DISTRIBUTION			NUMBER OF ACUTE CONDITIONS PER 100 PERSONS PER YEAR		
ALL ACUTE CONDITIONS--------	360,448	170,046	190,402	100.0	100.0	100.0	175.1	171.3	178.7
INFECTIVE AND PARASITIC DISEASES---	40,003	18,794	21,209	11.1	11.1	11.1	19.4	18.9	19.9
COMMON CHILDHOOD DISEASES--------	5,002	2,507	2,496	1.4	1.5	1.3	2.4	2.5	2.3
VIRUS, N.O.S.-------------------	14,300	7,015	7,284	4.0	4.1	3.8	6.9	7.1	6.8
OTHER INFECTIVE AND PARASITIC DISEASES---------------------	20,701	9,272	11,430	5.7	5.5	6.0	10.1	9.3	10.7
RESPIRATORY CONDITIONS------------	188,817	86,814	102,003	52.4	51.1	53.6	91.7	87.5	95.7
UPPER RESPIRATORY CONDITIONS-----	100,578	46,289	54,289	27.9	27.2	28.5	48.9	46.6	50.9
COMMON COLD--------------------	73,176	32,820	40,357	20.3	19.3	21.2	35.6	33.1	37.9
OTHER UPPER RESPIRATORY CONDITIONS--------------------	27,401	13,469	13,932	7.6	7.9	7.3	13.3	13.6	13.1
INFLUENZA----------------------	79,143	36,768	42,375	22.0	21.6	22.3	38.5	37.0	39.8
INFLUENZA WITH DIGESTIVE MANIFESTATIONS---------------	12,709	5,825	6,884	3.5	3.4	3.6	5.9	5.9	6.5
OTHER INFLUENZA---------------	66,434	30,943	35,491	18.4	18.2	18.6	32.3	31.2	33.3
OTHER RESPIRATORY CONDITIONS-----	9,097	3,758	5,339	2.5	2.2	2.8	4.4	3.8	5.0
PNEUMONIA---------------------	1,900	939	991	0.5	0.5	0.5	0.9	0.9	0.9
BRONCHITIS--------------------	3,977	1,531	2,447	1.1	0.9	1.3	1.9	1.5	2.3
OTHER RESPIRATORY CONDITIONS---	3,219	1,318	1,902	0.9	0.8	1.0	1.6	1.3	1.8
DIGESTIVE SYSTEM CONDITIONS--------	17,205	8,927	8,278	4.8	5.2	4.3	8.4	9.0	7.8
DENTAL CONDITIONS----------------	3,558	2,150	1,408	1.0	1.3	0.7	1.7	2.2	1.3
FUNCTIONAL AND SYMPTOMATIC UPPER GASTROINTESTINAL DISORDERS, N.E.C.-------------------------	7,411	3,933	3,479	2.1	2.3	1.8	3.6	4.0	3.3
OTHER DIGESTIVE SYSTEM CONDITIONS---------------------	6,236	2,845	3,391	1.7	1.7	1.8	3.0	2.9	3.2
INJURIES-------------------------	63,233	36,561	26,672	17.5	21.5	14.0	30.7	36.8	25.0
FRACTURES, DISLOCATIONS, SPRAINS, AND STRAINS--------------------	19,159	10,871	8,287	5.3	6.4	4.4	9.3	11.0	7.8
FRACTURES AND DISLOCATIONS-----	6,353	3,161	3,192	1.8	1.9	1.7	3.1	3.2	3.0
SPRAINS AND STRAINS------------	12,806	7,711	5,095	3.6	4.5	2.7	6.2	7.8	4.8
OPEN WOUNDS AND LACERATIONS------	17,549	11,416	6,133	4.9	6.7	3.2	8.5	11.5	5.8
CONTUSIONS AND SUPERFICIAL INJURIES----------------------	12,726	7,119	5,607	3.5	4.2	2.9	6.2	7.2	5.3
OTHER CURRENT INJURIES-----------	13,800	7,155	6,644	3.8	4.2	3.5	6.7	7.2	6.2
ALL OTHER ACUTE CONDITIONS---------	51,190	18,950	32,240	14.2	11.1	16.9	24.9	19.1	30.3
DISEASES OF THE EAR-------------	11,827	6,070	5,757	3.3	3.6	3.0	5.7	6.1	5.4
HEADACHES-----------------------	2,715	925	1,791	0.8	0.5	0.9	1.3	0.9	1.7
GENITOURINARY DISORDERS----------	9,354	1,223	8,130	2.6	0.7	4.3	4.5	1.2	7.6
DELIVERIES AND DISORDERS OF PREGNANCY AND THE PUERPERIUM----	2,544	...	2,544	0.7	...	1.3	1.2	...	2.4
DISEASES OF THE SKIN------------	3,327	1,477	1,850	0.9	0.9	1.0	1.6	1.5	1.7
DISEASES OF THE MUSCULOSKELETAL SYSTEM-------------------------	5,013	2,089	2,924	1.4	1.2	1.5	2.4	2.1	2.7
ALL OTHER ACUTE CONDITIONS-------	16,410	7,166	9,244	4.6	4.2	4.9	8.0	7.2	8.7

NOTE: Excluded from these statistics are all conditions involving neither restricted activity nor medical attention.

N.O.S.--not otherwise specified; N.E.C.--not elsewhere classified.

Table 5. Incidence of acute conditions and number of acute conditions per 100 persons per year, by age, sex, and condition group: United States, 1973 (Data are based on household interviews of the civilian, noninstitutionalized population)

SEX AND CONDITION GROUP	ALL AGES	UNDER 6 YEARS	6-16 YEARS	17-44 YEARS	45 YEARS & OVER	ALL AGES	UNDER 6 YEARS	6-16 YEARS	17-44 YEARS	45 YEARS & OVER
BOTH SEXES	INCIDENCE OF ACUTE CONDITIONS IN THOUSANDS					NUMBER OF ACUTE CONDITIONS PER 100 PERSONS PER YEAR				
ALL ACUTE CONDITIONS-	360,448	62,089	100,432	136,560	61,368	175.1	304.5	230.3	172.8	97.7
INFECTIVE AND PARASITIC DISEASES----------------	40,003	9,943	13,534	12,441	4,085	19.4	48.8	31.0	15.7	6.5
RESPIRATORY CONDITIONS---	188,817	33,222	53,128	70,510	31,957	91.7	162.9	121.8	89.2	50.9
UPPER RESPIRATORY CONDITIONS----------	100,578	22,542	31,869	32,746	13,420	48.9	110.5	73.1	41.4	21.4
INFLUENZA-------------	79,143	8,653	19,051	35,049	16,390	38.5	42.4	43.7	44.4	26.1
OTHER RESPIRATORY CONDITIONS----------	9,097	2,027	2,209	2,714	2,147	4.4	9.9	5.1	3.4	3.4
DIGESTIVE SYSTEM CONDITIONS--------------	17,205	2,394	4,959	6,849	3,003	8.4	11.7	11.4	8.7	4.8
INJURIES----------------	63,233	7,205	16,874	26,738	12,416	30.7	35.3	38.7	33.8	19.8
ALL OTHER ACUTE CONDITIONS--------------	51,190	9,325	11,936	20,023	9,906	24.9	45.7	27.4	25.3	15.8
MALE										
ALL ACUTE CONDITIONS-	170,046	33,601	50,296	60,220	25,929	171.3	318.8	228.0	158.1	90.8
INFECTIVE AND PARASITIC DISEASES----------------	18,794	5,308	6,703	5,293	1,490	18.9	50.4	30.4	13.9	5.2
RESPIRATORY CONDITIONS---	86,814	17,581	25,462	29,906	13,865	87.5	166.8	115.4	78.5	48.6
UPPER RESPIRATORY CONDITIONS----------	46,289	11,567	15,525	13,240	5,957	46.6	109.7	70.4	34.8	20.9
INFLUENZA-------------	36,768	5,021	9,005	15,769	6,972	37.0	47.6	40.8	41.4	24.4
OTHER RESPIRATORY CONDITIONS----------	3,758	993	932	896	937	3.8	9.4	4.2	2.4	3.3
DIGESTIVE SYSTEM CONDITIONS--------------	8,927	1,305	2,554	3,632	1,436	9.0	12.4	11.6	9.5	5.0
INJURIES----------------	36,561	4,397	10,198	16,390	5,575	36.8	41.7	46.2	43.0	19.5
ALL OTHER ACUTE CONDITIONS--------------	18,950	5,010	5,379	4,999	3,562	19.1	47.5	24.4	13.1	12.5
FEMALE										
ALL ACUTE CONDITIONS-	190,402	28,488	50,135	76,340	35,439	178.7	289.2	232.7	186.5	103.5
INFECTIVE AND PARASITIC DISEASES----------------	21,209	4,635	6,832	7,148	2,595	19.9	47.0	31.7	17.5	7.6
RESPIRATORY CONDITIONS---	102,003	15,642	27,666	40,604	18,092	95.7	158.8	128.4	99.2	52.8
UPPER RESPIRATORY CONDITIONS----------	54,289	10,976	16,344	19,506	7,464	50.9	111.4	75.9	47.7	21.8
INFLUENZA-------------	42,375	3,632	10,045	19,280	9,418	39.8	36.9	46.6	47.1	27.5
OTHER RESPIRATORY CONDITIONS----------	5,339	1,034	1,277	1,818	1,211	5.0	10.5	5.9	4.4	3.5
DIGESTIVE SYSTEM CONDITIONS--------------	8,278	1,089	2,405	3,217	1,567	7.8	11.1	11.2	7.9	4.6
INJURIES----------------	26,672	2,807	6,676	10,348	6,841	25.0	28.5	31.0	25.3	20.0
ALL OTHER ACUTE CONDITIONS--------------	32,240	4,315	6,557	15,024	6,344	30.3	43.8	30.4	36.7	18.5

NOTE: Excluded from these statistics are all conditions involving neither restricted activity nor medical attention.

Table 6.   Prevalence of heart conditions reported in health interviews and number of conditions per 1000 persons, by age and selected characteristics: United States, 1972 (Data are based on household interviews of the civilian, noninstitutionalized population)

Selected characteristic	Prevalence of conditions in thousands					Number per 1,000 persons				
	All ages	Under 17 years	17-44 years	45-64 years	65 years and over	All ages	Under 17 years	17-44 years	45-64 years	65 years and over
Total[1]	10,291	683	1,900	3,749	3,959	50.4	10.5	24.6	88.8	198.7
Sex										
Male	4,725	393	724	1,953	1,654	48.0	11.9	19.5	97.4	199.3
Female	5,566	290	1,176	1,796	2,305	52.7	9.1	29.3	81.0	198.3
Color										
White	9,237	593	1,639	3,370	3,635	51.7	10.8	24.2	88.4	200.0
All other	1,055	90	262	378	324	41.5	9.0	27.5	91.6	185.2
Family income										
Less than $3,000	2,244	39	183	588	1,435	114.1	9.1	32.6	162.7	233.6
$3,000-$4,999	1,651	58	209	461	923	78.0	9.4	32.4	117.8	199.6
$5,000-$6,999	1,335	119	230	478	509	54.5	15.1	25.2	98.7	190.7
$7,000-$9,999	1,381	103	310	608	361	39.9	8.8	22.0	88.2	188.9
$10,000-$14,999	1,676	210	478	743	245	32.8	11.5	22.5	74.3	158.9
$15,000 or more	1,442	109	406	665	262	35.2	8.5	24.3	66.6	174.8
Education of head of family										
Less than 9 years	3,803	116	299	1,279	2,108	82.3	9.6	25.4	102.5	213.1
9-11 years	1,732	113	337	730	552	49.4	9.4	27.2	95.9	179.5
12 years	2,468	243	614	975	637	37.5	10.7	22.4	79.7	183.0
13 years or more	2,123	197	623	735	568	38.9	11.3	25.2	78.4	186.7
Usual activity										
Preschool (under 6 years)	218	218	...	...	...	10.5	10.5	...	...	...
School-age (6-16 years)	465	465	...	...	...	10.5	10.5	...	...	...
Usually working (17 years and over)	3,129	...	954	1,824	351	41.7	...	21.1	67.7	125.7
Usually keeping house (female, 17 years and over)	3,684	...	647	1,154	1,883	92.6	...	35.8	94.7	197.3
Retired (45 years and over)	1,929	...	...	508	1,420	233.6	...	...	294.7	217.4
Other (17 years and over)	866	...	300	262	305	53.3	...	21.7	192.2	289.4
Place of residence										
All SMSA	6,503	485	1,300	2,372	2,347	49.6	11.9	25.7	86.1	192.3
Central city	3,159	204	589	1,156	1,211	55.0	12.1	26.9	94.6	187.2
Not central city	3,344	281	711	1,216	1,136	45.4	11.7	24.9	79.3	198.0
Outside SMSA										
Nonfarm	3,370	174	556	1,199	1,440	51.9	8.1	23.1	94.9	211.4
Farm	418	*	44	177	172	51.6	*	17.3	86.3	190.5
Geographic region										
Northeast	2,506	178	429	899	1,000	52.2	12.4	24.4	82.3	192.9
North Central	2,629	171	477	948	1,033	47.0	9.4	22.7	84.8	187.6
South	3,297	176	589	1,228	1,305	51.4	8.5	24.0	96.0	212.6
West	1,859	158	405	674	621	51.6	13.6	29.0	91.7	200.6

[1]Includes unknown income and education.

157

Table 7. Prevalence of hypertensive heart disease reported in health interviews and number of conditions per 1000 persons, by age and selected characteristics: United States, 1972 (Data are based on household interviews of the civilian, noninstitutionalized population)

Selected characteristic	All ages	Under 45 years	45-64 years	65 years and over	All ages	Under 45 years	45-64 years	65 years and over
	Prevalence of conditions in thousands				Number per 1,000 persons			
Total[1] --------------------	2,142	252	839	1,051	10.5	1.8	19.9	52.8
Sex								
Male--------------------------------	732	105	323	304	7.4	1.5	16.1	36.6
Female------------------------------	1,410	147	516	748	13.3	2.0	23.3	64.4
Color								
White-------------------------------	1,707	185	655	866	9.6	1.5	17.2	47.7
All other---------------------------	436	67	184	185	17.2	3.4	44.6	105.8
Family income								
Less than $3,000--------------------	787	41	245	500	40.0	4.1	67.8	81.4
$3,000-$4,999-----------------------	388	43	114	231	18.3	3.4	29.1	49.9
$5,000-$6,999-----------------------	220	*	109	90	9.0	*	22.5	33.7
$7,000-$9,999-----------------------	242	*	127	82	7.0	*	18.4	42.9
$10,000-$14,999---------------------	221	58	121	42	4.3	1.5	12.1	27.2
$15,000 or more---------------------	182	44	84	54	4.4	1.5	8.4	36.0
Education of head of family								
Less than 9 years-------------------	1,093	57	400	635	23.7	2.4	32.1	64.2
9-11 years--------------------------	357	71	167	120	10.2	2.9	21.9	39.0
12 years----------------------------	372	56	166	150	5.7	1.1	13.6	43.1
13 years or more--------------------	280	62	97	121	5.1	1.5	10.3	39.8
Usual activity								
Usually working (17 years and over)--	490	122	299	69	6.5	2.7	11.1	24.7
Usually keeping house (female, 17 years and over)--------------------	1,098	92	368	638	27.6	5.1	30.2	66.8
Retired (45 years and over)----------	375	...	114	261	45.4	...	66.1	40.0
Place of residence								
All SMSA----------------------------	1,257	182	506	569	9.6	2.0	18.4	46.6
Central city------------------------	703	102	272	329	12.2	2.6	22.3	50.9
Not central city-------------------	553	79	234	240	7.5	1.5	15.3	41.8
Outside SMSA								
Nonfarm-----------------------------	780	65	288	426	12.0	1.4	22.8	62.5
Farm--------------------------------	106	*	45	56	13.1	*	22.0	62.0
Geographic region								
Northeast---------------------------	480	64	201	215	10.0	2.0	18.4	41.5
North Central-----------------------	535	66	175	294	9.6	1.7	15.7	53.4
South-------------------------------	804	71	328	405	12.5	1.6	25.7	66.0
West--------------------------------	324	52	135	138	9.0	2.0	18.4	44.6

[1]Includes unknown income and education.

Table 8. Prevalence of coronary heart disease reported in health interviews and number of conditions per 1000 persons, by age and selected characteristics: United States, 1972 (Data are based on household interviews of the civilian, noninstitutionalized population)

Selected characteristic	All ages	Under 45 years	45-64 years	65 years and over	All ages	Under 45 years	45-64 years	65 years and over
	Prevalence of conditions in thousands				Number per 1,000 persons			
Total[1] -------------------	3,307	167	1,466	1,674	16.2	1.2	34.7	84.0
Sex								
Male---------------------------------	1,869	110	965	794	19.0	1.6	48.1	95.7
Female-------------------------------	1,439	57	502	880	13.6	0.8	22.6	75.7
Color								
White--------------------------------	3,178	144	1,403	1,631	17.8	1.2	36.8	89.7
All other----------------------------	129	*	64	43	5.1	*	15.5	24.6
Family income								
Less than $3,000--------------------	638	*	132	498	32.4	*	36.5	81.1
$3,000-$4,999-----------------------	600	*	171	411	28.4	*	43.7	88.9
$5,000-$6,999-----------------------	458	*	193	245	18.7	*	39.8	91.8
$7,000-$9,999-----------------------	432	*	243	161	12.5	*	35.2	84.2
$10,000-$14,999---------------------	495	44	321	131	9.7	1.1	32.1	85.0
$15,000 or more---------------------	492	41	321	130	12.0	1.4	32.1	86.7
Education of head of family								
Less than 9 years-------------------	1,258	*	410	815	27.2	*	32.9	82.4
9-11 years--------------------------	574	*	291	261	16.4	*	38.2	84.9
12 years----------------------------	767	52	425	290	11.7	1.0	34.8	83.3
13 years or more--------------------	660	59	327	274	12.1	1.4	34.9	90.0
Usual activity								
Usually working (17 years and over)-	1,095	107	823	165	14.6	2.4	30.5	59.1
Usually keeping house (female, 17 years and over)--------------------	1,057	*	321	703	26.6	*	26.3	73.7
Retired (45 years and over)---------	883	...	219	664	106.9	...	127.0	101.6
Place of residence								
All SMSA----------------------------	2,130	103	988	1,038	16.2	1.1	35.9	85.0
Central city-----------------------	1,016	47	432	537	17.7	1.2	35.4	83.0
Not central city-------------------	1,114	56	556	501	15.1	1.1	36.3	87.3
Outside SMSA								
Nonfarm----------------------------	1,079	57	431	591	16.6	1.3	34.1	86.7
Farm-------------------------------	99	*	47	45	12.2	*	22.9	49.8
Geographic region								
Northeast---------------------------	899	35	388	475	18.7	1.1	35.5	91.6
North Central-----------------------	853	46	385	423	15.2	1.2	34.5	76.8
South-------------------------------	1,012	51	454	507	15.8	1.1	35.5	82.6
West--------------------------------	543	*	239	269	15.1	*	32.5	86.9

[1]Includes unknown income and education.

Table 9. Prevalence of hemorrhoids reported in health interviews and number of conditions per 1000 persons, by age and selected characteristics: United States, 1972 (Data are based on household interviews of the civilian, noninstitutionalized population)

Selected characteristic	All ages	Under 17 years	17-44 years	45-64 years	65 years and over	All ages	Under 17 years	17-44 years	45-64 years	65 years and over
	Prevalence of conditions in thousands					Number per 1,000 persons				
Total[1] ---------------------------	9,744	61	4,838	3,369	1,476	47.7	0.9	62.7	79.8	74.1
Sex										
Male--------------------------------	4,106	*	1,954	1,585	543	41.7	*	52.7	79.1	65.4
Female------------------------------	5,638	37	2,884	1,784	933	53.3	1.2	72.0	80.4	80.3
Color										
White-------------------------------	9,022	53	4,444	3,150	1,375	50.5	1.0	65.7	82.7	75.7
All other---------------------------	722	*	394	219	101	28.4	*	41.4	53.1	57.7
Family income										
Less than $3,000-----------------------	1,258	*	317	363	573	63.9	*	56.5	100.4	93.3
$3,000-$4,999--------------------------	1,019	*	335	322	359	48.2	*	51.9	82.3	77.6
$5,000-$6,999--------------------------	1,215	*	568	437	200	49.6	*	62.2	90.2	74.9
$7,000-$9,999--------------------------	1,662	*	940	599	118	48.0	*	66.9	86.9	61.7
$10,000-$14,999------------------------	2,370	*	1,503	769	84	46.4	*	70.7	76.9	54.5
$15,000 or more-----------------------	1,826	*	1,017	707	81	44.6	*	60.8	70.8	54.0
Education of head of family										
Less than 9 years---------------------	2,420	*	581	1,057	775	52.4	*	49.3	84.7	78.4
9-11 years----------------------------	1,696	*	837	631	220	48.4	*	67.6	82.9	71.5
12 years-----------------------------	2,909	*	1,760	886	244	44.2	*	64.3	72.5	70.1
13 years or more---------------------	2,616	*	1,626	750	213	47.9	*	65.6	80.0	70.0
Usual activity										
School-age (6-16 years)-----------------	50	50	...	...	...	1.1	1.1	...	...	...
Usually working (17 years and over)----	4,872	...	2,752	1,971	149	65.0	...	60.8	73.1	53.3
Usually keeping house (female, 17 years and over)------------------------------	3,730	...	1,852	1,095	783	93.7	...	102.5	89.9	82.0
Retired (45 years and over)------------	641	...	...	183	458	77.6	...	...	106.1	70.1
Place of residence										
All SMSA-----------------------------	6,146	*	3,199	2,101	816	46.9	*	63.3	76.3	66.8
Central city------------------------	2,568	*	1,244	878	438	44.7	*	56.8	71.9	67.7
Not central city-------------------	3,578	*	1,954	1,223	378	48.5	*	68.4	79.8	65.9
Outside SMSA										
Nonfarm------ -----------------------	3,252	*	1,509	1,116	597	50.1	*	62.6	88.3	87.6
Farm--------------------------------	346	*	130	152	63	42.7	*	51.2	74.1	69.8
Geographic region										
Northeast---------------------------	2,182	*	1,070	811	286	45.4	*	60.9	74.3	55.2
North Central-----------------------	2,645	*	1,384	858	388	47.3	*	65.8	76.8	70.5
South-------------------------------	3,115	*	1,491	1,040	561	48.6	*	60.7	81.3	91.4
West--------------------------------	1,801	*	892	660	241	50.0	*	63.8	89.8	77.9

[1] Includes unknown income and education.

160

Table 10. Average number of persons with limitation of activity by selected chronic conditions causing limitation, by sex and age: United States, 1969–1970 (Data are based on household interviews of the civilian, noninstitutionalized population)

Selected chronic conditions	Both sexes				Male				Female			
	All ages	Under 45 years	45-64 years	65 years and over	All ages	Under 45 years	45-64 years	65 years and over	All ages	Under 45 years	45-64 years	65 years and over
	Average number of persons in thousands[1]											
Persons limited in activity-----------	23,237	7,293	7,987	7,958	11,740	3,940	4,113	3,686	11,498	3,353	3,873	4,271
Tuberculosis, all forms----	156	50	76	30	94	*	54	*	62	31	*	*
Malignant neoplasms--------	358	54	178	125	161	*	80	63	197	36	98	62
Benign and unspecified neoplasms-----------------	204	86	72	45	63	*	*	*	141	67	46	*
Diabetes-------------------	865	115	396	354	356	59	157	140	509	56	238	215
Mental and nervous conditions----------------	1,033	389	403	241	477	188	192	97	556	200	212	144
Heart conditions-----------	3,609	461	1,520	1,628	1,937	216	917	804	1,672	245	603	824
Cerebrovascular disease----	604	*	206	376	335	*	127	197	270	*	79	179
Hypertension without heart involvement----------------	1,059	132	416	510	351	51	152	147	708	81	264	363
Varicose veins-------------	169	33	93	43	47	*	*	*	122	31	66	*
Hemorrhoids----------------	44	*	*	*	*	*	*	*	*	*	*	*
Other conditions of circulatory system--------	694	114	242	338	324	47	126	151	370	67	115	188
Chronic bronchitis---------	219	91	66	62	138	48	40	50	81	43	*	*
Emphysema------------------	566	31	252	282	455	*	201	238	111	*	51	44
Asthma, with or without hay fever-----------------	1,010	595	260	154	574	343	133	98	435	252	127	56
Hay fever, without asthma--	149	100	35	*	76	59	*	*	73	41	*	*
Chronic sinusitis----------	105	40	44	*	51	*	*	*	55	*	*	*
Other conditions of respiratory system--------	451	157	143	152	307	95	104	108	144	61	38	44
Peptic ulcer---------------	320	79	157	84	218	52	106	60	102	*	51	*
Hernia---------------------	434	81	188	165	268	54	110	104	166	*	78	61
Other conditions of digestive system----------	589	147	213	230	259	67	101	91	330	79	112	139
Diseases of kidney and ureter-------------------	243	105	70	69	94	39	*	*	150	66	41	42
Other conditions of genitourinary system------	357	129	126	102	118	*	38	59	239	108	88	43
Arthritis and rheumatism---	3,265	321	1,254	1,691	1,096	122	442	532	2,170	199	812	1,159
Other musculoskeletal disorders-----------------	914	353	421	140	436	194	192	50	478	159	228	90
Visual impairments---------	1,115	259	302	554	623	188	178	257	492	70	125	297
Hearing impairments--------	431	211	101	119	267	140	64	63	165	71	38	56
Paralysis, complete or partial-------------------	817	279	254	284	470	168	146	156	347	111	108	128
Impairments (except paralysis) of back or spine---------------------	1,613	771	622	220	859	410	363	86	754	361	258	134
Impairments (except paralysis and absence) of upper extremities and shoulders-----------------	431	196	156	80	285	145	105	35	146	50	50	45
Impairments (except paralysis and absence) of lower extremities and hips---------------------	1,551	648	480	423	887	449	281	157	664	199	199	266

[1]Summations of conditions causing limitation may be greater than the number of persons limited because a person can report more than one condition as a cause of his limitation; on the other hand, they may be less because only selected conditions are shown.

161

Table 11. Applying cancer statistics locally

Community population	Estimated number who are alive, cured of cancer	Estimated number cancer cases under medical care in 1973	Estimated number who will die of cancer in 1973	Estimated number of new cases in 1973	Estimated number who will be saved from cancer in 1973	Estimated number who will eventually develop cancer	Estimated number who will die of cancer if present rates continue
1,000	7	4	1	3	1	250	150
2,000	15	9	3	6	2	500	300
3,000	22	13	4	8	3	750	450
4,000	30	18	6	11	4	1,000	600
5,000	37	21	7	14	5	1,250	750
10,000	74	43	15	28	9	2,500	1,500
25,000	185	107	37	70	23	6,250	3,750
50,000	370	215	75	140	47	12,500	7,500
100,000	740	430	150	280	93	25,000	15,000
200,000	1,480	860	300	560	186	50,000	30,000
500,000	3,700	2,150	750	1,400	465	125,000	75,000

The figures can only be the roughest approximation of actual data for your community. It is suggested that every effort be made to obtain actual data from a Registry source.

Table 12.   New York State List of Reportable Diseases (1973)

Common	Rare
Chickenpox	Amebiasis
Central nervous system infections	Anthrax
(specify site and agent if known)	Botulism
Bacterial	Brucellosis
Nonbacterial	Chancroid
Food poisoning (specify agent if known)	Cholera
Gonorrhea	Diphtheria
Genitourinary	Granuloma inguinale
Ophthalmia	Histoplasmosis (new cases)
Other (specify)	Leprosy
Hepatitis, viral	Leptospirosis
Infectious (A)	Lymphogranuloma venereum
Serum (B)	Malaria
Hospital associated infections (including	Plague
diarrhea and conjunctivitis of newborn)	Poliomyelitis
Infectious mononucleosis	Psittacosis
Measles	Rabies
Mumps	Relapsing fever
Rubella (including congenital rubella syndrome)	Rocky mountain spotted fever
Salmonellosis	Smallpox
Shigellosis	Tetanus
Streptococcal sore throat (including	Trichinosis
scarlet fever, dairy farms only)	Tularemia
Syphilis	Typhoid
Tuberculosis, new active and reactivations	Typhus
(specify site, extent, activity)	Whooping cough
	Yellow fever

necessary to obtain a more reliable estimate of disease frequency. In estimating disease frequency, it seems wise to guess high. If the test performs poorly under these conditions, then there is no point in going any further.

The list below consists of Schools of Public Health in the United States which are accredited by the American Public Health Association. It is presented with the hope of facilitating communication between laboratory scientists and epidemiologists, a relationship that is likely to be a positive experience for both.

University of California, School of Public Health
Earl Warren Hall, Berkeley, California 94720

University of California at Los Angeles, School of Public Health
Los Angeles, California 90024

Columbia University, School of Public Health and Administrative Medicine
600 West 168th Street, New York, New York 10032

Harvard University, School of Public Health
55 Shattuck Street, Boston Massachusetts 02115

University of Hawaii, School of Public Health
2540 Maila Way, Honolulu, Hawaii 96822

University of Illinois, School of Public Health
Chicago, Illinois 60680

Johns Hopkins University, School of Hygiene and Public Health
615 North Wolfe Street, Baltimore, Maryland 21203

Loma Linda University, School of Public Health
Loma Linda, California 92354

University of Michigan, School of Public Health
Ann Arbor, Michigan 48104

University of Minnesota, School of Public Health
1325 May Memorial Building, Minneapolis, Minnesota 55455

University of North Carolina, School of Public Health
Chapel Hill, North Carolina 27515

University of Oklahoma, School of Public Health
800 N.E. Thirteenth Street, Oklahoma City, Oklahoma 73104

University of Pittsburgh, Graduate School of Public Health
4200 Fifth Avenue, Pittsburgh, Pennsylvania 15213

University of Puerto Rico, School of Medicine
San Juan, Puerto Rico 00905

University of Texas at Houston, School of Public Health, Texas Medical Center
P.O. Box 2018, Astrodome Station, Houston, Texas 77023

Tulane University, School of Public Health and Tropical Medicine
1430 Tulane Avenue, New Orleans, Louisiana 70112

Yale University, School of Medicine, Department of Epidemiology and Public Health
Sixty College Street, New Haven, Connecticut 06510

REFERENCES

1. MacMahon, Brian and Pugh, Thomas F. *Epidemiology: Principles and Methods.* Little, Brown, Boston, Mass., 1970.

2. *Morbidity and Mortality: Reported Morbidity and Mortality in the United States, 1973, U.S. Department Health, Education, and Welfare,* Public Health Service, Center for *Disease Control,* Vol. 22, No. 53, Atlanta, Georgia, 1974.

3. *Current Estimates from the Health Interview Survey, United States, 1973.* Vital and Health Statistics, Series 10: Data from the National Health Survey, No. 95. U.S. Department Health, Education, and Welfare, Public Health Service, Health Resources Administration. National Center for Health Statistics, Washington, D.C., 1974.

4. *Prevalence of Chronic Circulatory Conditions, United States, 1972.* Vital and Health Statistics, Series 10: Data from the National Health Survey, No. 94, U.S. Department Health, Education, and Welfare, Public Health Service, Health Resources Administration. National Center for Health Statistics, Washington, D.C. 1974.

5. *Limitation of Activity Due to Chronic Conditions, United States, 1969 and 1970.* Vital and Health Statistics, Series 10: Data from the National Health Survey, No. 80. U.S. Department Health, Education, and Welfare, Public Health Service, Health Resources Administration. National Center for Health Statistics, Washington, D.C. 1973.

6. *Cancer Facts and Figures, 1973.* American Cancer Society, New York, 1973.

APPENDIX IX   RISK FACTORS AND LABORATORY TESTS

Relative risk is defined by the following ratio:

$$\frac{\text{incidence of a disease among those exposed to a factor}}{\text{incidence among those not exposed}}$$

When a causal relationship exists between the exposure to a factor and a particular disease, then the particular exposure factor is referred to as a "risk factor."[1] Risk factors may be blood constituents, such as serum cholesterol, which are measured in the laboratory.

Can risk factors serve as useful laboratory tests? The answer depends on the predictive value of the risk factor *if it is used as a laboratory test*. There is much confusion in the literature because many physicians believe that a well-defined risk factor can be used to predict the occurrence of disease. As an example of this confusion we cite the following criticism by Dr. Stephen M. Brown of the Epidemiology Research Unit at Berkeley[2] of the application of our predictive value model to a study of food antibodies in myocardial infarction[3,4] (see also Chapter 5):

> Sir—Dr. Galen criticized the results of Dr. Davies and his colleagues, who demonstrated a nearly threefold relative risk of death from coronary heart disease (C.H.D.) among persons with antibody to cow's milk and egg protein. The basis of his criticism is first, that there are too many false positives, and, second, that those with this risk factor account for only one-fourth of the entire burden of mortality.
>
> From an epidemilogical point of view, possession of a risk factor ought not be merely judged *vis-à-vis* its usefulness as a screening test, but also must be considered from the position of public health and preventative medicine. The example of smoking and lung cancer, too often cited, must again be considered. Clearly, the fact that one is a smoker is not intended to serve as a screening test. The argument of Dr. Galen about false positives and relative efficiency of the "screening test" could equally well have been leveled against smoking. More than 99% of smokers never develop malignancies of the trachea, lung, or bronchus. Are we then to take this as an argument against the usefulness of smoking status in predicting the occurrence of lung cancer?

Our answer to Dr. Brown's last question is a resounding *yes*. Let us create a hypothetical data base and explore the problem further. We assume that the prevalence of lung cancer in the population is 100/100,000 and that 33.3% of the population smokes ciagarettes. We also assume that our study revealed the data in Table 1

Table 1.   **Hypothetical data base**

	Positive for smoking	Negative for smoking	Totals
Lung cancer	100	None	100
No lung cancer	33,233	66,667	99,900
Totals	33,333	66,667	100,000

This data might support an argument that cigarette smoking is a risk factor for cancer of the lung; and such an argument would be very reasonable since *all* of the cases of lung cancer occurred in cigarette smokers. *But is cigarette smoking highly predictive of lung cancer as suggested by Dr. Brown?* The answer has to be no, because the predictive value of a positive history of cigarette smoking is only 0.3 % (100/33,333)! Ninety-nine and seven tenths percent of smokers do *not* develop lung cancer. Although we want to discourage smoking, because of its status as a risk factor, we do not want to subject smokers to any additional expensive or possibly injurious diagnostic procedures on the off chance that we may discover an occult carcinoma. There is a big difference between a risk factor and a test. Although some risk factors may indeed be tests, there are many risks factors that are not useful tests; and, conversely, there are many laboratory tests that do not serve as measures of risk.

Fortunately, no one has suggested that we use smoking status as a laboratory test, but other risk factors have found their way into our testing regimens. One of the most disturbing examples of this is the measurement of serum cholesterol. Serum cholesterol is assayed routinely on the assumption that it is an important risk factor, and that its measurement is useful in predicting the possible occurrence of coronary atherosclerosis. But how good a risk factor is it? If it were possible to lower everyone's serum cholesterol to a level that would eliminate cholseterol as a risk factor, what effect would that have on the incidence of ischemic heart disease? Lars Werko reports the following:

> The 10-year incidence of ischemic heart disease would then decrease about 10 % in one-third of the population. The total effect of a successful attack of hypercholesterolemia would be only a reduction of new events from 14 in 100 men to 11 in 100 in 10 years' time. This provided you get full cooperation, that you can lower serum cholesterol effectively, and that this itself will decrease the incidence of disease. All these provisions are open to doubt.[5]

Although serum cholesterol is measured routinely *in order to identify and quantitate a risk factor for ischemic heart disease*, it is not a very powerful risk factor. Therefore, we question the current effectiveness of performing this test on a routine basis at this time.

REFERENCES

---

1. MacMahon, Brian and Pugh, Thomas F. *Epidemiology: Principles and Methods.* Little, Brown, Boston, Mass., 1970.
2. Brown, Stephen M. Food antibodies and myocardial infarction. *Lancet* **ii:** 1147–1148, 1974.
3. Davies, D. F., Rees, B. W. G., Johnson, A. P. Elwood, P. C., and Abernethy, M. Food antibodies and myocardial infarction. *Lancet* **i:** 1012–1014, 1974.
4. Galen, R. S. Food antibodies and myocardial infarction. *Lancet* **ii:** 832, 1974.
5. Werko, Lars. Can we prevent heart disease? *Ann. Intern. Med.* 278–288, 1971.

PREDICTIVE VALUE AND EFFICIENCY TABLES

PREDICTIVE VALUE OF A POSITIVE TEST BASED ON
TEST SENSITIVITY, SPECIFICITY, AND DISEASE PREVALENCE*

Three relationships are possible between sensitivity and specificity for any test. The sensitivity may be greater than the specificity, the sensitivity may be equal to the specificity, or the sensitivity may be less than the specificity. Let us review what happens to the predictive value of a positive test under each of these circumstances in the face of fixed as well as increasing disease prevalence:

At a given prevalence, an incremental increase in specificity results in a greater increase in the predictive value of a positive test than the same incremental increase in sensitivity. As prevalence increases, the predictive value of a positive test increases regardless of the relationship between sensitivity and specificity.

Table 1

PREDICTIVE VALUE OF POSITIVES (IN PERCENT)
PREVALENCE=   1 PER 100,000

		SENSITIVITY (%)															
		50	60	70	80	85	90	91	92	93	94	95	96	97	98	99	100
	50.00	0	0	0	0	0	0	0	0	0	0	0	0	0	0	0	0
	60.00	0	0	0	0	0	0	0	0	0	0	0	0	0	0	0	0
	70.00	0	0	0	0	0	0	0	0	0	0	0	0	0	0	0	0
SPECI-	80.00	0	0	0	0	0	0	0	0	0	0	0	0	0	0	0	0
FICITY	90.00	0	0	0	0	0	0	0	0	0	0	0	0	0	0	0	0
(%)	91.00	0	0	0	0	0	0	0	0	0	0	0	0	0	0	0	0
	93.00	0	0	0	0	0	0	0	0	0	0	0	0	0	0	0	0
	95.00	0	0	0	0	0	0	0	0	0	0	0	0	0	0	0	0
	97.00	0	0	0	0	0	0	0	0	0	0	0	0	0	0	0	0
	99.00	0	0	0	0	0	0	0	0	0	0	0	0	0	0	0	0
	99.10	0	0	0	0	0	0	0	0	0	0	0	0	0	0	0	0
	99.30	0	0	0	0	0	0	0	0	0	0	0	0	0	0	0	0
	99.50	0	0	0	0	0	0	0	0	0	0	0	0	0	0	0	0
	99.70	0	0	0	0	0	0	0	0	0	0	0	0	0	0	0	0
	99.90	0	1	1	1	1	1	1	1	1	1	1	1	1	1	1	1
	99.91	1	1	1	1	1	1	1	1	1	1	1	1	1	1	1	1
	99.92	1	1	1	1	1	1	1	1	1	1	1	1	1	1	1	1
	99.93	1	1	1	1	1	1	1	1	1	1	1	1	1	1	1	1
	99.94	1	1	1	1	1	1	1	2	2	2	2	2	2	2	2	2
	99.95	1	1	1	2	2	2	2	2	2	2	2	2	2	2	2	2
	99.96	1	1	2	2	2	2	2	2	2	2	2	2	2	2	2	2
	99.97	2	2	2	3	3	3	3	3	3	3	3	3	3	3	3	3
	99.98	2	3	3	4	4	4	4	4	4	4	5	5	5	5	5	5
	99.99	5	6	7	7	8	8	8	8	9	9	9	9	9	9	9	9
	100.00	100	100	100	100	100	100	100	100	100	100	100	100	100	100	100	100

* © 1972 by Robert S. Galen, M.D., M.P.H. Galen Tables of the predictive value of clinical laboratory tests: 72-386841.

Table 2

PREDICTIVE VALUE OF POSITIVES (IN PERCENT)
PREVALENCE=   2 PER 100,000

		SENSITIVITY (%)															
		50	60	70	80	85	90	91	92	93	94	95	96	97	98	99	100
	50.00	0	0	0	0	0	0	0	0	0	0	0	0	0	0	0	0
	60.00	0	0	0	0	0	0	0	0	0	0	0	0	0	0	0	0
	70.00	0	0	0	0	0	0	0	0	0	0	0	0	0	0	0	0
SPECI-	80.00	0	0	0	0	0	0	0	0	0	0	0	0	0	0	0	0
FICITY	90.00	0	0	0	0	0	0	0	0	0	0	0	0	0	0	0	0
(%)	91.00	0	0	0	0	0	0	0	0	0	0	0	0	0	0	0	0
	93.00	0	0	0	0	0	0	0	0	0	0	0	0	0	0	0	0
	95.00	0	0	0	0	0	0	0	0	0	0	0	0	0	0	0	0
	97.00	0	0	0	0	0	0	0	0	0	0	0	0	0	0	0	0
	99.00	0	0	0	0	0	0	0	0	0	0	0	0	0	0	0	0
	99.10	0	0	0	0	0	0	0	0	0	0	0	0	0	0	0	0
	99.30	0	0	0	0	0	0	0	0	0	0	0	0	0	0	0	0
	99.50	0	0	0	0	0	0	0	0	0	0	0	0	0	0	0	0
	99.70	0	0	0	1	1	1	1	1	1	1	1	1	1	1	1	1
	99.90	1	1	1	2	2	2	2	2	2	2	2	2	2	2	2	2
	99.91	1	1	2	2	2	2	2	2	2	2	2	2	2	2	2	2
	99.92	1	1	2	2	2	2	2	2	2	2	2	2	2	2	2	2
	99.93	1	2	2	2	2	3	3	3	3	3	3	3	3	3	3	3
	99.94	2	2	2	3	3	3	3	3	3	3	3	3	3	3	3	3
	99.95	2	2	3	3	3	3	4	4	4	4	4	4	4	4	4	4
	99.96	2	3	3	4	4	4	4	4	4	4	5	5	5	5	5	5
	99.97	3	4	4	5	5	6	6	6	6	6	6	6	6	6	6	6
	99.98	5	6	7	7	8	8	8	8	9	9	9	9	9	9	9	9
	99.99	9	11	12	14	15	15	15	16	16	16	16	16	16	16	17	17
	100.00	100	100	100	100	100	100	100	100	100	100	100	100	100	100	100	100

Table 3

PREDICTIVE VALUE OF POSITIVES (IN PERCENT)
PREVALENCE=   3 PER 100,000

		SENSITIVITY (%)															
		50	60	70	80	85	90	91	92	93	94	95	96	97	98	99	100
	50.00	0	0	0	0	0	0	0	0	0	0	0	0	0	0	0	0
	60.00	0	0	0	0	0	0	0	0	0	0	0	0	0	0	0	0
	70.00	0	0	0	0	0	0	0	0	0	0	0	0	0	0	0	0
SPECI-	80.00	0	0	0	0	0	0	0	0	0	0	0	0	0	0	0	0
FICITY	90.00	0	0	0	0	0	0	0	0	0	0	0	0	0	0	0	0
(%)	91.00	0	0	0	0	0	0	0	0	0	0	0	0	0	0	0	0
	93.00	0	0	0	0	0	0	0	0	0	0	0	0	0	0	0	0
	95.00	0	0	0	0	0	0	0	0	0	0	0	0	0	0	0	0
	97.00	0	0	0	0	0	0	0	0	0	0	0	0	0	0	0	0
	99.00	0	0	0	0	0	0	0	0	0	0	0	0	0	0	0	0
	99.10	0	0	0	0	0	0	0	0	0	0	0	0	0	0	0	0
	99.30	0	0	0	0	0	0	0	0	0	0	0	0	0	0	0	0
	99.50	0	0	0	0	1	1	1	1	1	1	1	1	1	1	1	1
	99.70	0	1	1	1	1	1	1	1	1	1	1	1	1	1	1	1
	99.90	1	2	2	2	2	3	3	3	3	3	3	3	3	3	3	3
	99.91	2	2	2	3	3	3	3	3	3	3	3	3	3	3	3	3
	99.92	2	2	3	3	3	3	3	3	3	3	3	3	4	4	4	4
	99.93	2	3	3	3	4	4	4	4	4	4	4	4	4	4	4	4
	99.94	2	3	3	4	4	4	4	4	4	4	5	5	5	5	5	5
	99.95	3	3	4	5	5	5	5	5	5	5	5	5	5	6	6	6
	99.96	4	4	5	6	6	6	6	6	7	7	7	7	7	7	7	7
	99.97	5	6	7	7	8	8	8	8	9	9	9	9	9	9	9	9
	99.98	7	8	10	11	11	12	12	12	12	12	12	13	13	13	13	13
	99.99	13	15	17	19	20	21	21	22	22	22	22	23	23	23	23	23
	100.00	100	100	100	100	100	100	100	100	100	100	100	100	100	100	100	100

Table 4

PREDICTIVE VALUE OF POSITIVES (IN PERCENT)
PREVALENCE=   4 PER 100,000

		SENSITIVITY (%)															
		50	60	70	80	85	90	91	92	93	94	95	96	97	98	99	100
	50.00	0	0	0	0	0	0	0	0	0	0	0	0	0	0	0	0
	60.00	0	0	0	0	0	0	0	0	0	0	0	0	0	0	0	0
	70.00	0	0	0	0	0	0	0	0	0	0	0	0	0	0	0	0
SPECI-	80.00	0	0	0	0	0	0	0	0	0	0	0	0	0	0	0	0
FICITY	90.00	0	0	0	0	0	0	0	0	0	0	0	0	0	0	0	0
(%)	91.00	0	0	0	0	0	0	0	0	0	0	0	0	0	0	0	0
	93.00	0	0	0	0	0	0	0	0	0	0	0	0	0	0	0	0
	95.00	0	0	0	0	0	0	0	0	0	0	0	0	0	0	0	0
	97.00	0	0	0	0	0	0	0	0	0	0	0	0	0	0	0	0
	99.00	0	0	0	0	0	0	0	0	0	0	0	0	0	0	0	0
	99.10	0	0	0	0	0	0	0	0	0	0	0	0	0	0	0	0
	99.30	0	0	0	0	0	1	1	1	1	1	1	1	1	1	1	1
	99.50	0	0	1	1	1	1	1	1	1	1	1	1	1	1	1	1
	99.70	1	1	1	1	1	1	1	1	1	1	1	1	1	1	1	1
	99.90	2	2	3	3	3	3	4	4	4	4	4	4	4	4	4	4
	99.91	2	3	3	3	4	4	4	4	4	4	4	4	4	4	4	4
	99.92	2	3	3	4	4	4	4	4	4	4	5	5	5	5	5	5
	99.93	3	3	4	4	5	5	5	5	5	5	5	5	5	5	5	5
	99.94	3	4	4	5	5	6	6	6	6	6	6	6	6	6	6	6
	99.95	4	5	5	6	6	7	7	7	7	7	7	7	7	7	7	7
	99.96	5	6	7	7	8	8	8	8	9	9	9	9	9	9	9	9
	99.97	6	7	9	10	10	11	11	11	11	11	11	11	11	12	12	12
	99.98	9	11	12	14	15	15	15	16	16	16	16	16	16	16	17	17
	99.99	17	19	22	24	25	26	27	27	27	27	28	28	28	28	28	29
	100.00	100	100	100	100	100	100	100	100	100	100	100	100	100	100	100	100

Table 5

PREDICTIVE VALUE OF POSITIVES (IN PERCENT)
PREVALENCE=   5 PER 100,000

		SENSITIVITY (%)															
		50	60	70	80	85	90	91	92	93	94	95	96	97	98	99	100
	50.00	0	0	0	0	0	0	0	0	0	0	0	0	0	0	0	0
	60.00	0	0	0	0	0	0	0	0	0	0	0	0	0	0	0	0
	70.00	0	0	0	0	0	0	0	0	0	0	0	0	0	0	0	0
SPECI-	80.00	0	0	0	0	0	0	0	0	0	0	0	0	0	0	0	0
FICITY	90.00	0	0	0	0	0	0	0	0	0	0	0	0	0	0	0	0
(%)	91.00	0	0	0	0	0	0	0	0	0	0	0	0	0	0	0	0
	93.00	0	0	0	0	0	0	0	0	0	0	0	0	0	0	0	0
	95.00	0	0	0	0	0	0	0	0	0	0	0	0	0	0	0	0
	97.00	0	0	0	0	0	0	0	0	0	0	0	0	0	0	0	0
	99.00	0	0	0	0	0	0	0	0	0	0	0	0	0	0	0	0
	99.10	0	0	0	0	0	0	1	1	1	1	1	1	1	1	1	1
	99.30	0	0	0	1	1	1	1	1	1	1	1	1	1	1	1	1
	99.50	0	1	1	1	1	1	1	1	1	1	1	1	1	1	1	1
	99.70	1	1	1	1	1	1	1	2	2	2	2	2	2	2	2	2
	99.90	2	3	3	4	4	4	4	4	4	4	5	5	5	5	5	5
	99.91	3	3	4	4	5	5	5	5	5	5	5	5	5	5	5	5
	99.92	3	4	4	5	5	5	5	5	5	6	6	6	6	6	6	6
	99.93	3	4	5	5	6	6	6	6	6	6	6	6	6	7	7	7
	99.94	4	5	6	6	7	7	7	7	7	7	7	7	7	8	8	8
	99.95	5	6	7	7	8	8	8	8	9	9	9	9	9	9	9	9
	99.96	6	7	8	9	10	10	10	10	10	11	11	11	11	11	11	11
	99.97	8	9	10	12	12	13	13	13	13	14	14	14	14	14	14	14
	99.98	11	13	15	17	18	18	19	19	19	19	19	19	20	20	20	20
	99.99	20	23	26	29	30	31	31	31	32	32	32	32	33	33	33	33
	100.00	100	100	100	100	100	100	100	100	100	100	100	100	100	100	100	100

Table 6

PREDICTIVE VALUE OF POSITIVES (IN PERCENT)
PREVALENCE=   10 PER 100,000

		SENSITIVITY (%)															
		50	60	70	80	85	90	91	92	93	94	95	96	97	98	99	100
	50.00	0	0	0	0	0	0	0	0	0	0	0	0	0	0	0	0
	60.00	0	0	0	0	0	0	0	0	0	0	0	0	0	0	0	0
	70.00	0	0	0	0	0	0	0	0	0	0	0	0	0	0	0	0
SPECI-	80.00	0	0	0	0	0	0	0	0	0	0	0	0	0	0	0	0
FICITY	90.00	0	0	0	0	0	0	0	0	0	0	0	0	0	0	0	0
(%)	91.00	0	0	0	0	0	0	0	0	0	0	0	0	0	0	0	0
	93.00	0	0	0	0	0	0	0	0	0	0	0	0	0	0	0	0
	95.00	0	0	0	0	0	0	0	0	0	0	0	0	0	0	0	0
	97.00	0	0	0	0	0	0	0	0	0	0	0	0	0	0	0	0
	99.00	0	1	1	1	1	1	1	1	1	1	1	1	1	1	1	1
	99.10	1	1	1	1	1	1	1	1	1	1	1	1	1	1	1	1
	99.30	1	1	1	1	1	1	1	1	1	1	1	1	1	1	1	1
	99.50	1	1	1	2	2	2	2	2	2	2	2	2	2	2	2	2
	99.70	2	2	2	3	3	3	3	3	3	3	3	3	3	3	3	3
	99.90	5	6	7	7	8	8	8	8	9	9	9	9	9	9	9	9
	99.91	5	6	7	8	9	9	9	9	9	9	10	10	10	10	10	10
	99.92	6	7	8	9	10	10	10	10	10	11	11	11	11	11	11	11
	99.93	7	8	9	10	11	11	12	12	12	12	12	12	12	12	12	12
	99.94	8	9	10	12	12	13	13	13	13	14	14	14	14	14	14	14
	99.95	9	11	12	14	15	15	15	16	16	16	16	16	16	16	17	17
	99.96	11	13	15	17	18	18	19	19	19	19	19	19	20	20	20	20
	99.97	14	17	19	21	22	23	23	24	24	24	24	24	24	25	25	25
	99.98	20	23	26	29	30	31	31	32	32	32	32	32	33	33	33	33
	99.99	33	37	41	44	46	47	48	48	48	48	49	49	49	49	50	50
	100.00	100	100	100	100	100	100	100	100	100	100	100	100	100	100	100	100

Table 7

PREDICTIVE VALUE OF POSITIVES (IN PERCENT)
PREVALENCE=   20 PER 100,000

		SENSITIVITY (%)															
		50	60	70	80	85	90	91	92	93	94	95	96	97	98	99	100
	50.00	0	0	0	0	0	0	0	0	0	0	0	0	0	0	0	0
	60.00	0	0	0	0	0	0	0	0	0	0	0	0	0	0	0	0
	70.00	0	0	0	0	0	0	0	0	0	0	0	0	0	0	0	0
SPECI-	80.00	0	0	0	0	0	0	0	0	0	0	0	0	0	0	0	0
FICITY	90.00	0	0	0	0	0	0	0	0	0	0	0	0	0	0	0	0
(%)	91.00	0	0	0	0	0	0	0	0	0	0	0	0	0	0	0	0
	93.00	0	0	0	0	0	0	0	0	0	0	0	0	0	0	0	0
	95.00	0	0	0	0	0	0	0	0	0	0	0	0	0	0	0	0
	97.00	0	0	0	1	1	1	1	1	1	1	1	1	1	1	1	1
	99.00	1	1	1	2	2	2	2	2	2	2	2	2	2	2	2	2
	99.10	1	1	2	2	2	2	2	2	2	2	2	2	2	2	2	2
	99.30	1	2	2	2	2	3	3	3	3	3	3	3	3	3	3	3
	99.50	2	2	3	3	3	3	4	4	4	4	4	4	4	4	4	4
	99.70	3	4	4	5	5	6	6	6	6	6	6	6	6	6	6	6
	99.90	9	11	12	14	15	15	15	16	16	16	16	16	16	16	17	17
	99.91	10	12	13	15	16	17	17	17	17	17	17	18	18	18	18	18
	99.92	11	13	15	17	18	18	19	19	19	19	19	19	20	20	20	20
	99.93	13	15	17	19	20	20	21	21	21	21	21	22	22	22	22	22
	99.94	14	17	19	21	22	23	23	23	24	24	24	24	24	25	25	25
	99.95	17	19	22	24	25	26	27	27	27	27	28	28	28	28	28	29
	99.96	20	23	26	29	30	31	31	32	32	32	32	32	33	33	33	33
	99.97	25	29	32	35	36	37	38	38	38	39	39	39	39	40	40	40
	99.98	33	37	41	44	46	47	48	48	48	48	49	49	49	49	50	50
	99.99	50	55	58	62	63	64	65	65	65	65	65	66	66	66	66	67
	100.00	100	100	100	100	100	100	100	100	100	100	100	100	100	100	100	100

170

Table 8

PREDICTIVE VALUE OF POSITIVES (IN PERCENT)
PREVALENCE= 30 PER 100,000

SPECI-FICITY (%)	SENSITIVITY (%)															
	50	60	70	80	85	90	91	92	93	94	95	96	97	98	99	100
50.00	0	0	0	0	0	0	0	0	0	0	0	0	0	0	0	0
60.00	0	C	0	0	0	0	0	0	0	0	0	0	0	0	0	0
70.00	0	0	0	0	0	0	0	0	0	0	0	0	0	0	C	0
80.00	0	0	0	0	0	0	0	0	0	0	0	0	0	0	0	0
90.00	0	0	0	0	0	0	0	0	0	0	0	0	0	0	C	0
91.00	0	0	0	0	0	0	0	0	0	0	0	0	0	0	0	0
93.00	C	0	0	0	0	0	0	0	0	0	0	0	0	0	0	0
95.00	0	0	0	0	1	1	1	1	1	1	1	1	1	1	1	1
97.00	0	1	1	1	1	1	1	1	1	1	1	1	1	1	1	1
99.00	1	2	2	2	2	3	3	3	3	3	3	3	3	3	3	3
99.10	2	2	2	3	3	3	3	3	3	3	3	3	3	3	3	3
99.30	2	3	3	3	4	4	4	4	4	4	4	4	4	4	4	4
99.50	3	3	4	5	5	5	5	5	5	5	5	5	6	6	6	6
99.70	5	6	7	7	8	8	8	8	9	9	9	9	9	9	9	9
99.90	13	15	17	19	20	21	21	22	22	22	22	22	23	23	23	23
99.91	14	17	19	21	22	23	23	23	24	24	24	24	24	25	25	25
99.92	16	18	21	23	24	25	25	26	26	26	26	26	27	27	27	27
99.93	18	20	23	26	27	28	28	28	29	29	29	29	29	30	30	30
99.94	20	23	26	29	30	31	31	32	32	32	32	32	33	33	33	33
99.95	23	26	30	32	34	35	35	36	36	36	36	36	37	37	37	38
99.96	27	31	34	38	39	40	41	41	41	41	42	42	42	42	43	43
99.97	33	37	41	44	46	47	48	48	48	48	49	49	49	49	50	50
99.98	43	47	51	55	56	57	58	58	58	59	59	59	59	60	60	60
99.99	60	64	68	71	72	73	73	73	74	74	74	74	74	75	75	75
100.00	100	100	100	100	100	100	100	100	100	100	100	100	100	100	100	100

Table 9

PREDICTIVE VALUE OF POSITIVES (IN PERCENT)
PREVALENCE= 40 PER 100,000

SPECI-FICITY (%)	SENSITIVITY (%)															
	50	60	70	80	85	90	91	92	93	94	95	96	97	98	99	100
50.00	0	0	0	0	0	0	0	0	0	0	0	0	0	0	0	0
60.00	C	0	0	0	0	0	0	0	0	0	0	0	0	0	0	0
70.00	0	0	0	0	0	0	0	0	0	0	0	0	0	0	0	0
80.00	0	0	0	0	0	0	0	0	0	0	0	0	0	0	0	0
90.00	0	0	0	0	0	0	C	0	0	0	0	0	0	0	0	0
91.00	0	0	0	0	0	0	0	0	0	0	0	0	0	0	0	0
93.00	0	0	0	0	0	1	1	1	1	1	1	1	1	1	1	1
95.00	0	0	1	1	1	1	1	1	1	1	1	1	1	1	1	1
97.00	1	1	1	1	1	1	1	1	1	1	1	1	1	1	1	1
99.00	2	2	3	3	3	3	4	4	4	4	4	4	4	4	4	4
99.10	2	3	3	3	4	4	4	4	4	4	4	4	4	4	4	4
99.30	3	3	4	4	5	5	5	5	5	5	5	5	5	5	5	5
99.50	4	5	5	6	6	7	7	7	7	7	7	7	7	7	7	7
99.70	6	7	9	10	10	11	11	11	11	11	11	11	11	12	12	12
99.90	17	19	22	24	25	26	27	27	27	27	28	28	28	28	28	29
99.91	18	21	24	26	27	29	29	29	29	29	30	30	30	30	31	31
99.92	20	23	26	29	30	31	31	32	32	32	32	32	33	33	33	33
99.93	22	26	29	31	33	34	34	34	35	35	35	35	36	36	36	36
99.94	25	29	32	35	36	38	38	38	38	39	39	39	39	40	40	40
99.95	29	32	36	39	40	42	42	42	43	43	43	43	44	44	44	44
99.96	33	38	41	44	46	47	48	48	48	48	49	49	49	49	50	50
99.97	40	44	48	52	53	55	55	55	55	56	56	56	56	57	57	57
99.98	50	55	58	62	63	64	65	65	65	65	66	66	66	66	66	67
99.99	67	71	74	76	77	78	78	79	79	79	79	79	79	80	80	80
100.00	100	100	100	100	100	100	100	100	100	100	100	100	100	100	100	100

Table 10

PREDICTIVE VALUE OF POSITIVES (IN PERCENT)
PREVALENCE=   50 PER 100,000

		SENSITIVITY (%)															
		50	60	70	80	85	90	91	92	93	94	95	96	97	98	99	100
	50.00	0	0	0	0	0	0	0	0	0	0	0	0	0	0	0	0
	60.00	0	0	0	0	0	0	0	0	0	0	0	0	0	0	0	0
	70.00	0	0	0	0	0	0	0	0	0	0	0	0	0	0	0	0
SPECI-	80.00	0	0	0	0	0	0	0	0	0	0	0	0	0	0	0	0
FICITY	90.00	0	0	0	0	0	0	0	0	0	0	0	0	0	0	0	0
(%)	91.00	0	0	0	0	0	0	1	1	1	1	1	1	1	1	1	1
	93.00	0	0	0	1	1	1	1	1	1	1	1	1	1	1	1	1
	95.00	0	1	1	1	1	1	1	1	1	1	1	1	1	1	1	1
	97.00	1	1	1	1	1	1	1	2	2	2	2	2	2	2	2	2
	99.00	2	3	3	4	4	4	4	4	4	4	5	5	5	5	5	5
	99.10	3	3	4	4	5	5	5	5	5	5	5	5	5	5	5	5
	99.30	3	4	5	5	6	6	6	6	6	6	6	6	6	7	7	7
	99.50	5	6	7	7	8	8	8	8	9	9	9	9	9	9	9	9
	99.70	8	9	10	12	12	13	13	13	13	14	14	14	14	14	14	14
	99.90	20	23	26	29	30	31	31	32	32	32	32	32	33	33	33	33
	99.91	22	25	28	31	32	33	34	34	34	34	35	35	35	35	35	36
	99.92	24	27	30	33	35	36	36	37	37	37	37	38	38	38	38	38
	99.93	26	30	33	36	38	39	39	40	40	40	40	41	41	41	41	42
	99.94	29	33	37	40	41	43	43	43	44	44	44	44	45	45	45	45
	99.95	33	38	41	44	46	47	48	48	48	48	49	49	49	50	50	50
	99.96	38	43	47	50	52	53	53	53	54	54	54	55	55	55	55	56
	99.97	45	50	54	57	59	60	60	61	61	61	62	62	62	62	62	63
	99.98	56	60	64	67	68	69	69	70	70	70	70	71	71	71	71	71
	99.99	71	75	78	80	81	82	82	82	82	82	83	83	83	83	83	83
	100.00	100	100	100	100	100	100	100	100	100	100	100	100	100	100	100	100

Table 11

PREDICTIVE VALUE OF POSITIVES (IN PERCENT)
PREVALENCE=   100 PER 100,000

		SENSITIVITY (%)															
		50	60	70	80	85	90	91	92	93	94	95	96	97	98	99	100
	50.00	0	0	0	0	0	0	0	0	0	0	0	0	0	0	0	0
	60.00	0	0	0	0	0	0	0	0	0	0	0	0	0	0	0	0
	70.00	0	0	0	0	0	0	0	0	0	0	0	0	0	0	0	0
SPECI-	80.00	0	0	0	0	0	0	0	0	0	0	0	0	0	0	0	0
FICITY	90.00	0	1	1	1	1	1	1	1	1	1	1	1	1	1	1	1
(%)	91.00	1	1	1	1	1	1	1	1	1	1	1	1	1	1	1	1
	93.00	1	1	1	1	1	1	1	1	1	1	1	1	1	1	1	1
	95.00	1	1	1	2	2	2	2	2	2	2	2	2	2	2	2	2
	97.00	2	2	2	3	3	3	3	3	3	3	3	3	3	3	3	3
	99.00	5	6	7	7	8	8	8	8	9	9	9	9	9	9	9	9
	99.10	5	6	7	8	9	9	9	9	9	9	10	10	10	10	10	10
	99.30	7	8	9	10	11	11	12	12	12	12	12	12	12	12	12	13
	99.50	9	11	12	14	15	15	15	16	16	16	16	16	16	16	17	17
	99.70	14	17	19	21	22	23	23	23	24	24	24	24	24	25	25	25
	99.90	33	38	41	44	46	47	48	48	48	48	49	49	49	50	50	50
	99.91	36	40	44	47	49	50	50	51	51	51	51	52	52	52	52	53
	99.92	38	43	47	50	52	53	53	54	54	54	54	55	55	55	55	56
	99.93	42	46	50	53	55	56	57	57	57	57	58	58	58	58	59	59
	99.94	45	50	54	57	59	60	60	61	61	61	61	62	62	62	62	63
	99.95	50	55	58	62	63	64	65	65	65	65	66	66	66	66	66	67
	99.96	56	60	64	67	68	69	69	70	70	70	70	71	71	71	71	71
	99.97	63	67	70	73	74	75	75	75	76	76	76	76	76	77	77	77
	99.98	71	75	78	80	81	82	82	82	82	82	83	83	83	83	83	83
	99.99	83	86	88	89	89	90	90	90	90	90	90	91	91	91	91	91
	100.00	100	100	100	100	100	100	100	100	100	100	100	100	100	100	100	100

Table 12

PREDICTIVE VALUE OF POSITIVES (IN PERCENT)
PREVALENCE= 200 PER 100,000

	SENSITIVITY (%)															
	50	60	70	80	85	90	91	92	93	94	95	96	97	98	99	100
50.00	0	0	0	0	0	0	0	0	0	0	0	0	0	0	0	0
60.00	0	0	0	0	0	0	0	0	0	0	0	0	0	0	0	0
70.00	0	0	0	1	1	1	1	1	1	1	1	1	1	1	1	1
SPECI- 80.00	0	1	1	1	1	1	1	1	1	1	1	1	1	1	1	1
FICITY 90.00	1	1	1	2	2	2	2	2	2	2	2	2	2	2	2	2
(%) 91.00	1	1	2	2	2	2	2	2	2	2	2	2	2	2	2	2
93.00	1	2	2	2	2	3	3	3	3	3	3	3	3	3	3	3
95.00	2	2	3	3	3	3	4	4	4	4	4	4	4	4	4	4
97.00	3	4	4	5	5	6	6	6	6	6	6	6	6	6	6	6
99.00	9	11	12	14	15	15	15	16	16	16	16	16	16	16	17	17
99.10	10	12	13	15	16	17	17	17	17	17	17	18	18	18	18	18
99.30	13	15	17	19	20	20	21	21	21	21	21	22	22	22	22	22
99.50	17	19	22	24	25	27	27	27	27	27	28	28	28	28	28	29
99.70	25	29	32	35	36	38	38	38	38	39	39	39	39	40	40	40
99.90	50	55	58	62	63	64	65	65	65	65	66	66	66	66	66	67
99.91	53	57	61	64	65	67	67	67	67	68	68	68	68	69	69	69
99.92	56	60	64	67	68	69	70	70	70	70	70	71	71	71	71	71
99.93	59	63	67	70	71	72	72	72	73	73	73	73	74	74	74	74
99.94	63	67	70	73	74	75	75	75	76	76	76	76	76	77	77	77
99.95	67	71	74	76	77	78	78	79	79	79	79	79	80	80	80	80
99.96	71	75	78	80	81	82	82	82	82	82	83	83	83	83	83	83
99.97	77	80	82	84	85	86	86	86	86	86	86	87	87	87	87	87
99.98	83	86	88	89	89	90	90	90	90	90	90	91	91	91	91	91
99.99	91	92	93	94	94	95	95	95	95	95	95	95	95	95	95	95
100.00	100	100	100	100	100	100	100	100	100	100	100	100	100	100	100	100

Table 13

PREDICTIVE VALUE OF POSITIVES (IN PERCENT)
PREVALENCE= 300 PER 100,000

	SENSITIVITY (%)															
	50	60	70	80	85	90	91	92	93	94	95	96	97	98	99	100
50.00	0	0	0	0	1	1	1	1	1	1	1	1	1	1	1	1
60.00	0	0	1	1	1	1	1	1	1	1	1	1	1	1	1	1
70.00	0	1	1	1	1	1	1	1	1	1	1	1	1	1	1	1
SPECI- 80.00	1	1	1	1	1	1	1	1	1	1	1	1	1	1	1	1
FICITY 90.00	1	2	2	2	2	3	3	3	3	3	3	3	3	3	3	3
(%) 91.00	2	2	2	3	3	3	3	3	3	3	3	3	3	3	3	3
93.00	2	3	3	3	4	4	4	4	4	4	4	4	4	4	4	4
95.00	3	3	4	5	5	5	5	5	5	5	5	5	6	6	6	6
97.00	5	6	7	7	8	8	8	8	9	9	9	9	9	9	9	9
99.00	13	15	17	19	20	21	21	22	22	22	22	22	23	23	23	23
99.10	14	17	19	21	22	23	23	24	24	24	24	24	24	25	25	25
99.30	18	21	23	26	27	28	28	28	29	29	29	29	29	30	30	30
99.50	23	27	30	32	34	35	35	36	36	36	36	37	37	37	37	38
99.70	33	38	41	45	46	47	48	48	48	49	49	49	49	50	50	50
99.90	60	64	68	71	72	73	73	73	74	74	74	74	74	75	75	75
99.91	63	67	70	73	74	75	75	75	76	76	76	76	76	77	77	77
99.92	65	69	72	75	76	77	77	78	78	78	78	78	78	79	79	79
99.93	68	72	75	77	79	79	80	80	80	80	80	80	81	81	81	81
99.94	71	75	78	80	81	82	82	82	82	82	83	83	83	83	83	83
99.95	75	78	81	83	84	84	85	85	85	85	85	85	85	86	86	86
99.96	79	82	84	86	86	87	87	87	87	88	88	88	88	88	88	88
99.97	83	86	88	89	89	90	90	90	90	90	90	91	91	91	91	91
99.98	88	90	91	92	93	93	93	93	93	93	93	94	94	94	94	94
99.99	94	95	95	96	96	96	96	97	97	97	97	97	97	97	97	97
100.00	100	100	100	100	100	100	100	100	100	100	100	100	100	100	100	100

Table 14

PREDICTIVE VALUE OF POSITIVES (IN PERCENT)
PREVALENCE= 400 PER 100,000

							SENSITIVITY (%)									
		50	60	70	80	85	90	91	92	93	94	95	96	97	98	99	100
	50.00	0	0	1	1	1	1	1	1	1	1	1	1	1	1	1	1
	60.00	0	1	1	1	1	1	1	1	1	1	1	1	1	1	1	1
	70.00	1	1	1	1	1	1	1	1	1	1	1	1	1	1	1	1
SPECI-	80.00	1	1	1	2	2	2	2	2	2	2	2	2	2	2	2	2
FICITY	90.00	2	2	3	3	3	3	4	4	4	4	4	4	4	4	4	4
(%)	91.00	2	3	3	3	4	4	4	4	4	4	4	4	4	4	4	4
	93.00	3	3	4	4	5	5	5	5	5	5	5	5	5	5	5	5
	95.00	4	5	5	6	6	7	7	7	7	7	7	7	7	7	7	7
	97.00	6	7	9	10	10	11	11	11	11	11	11	11	11	12	12	12
	99.00	17	19	22	24	25	27	27	27	27	27	28	28	28	28	28	29
	99.10	18	21	24	26	27	29	29	29	29	30	30	30	30	30	31	31
	99.30	22	26	29	31	33	34	34	35	35	35	35	36	36	36	36	36
	99.50	29	33	36	39	41	42	42	42	43	43	43	44	44	44	44	45
	99.70	40	45	48	52	53	55	55	55	55	56	56	56	56	57	57	57
	99.90	67	71	74	76	77	78	79	79	79	79	79	79	80	80	80	80
	99.91	69	73	76	78	79	80	80	80	81	81	81	81	81	81	82	82
	99.92	72	75	78	80	81	82	82	82	82	83	83	83	83	83	83	83
	99.93	74	77	80	82	83	84	84	84	84	84	85	85	85	85	85	85
	99.94	77	80	82	84	85	86	86	86	86	86	86	87	87	87	87	87
	99.95	80	83	85	87	87	88	88	88	88	88	88	89	89	89	89	89
	99.96	83	86	88	89	90	90	90	90	90	90	91	91	91	91	91	91
	99.97	87	89	90	91	92	92	92	92	93	93	93	93	93	93	93	93
	99.98	91	92	93	94	94	95	95	95	95	95	95	95	95	95	95	95
	99.99	95	96	97	97	97	97	97	97	97	97	97	97	97	98	98	98
	100.00	100	100	100	100	100	100	100	100	100	100	100	100	100	100	100	100

Table 15

PREDICTIVE VALUE OF POSITIVES (IN PERCENT)
PREVALENCE= 500 PER 100,000

							SENSITIVITY (%)									
		50	60	70	80	85	90	91	92	93	94	95	96	97	98	99	100
	50.00	1	1	1	1	1	1	1	1	1	1	1	1	1	1	1	1
	60.00	1	1	1	1	1	1	1	1	1	1	1	1	1	1	1	1
	70.00	1	1	1	1	1	1	2	2	2	2	2	2	2	2	2	2
SPECI-	80.00	1	1	2	2	2	2	2	2	2	2	2	2	2	2	2	2
FICITY	90.00	2	3	3	4	4	4	4	4	4	5	5	5	5	5	5	5
(%)	91.00	3	3	4	4	5	5	5	5	5	5	5	5	5	5	5	5
	93.00	3	4	5	5	6	6	6	6	6	6	6	6	7	7	7	7
	95.00	5	6	7	7	8	8	8	8	9	9	9	9	9	9	9	9
	97.00	8	9	10	12	12	13	13	13	13	14	14	14	14	14	14	14
	99.00	20	23	26	29	30	31	31	32	32	32	32	33	33	33	33	33
	99.10	22	25	28	31	32	33	34	34	34	34	35	35	35	35	36	36
	99.30	26	30	33	36	38	39	40	40	40	40	41	41	41	41	42	42
	99.50	33	38	41	45	46	47	48	48	48	49	49	49	49	50	50	50
	99.70	46	50	54	57	59	60	60	61	61	61	61	62	62	62	62	63
	99.90	72	75	78	80	81	82	82	82	82	83	83	83	83	83	83	83
	99.91	74	77	80	82	83	83	84	84	84	84	84	84	84	85	85	85
	99.92	76	79	81	83	84	85	85	85	85	86	86	86	86	86	86	86
	99.93	78	81	83	85	86	87	87	87	87	87	87	87	87	88	88	88
	99.94	81	83	85	87	88	88	88	89	89	89	89	89	89	89	89	89
	99.95	83	86	88	89	90	90	90	90	90	90	91	91	91	91	91	91
	99.96	86	88	90	91	91	92	92	92	92	92	92	92	92	92	93	93
	99.97	89	91	92	93	93	94	94	94	94	94	94	94	94	94	94	94
	99.98	93	94	95	95	96	96	96	96	96	96	96	96	96	96	96	96
	99.99	96	97	97	98	98	98	98	98	98	98	98	98	98	98	98	98
	100.00	100	100	100	100	100	100	100	100	100	100	100	100	100	100	100	100

Table 16

PREDICTIVE VALUE OF POSITIVES (IN PERCENT)
PREVALENCE= 1000 PER 100,000

		SENSITIVITY (%)															
		50	60	70	80	85	90	91	92	93	94	95	96	97	98	99	100
	50.00	1	1	1	2	2	2	2	2	2	2	2	2	2	2	2	2
	60.00	1	1	2	2	2	2	2	2	2	2	2	2	2	2	2	2
	70.00	2	2	2	3	3	3	3	3	3	3	3	3	3	3	3	3
SPECI-	80.00	2	3	3	4	4	4	4	4	4	5	5	5	5	5	5	5
FICITY	90.00	5	6	7	7	8	8	8	9	9	9	9	9	9	9	9	9
(%)	91.00	5	6	7	8	9	9	9	9	9	10	10	10	10	10	10	10
	93.00	7	8	9	10	11	11	12	12	12	12	12	12	12	12	13	13
	95.00	9	11	12	14	15	15	16	16	16	16	16	16	16	17	17	17
	97.00	14	17	19	21	22	23	23	24	24	24	24	24	25	25	25	25
	99.00	34	38	41	45	46	48	48	48	48	49	49	49	49	50	50	50
	99.10	36	40	44	47	49	50	51	51	51	51	52	52	52	52	53	53
	99.30	42	46	50	54	55	56	57	57	57	58	58	58	58	59	59	59
	99.50	50	55	59	62	63	65	65	65	65	66	66	66	66	66	67	67
	99.70	63	67	70	73	74	75	75	76	76	76	76	76	77	77	77	77
	99.90	83	86	88	89	90	90	90	90	90	90	91	91	91	91	91	91
	99.91	85	87	89	90	91	91	91	91	91	91	91	92	92	92	92	92
	99.92	86	88	90	91	91	92	92	92	92	92	92	92	92	93	93	93
	99.93	88	90	91	92	92	93	93	93	93	93	93	93	93	93	93	94
	99.94	89	91	92	93	93	94	94	94	94	94	94	94	94	94	94	94
	99.95	91	92	93	94	94	95	95	95	95	95	95	95	95	95	95	95
	99.96	93	94	95	95	96	96	96	96	96	96	96	96	96	96	96	96
	99.97	94	95	96	96	97	97	97	97	97	97	97	97	97	97	97	97
	99.98	96	97	97	98	98	98	98	98	98	98	98	98	98	98	98	98
	99.99	98	98	99	99	99	99	99	99	99	99	99	99	99	99	99	99
	100.00	100	100	100	100	100	100	100	100	100	100	100	100	100	100	100	100

Table 17

PREDICTIVE VALUE OF POSITIVES (IN PERCENT)
PREVALENCE= 2000 PER 100,000

		SENSITIVITY (%)															
		50	60	70	80	85	90	91	92	93	94	95	96	97	98	99	100
	50.00	2	2	3	3	3	4	4	4	4	4	4	4	4	4	4	4
	60.00	2	3	3	4	4	4	4	4	5	5	5	5	5	5	5	5
	70.00	3	4	5	5	5	6	6	6	6	6	6	6	6	6	6	6
SPECI-	80.00	5	6	7	8	8	8	8	9	9	9	9	9	9	9	9	9
FICITY	90.00	9	11	13	14	15	16	16	16	16	16	16	16	17	17	17	17
(%)	91.00	10	12	14	15	16	17	17	17	17	18	18	18	18	18	18	18
	93.00	13	15	17	19	20	21	21	21	21	22	22	22	22	22	22	23
	95.00	17	20	22	25	26	27	27	27	28	28	28	28	28	29	29	29
	97.00	25	29	32	35	37	38	38	38	39	39	39	40	40	40	40	40
	99.00	51	55	59	62	63	65	65	65	65	66	66	66	66	67	67	67
	99.10	53	58	61	64	66	67	67	68	68	68	68	69	69	69	69	69
	99.30	59	64	67	70	71	72	73	73	73	73	73	74	74	74	74	74
	99.50	67	71	74	77	78	79	79	79	79	79	79	80	80	80	80	80
	99.70	77	80	83	84	85	86	86	86	86	86	87	87	87	87	87	87
	99.90	91	92	93	94	95	95	95	95	95	95	95	95	95	95	95	95
	99.91	92	93	94	95	95	95	95	95	95	96	96	96	96	96	96	96
	99.92	93	94	95	95	96	96	96	96	96	96	96	96	96	96	96	96
	99.93	94	95	95	96	96	96	96	96	96	96	97	97	97	97	97	97
	99.94	94	95	96	96	97	97	97	97	97	97	97	97	97	97	97	97
	99.95	95	96	97	97	97	97	97	97	97	97	97	98	98	98	98	98
	99.96	96	97	97	98	98	98	98	98	98	98	98	98	98	98	98	98
	99.97	97	98	98	98	98	98	98	98	98	98	98	98	99	99	99	99
	99.98	98	98	99	99	99	99	99	99	99	99	99	99	99	99	99	99
	99.99	99	99	99	99	99	99	99	99	99	99	99	99	99	100	100	100
	100.00	100	100	100	100	100	100	100	100	100	100	100	100	100	100	100	100

Table 18

PREDICTIVE VALUE OF POSITIVES (IN PERCENT)
PREVALENCE= 3000 PER 100,000

		SENSITIVITY (%)														
		50	60	70	80	85	90	91	92	93	94	95	96	97	98	99	100
	50.00	3	4	4	5	5	5	5	5	5	5	6	6	6	6	6	6
	60.00	4	4	5	6	6	7	7	7	7	7	7	7	7	7	7	7
	70.00	5	6	7	8	8	8	9	9	9	9	9	9	9	9	9	9
SPECI-	80.00	7	8	10	11	12	12	12	12	13	13	13	13	13	13	13	13
FICITY	90.00	13	16	18	20	21	22	22	22	22	23	23	23	23	23	23	24
(%)	91.00	15	17	19	22	23	24	24	24	24	24	25	25	25	25	25	26
	93.00	18	21	24	26	27	28	29	29	29	29	30	30	30	30	30	31
	95.00	24	27	30	33	34	36	36	36	37	37	37	37	38	38	38	38
	97.00	34	38	42	45	47	48	48	49	49	49	49	50	50	50	51	51
	99.00	61	65	68	71	72	74	74	74	74	74	75	75	75	75	75	76
	99.10	63	67	71	73	74	76	76	76	76	76	77	77	77	77	77	77
	99.30	69	73	76	78	79	80	80	80	80	81	81	81	81	81	81	82
	99.50	76	79	81	83	84	85	85	85	85	85	85	86	86	86	86	86
	99.70	84	86	88	89	90	90	90	90	91	91	91	91	91	91	91	91
	99.90	94	95	96	96	96	97	97	97	97	97	97	97	97	97	97	97
	99.91	94	95	96	96	97	97	97	97	97	97	97	97	97	97	97	97
	99.92	95	96	96	97	97	97	97	97	97	97	97	97	97	97	97	97
	99.93	96	96	97	97	97	98	98	98	98	98	98	98	98	98	98	98
	99.94	96	97	97	98	98	98	98	98	98	98	98	98	98	98	98	98
	99.95	97	97	98	98	98	98	98	98	98	98	98	98	98	98	98	98
	99.96	97	98	98	98	99	99	99	99	99	99	99	99	99	99	99	99
	99.97	98	98	99	99	99	99	99	99	99	99	99	99	99	99	99	99
	99.98	99	99	99	99	99	99	99	99	99	99	99	99	99	99	99	99
	99.99	99	99	100	100	100	100	100	100	100	100	100	100	100	100	100	100
	100.00	100	100	100	100	100	100	100	100	100	100	100	100	100	100	100	100

Table 19

PREDICTIVE VALUE OF POSITIVES (IN PERCENT)
PREVALENCE= 4000 PER 100,000

		SENSITIVITY (%)														
		50	60	70	80	85	90	91	92	93	94	95	96	97	98	99	100
	50.00	4	5	6	6	7	7	7	7	7	7	7	7	7	8	8	8
	60.00	5	6	7	8	8	9	9	9	9	9	9	9	9	9	9	9
	70.00	6	8	9	10	11	11	11	11	11	12	12	12	12	12	12	12
SPECI-	80.00	9	11	13	14	15	16	16	16	16	16	17	17	17	17	17	17
FICITY	90.00	17	20	23	25	26	27	27	28	28	28	28	29	29	29	29	29
(%)	91.00	19	22	24	27	28	29	30	30	30	30	31	31	31	31	31	32
	93.00	23	26	29	32	34	35	35	35	36	36	36	36	37	37	37	37
	95.00	29	33	37	40	41	43	43	43	44	44	44	44	45	45	45	45
	97.00	41	45	49	53	54	56	56	56	57	57	57	57	58	58	58	58
	99.00	68	71	74	77	78	79	79	79	79	80	80	80	80	80	80	81
	99.10	70	74	76	79	80	81	81	81	81	81	81	82	82	82	82	82
	99.30	75	78	81	83	83	84	84	85	85	85	85	85	85	85	85	86
	99.50	81	83	85	87	88	88	88	88	89	89	89	89	89	89	89	89
	99.70	87	89	91	92	92	93	93	93	93	93	93	93	93	93	93	93
	99.90	95	96	97	97	97	97	97	97	97	98	98	98	98	98	98	98
	99.91	96	97	97	97	98	98	98	98	98	98	98	98	98	98	98	98
	99.92	96	97	97	98	98	98	98	98	98	98	98	98	98	98	98	98
	99.93	97	97	98	98	98	98	98	98	98	98	98	98	98	98	98	98
	99.94	97	98	98	98	98	98	98	98	98	98	99	99	99	99	99	99
	99.95	98	98	98	99	99	99	99	99	99	99	99	99	99	99	99	99
	99.96	98	98	99	99	99	99	99	99	99	99	99	99	99	99	99	99
	99.97	99	99	99	99	99	99	99	99	99	99	99	99	99	99	99	99
	99.98	99	99	99	99	99	99	99	99	99	99	99	100	100	100	100	100
	99.99	100	100	100	100	100	100	100	100	100	100	100	100	100	100	100	100
	100.00	100	100	100	100	100	100	100	100	100	100	100	100	100	100	100	100

Table 20

PREDICTIVE VALUE OF POSITIVES (IN PERCENT)
PREVALENCE= 5000 PER 100,000

SENSITIVITY (%)

SPECIFICITY (%)	50	60	70	80	85	90	91	92	93	94	95	96	97	98	99	100
50.00	5	6	7	8	8	9	9	9	9	9	9	9	9	9	9	10
60.00	6	7	8	10	10	11	11	11	11	11	11	11	11	11	12	12
70.00	8	10	11	12	13	14	14	14	14	14	14	15	15	15	15	15
80.00	12	14	16	17	18	19	19	19	20	20	20	20	20	21	21	21
90.00	21	24	27	30	31	32	32	33	33	33	33	34	34	34	34	34
91.00	23	26	29	32	33	34	35	35	35	35	36	36	36	36	37	37
93.00	27	31	34	38	39	40	41	41	41	41	42	42	42	42	43	43
95.00	34	39	42	46	47	49	49	49	49	50	50	50	51	51	51	51
97.00	47	51	55	58	60	61	61	62	62	62	63	63	63	63	63	64
99.00	72	76	79	81	82	83	83	83	83	83	83	83	84	84	84	84
99.10	75	78	80	82	83	84	84	84	84	85	85	85	85	85	85	85
99.30	79	82	84	86	86	87	87	87	87	88	88	88	88	88	88	88
99.50	84	86	88	89	90	90	91	91	91	91	91	91	91	91	91	91
99.70	90	91	92	93	94	94	94	94	94	94	94	94	94	95	95	95
99.90	96	97	97	98	98	98	98	98	98	98	98	98	98	98	98	98
99.91	97	97	98	98	98	98	98	98	98	98	98	98	98	98	98	98
99.92	97	98	98	98	98	98	98	98	98	98	98	98	98	98	98	99
99.93	97	98	98	98	98	99	99	99	99	99	99	99	99	99	99	99
99.94	98	98	98	99	99	99	99	99	99	99	99	99	99	99	99	99
99.95	98	98	99	99	99	99	99	99	99	99	99	99	99	99	99	99
99.96	99	99	99	99	99	99	99	99	99	99	99	99	99	99	99	99
99.97	99	99	99	99	99	99	99	99	99	99	99	99	99	99	99	99
99.98	99	99	99	100	100	100	100	100	100	100	100	100	100	100	100	100
99.99	100	100	100	100	100	100	100	100	100	100	100	100	100	100	100	100
100.00	100	100	100	100	100	100	100	100	100	100	100	100	100	100	100	100

Table 21

PREDICTIVE VALUE OF POSITIVES (IN PERCENT)
PREVALENCE=10000 PER 100,000

SENSITIVITY (%)

SPECIFICITY (%)	50	60	70	80	85	90	91	92	93	94	95	96	97	98	99	100
50.00	10	12	13	15	16	17	17	17	17	17	17	18	18	18	18	18
60.00	12	14	16	18	19	20	20	20	21	21	21	21	21	21	22	22
70.00	16	18	21	23	24	25	25	25	26	26	26	26	26	27	27	27
80.00	22	25	28	31	32	33	34	34	34	34	35	35	35	35	35	36
90.00	36	40	44	47	49	50	50	51	51	51	51	52	52	52	52	53
91.00	38	43	46	50	51	53	53	53	53	54	54	54	54	55	55	55
93.00	44	49	53	56	57	59	59	59	60	60	60	60	61	61	61	61
95.00	53	57	61	64	65	67	67	67	68	68	68	68	69	69	69	69
97.00	65	69	72	75	76	77	77	77	78	78	78	78	78	78	79	79
99.00	85	87	89	90	90	91	91	91	91	91	91	91	92	92	92	92
99.10	86	88	90	91	91	92	92	92	92	92	92	92	92	92	92	93
99.30	89	90	92	93	93	93	94	94	94	94	94	94	94	94	94	94
99.50	92	93	94	95	95	95	95	95	95	95	95	96	96	96	96	96
99.70	95	96	96	97	97	97	97	97	97	97	97	97	97	97	97	97
99.90	98	99	99	99	99	99	99	99	99	99	99	99	99	99	99	99
99.91	98	99	99	99	99	99	99	99	99	99	99	99	99	99	99	99
99.92	99	99	99	99	99	99	99	99	99	99	99	99	99	99	99	99
99.93	99	99	99	99	99	99	99	99	99	99	99	99	99	99	99	99
99.94	99	99	99	99	99	99	99	99	99	99	99	99	99	99	99	99
99.95	99	99	99	99	99	100	100	100	100	100	100	100	100	100	100	100
99.96	99	99	99	100	100	100	100	100	100	100	100	100	100	100	100	100
99.97	99	100	100	100	100	100	100	100	100	100	100	100	100	100	100	100
99.98	100	100	100	100	100	100	100	100	100	100	100	100	100	100	100	100
99.99	100	100	100	100	100	100	100	100	100	100	100	100	100	100	100	100
100.00	100	100	100	100	100	100	100	100	100	100	100	100	100	100	100	100

Table 22

PREDICTIVE VALUE OF POSITIVES (IN PERCENT)
PREVALENCE=15000 PER 100,000

					SENSITIVITY (%)											
		50	60	70	80	85	90	91	92	93	94	95	96	97	98	99	100
	50.00	15	17	20	22	23	24	24	25	25	25	25	25	26	26	26	26
	60.00	18	21	24	26	27	28	29	29	29	29	30	30	30	30	30	31
	70.00	23	26	29	32	33	35	35	35	35	36	36	36	36	37	37	37
SPECI-	80.00	31	35	38	41	43	44	45	45	45	45	46	46	46	46	47	47
FICITY	90.00	47	51	55	59	60	61	62	62	62	62	63	63	63	63	64	64
(%)	91.00	50	54	58	61	63	64	64	64	65	65	65	65	66	66	66	66
	93.00	56	60	64	67	68	69	70	70	70	70	71	71	71	71	71	72
	95.00	64	68	71	74	75	76	76	76	77	77	77	77	77	78	78	78
	97.00	75	78	80	82	83	84	84	84	85	85	85	85	85	85	85	85
	99.00	90	91	93	93	94	94	94	94	94	94	94	94	94	95	95	95
	99.10	91	92	93	94	94	95	95	95	95	95	95	95	95	95	95	95
	99.30	93	94	95	95	96	96	96	96	96	96	96	96	96	96	96	96
	99.50	95	95	96	97	97	97	97	97	97	97	97	97	97	97	97	97
	99.70	97	97	98	98	98	98	98	98	98	98	98	98	98	98	98	98
	99.90	99	99	99	99	99	99	99	99	99	99	99	99	99	99	99	99
	99.91	99	99	99	99	99	99	99	99	99	99	99	99	99	99	99	99
	99.92	99	99	99	99	99	99	100	100	100	100	100	100	100	100	100	100
	99.93	99	99	99	100	100	100	100	100	100	100	100	100	100	100	100	100
	99.94	99	99	100	100	100	100	100	100	100	100	100	100	100	100	100	100
	99.95	99	100	100	100	100	100	100	100	100	100	100	100	100	100	100	100
	99.96	100	100	100	100	100	100	100	100	100	100	100	100	100	100	100	100
	99.97	100	100	100	100	100	100	100	100	100	100	100	100	100	100	100	100
	99.98	100	100	100	100	100	100	100	100	100	100	100	100	100	100	100	100
	99.99	100	100	100	100	100	100	100	100	100	100	100	100	100	100	100	100
	100.00	100	100	100	100	100	100	100	100	100	100	100	100	100	100	100	100

Table 23

PREDICTIVE VALUE OF POSITIVES (IN PERCENT)
PREVALENCE=20000 PER 100,000

						SENSITIVITY (%)											
		50	60	70	80	85	90	91	92	93	94	95	96	97	98	99	100
	50.00	20	23	26	29	30	31	31	32	32	32	32	32	33	33	33	33
	60.00	24	27	30	33	35	36	36	37	37	37	37	38	38	38	38	38
	70.00	29	33	37	40	41	43	43	43	44	44	44	44	45	45	45	45
SPECI-	80.00	38	43	47	50	52	53	53	53	54	54	54	55	55	55	55	56
FICITY	90.00	56	60	64	67	68	69	69	70	70	70	70	71	71	71	71	71
(%)	91.00	58	63	66	69	70	71	72	72	72	72	73	73	73	73	73	74
	93.00	64	68	71	74	75	76	76	77	77	77	77	77	78	78	78	78
	95.00	71	75	78	80	81	82	82	82	82	82	83	83	83	83	83	83
	97.00	81	83	85	87	88	88	88	88	89	89	89	89	89	89	89	89
	99.00	93	94	95	95	96	96	96	96	96	96	96	96	96	96	96	96
	99.10	93	94	95	96	96	96	96	96	96	96	96	96	96	96	96	97
	99.30	95	96	96	97	97	97	97	97	97	97	97	97	97	97	97	97
	99.50	96	97	97	98	98	98	98	98	98	98	98	98	98	98	98	98
	99.70	98	98	98	99	99	99	99	99	99	99	99	99	99	99	99	99
	99.90	99	99	99	100	100	100	100	100	100	100	100	100	100	100	100	100
	99.91	99	99	99	100	100	100	100	100	100	100	100	100	100	100	100	100
	99.92	99	99	100	100	100	100	100	100	100	100	100	100	100	100	100	100
	99.93	99	100	100	100	100	100	100	100	100	100	100	100	100	100	100	100
	99.94	100	100	100	100	100	100	100	100	100	100	100	100	100	100	100	100
	99.95	100	100	100	100	100	100	100	100	100	100	100	100	100	100	100	100
	99.96	100	100	100	100	100	100	100	100	100	100	100	100	100	100	100	100
	99.97	100	100	100	100	100	100	100	100	100	100	100	100	100	100	100	100
	99.98	100	100	100	100	100	100	100	100	100	100	100	100	100	100	100	100
	99.99	100	100	100	100	100	100	100	100	100	100	100	100	100	100	100	100
	100.00	100	100	100	100	100	100	100	100	100	100	100	100	100	100	100	100

Table 24

PREDICTIVE VALUE OF POSITIVES (IN PERCENT)
PREVALENCE=25000 PER 100,000

		SENSITIVITY (%)

		50	60	70	80	85	90	91	92	93	94	95	96	97	98	99	100
	50.00	25	29	32	35	36	37	38	38	38	39	39	39	39	40	40	40
	60.00	29	33	37	40	41	43	43	43	44	44	44	44	45	45	45	45
	70.00	36	40	44	47	49	50	50	51	51	51	51	52	52	52	52	53
SPECI-	80.00	45	50	54	57	59	60	60	61	61	61	61	62	62	62	62	62
FICITY	90.00	63	67	70	73	74	75	75	75	76	76	76	76	76	77	77	77
(%)	91.00	65	69	72	75	76	77	77	77	77	78	78	78	78	78	79	79
	93.00	70	74	77	79	80	81	81	81	82	82	82	82	82	82	82	83
	95.00	77	80	82	84	85	86	86	86	86	86	86	86	87	87	87	87
	97.00	85	87	89	90	90	91	91	91	91	91	91	91	92	92	92	92
	99.00	94	95	96	96	97	97	97	97	97	97	97	97	97	97	97	97
	99.10	95	96	96	97	97	97	97	97	97	97	97	97	97	97	97	97
	99.30	96	97	97	97	98	98	98	98	98	98	98	98	98	98	98	98
	99.50	97	98	98	98	98	98	98	98	98	98	98	98	98	98	99	99
	99.70	98	99	99	99	99	99	99	99	99	99	99	99	99	99	99	99
	99.90	99	100	100	100	100	100	100	100	100	100	100	100	100	100	100	100
	99.91	99	100	100	100	100	100	100	100	100	100	100	100	100	100	100	100
	99.92	100	100	100	100	100	100	100	100	100	100	100	100	100	100	100	100
	99.93	100	100	100	100	100	100	100	100	100	100	100	100	100	100	100	100
	99.94	100	100	100	100	100	100	100	100	100	100	100	100	100	100	100	100
	99.95	100	100	100	100	100	100	100	100	100	100	100	100	100	100	100	100
	99.96	100	100	100	100	100	100	100	100	100	100	100	100	100	100	100	100
	99.97	100	100	100	100	100	100	100	100	100	100	100	100	100	100	100	100
	99.98	100	100	100	100	100	100	100	100	100	100	100	100	100	100	100	100
	99.99	100	100	100	100	100	100	100	100	100	100	100	100	100	100	100	100
	100.00	100	100	100	100	100	100	100	100	100	100	100	100	100	100	100	100

Table 25

PREDICTIVE VALUE OF POSITIVES (IN PERCENT)
PREVALENCE=50000 PER 100,000

SENSITIVITY (%)

		50	60	70	80	85	90	91	92	93	94	95	96	97	98	99	100
	50.00	50	55	58	62	63	64	65	65	65	65	66	66	66	66	66	67
	60.00	56	60	64	67	68	69	69	70	70	70	70	71	71	71	71	71
	70.00	62	67	70	73	74	75	75	75	76	76	76	76	77	77	77	77
SPECI-	80.00	71	75	78	80	81	82	82	82	82	82	83	83	83	83	83	83
FICITY	90.00	83	86	88	89	89	90	90	90	90	90	90	91	91	91	91	91
(%)	91.00	85	87	89	90	90	91	91	91	91	91	91	91	92	92	92	92
	93.00	88	90	91	92	92	93	93	93	93	93	93	93	93	93	93	93
	95.00	91	92	93	94	94	95	95	95	95	95	95	95	95	95	95	95
	97.00	94	95	96	96	97	97	97	97	97	97	97	97	97	97	97	97
	99.00	98	98	99	99	99	99	99	99	99	99	99	99	99	99	99	99
	99.10	98	99	99	99	99	99	99	99	99	99	99	99	99	99	99	99
	99.30	99	99	99	99	99	99	99	99	99	99	99	99	99	99	99	99
	99.50	99	99	99	99	99	99	99	99	99	99	99	99	99	99	99	100
	99.70	99	100	100	100	100	100	100	100	100	100	100	100	100	100	100	100
	99.90	100	100	100	100	100	100	100	100	100	100	100	100	100	100	100	100
	99.91	100	100	100	100	100	100	100	100	100	100	100	100	100	100	100	100
	99.92	100	100	100	100	100	100	100	100	100	100	100	100	100	100	100	100
	99.93	100	100	100	100	100	100	100	100	100	100	100	100	100	100	100	100
	99.94	100	100	100	100	100	100	100	100	100	100	100	100	100	100	100	100
	99.95	100	100	100	100	100	100	100	100	100	100	100	100	100	100	100	100
	99.96	100	100	100	100	100	100	100	100	100	100	100	100	100	100	100	100
	99.97	100	100	100	100	100	100	100	100	100	100	100	100	100	100	100	100
	99.98	100	100	100	100	100	100	100	100	100	100	100	100	100	100	100	100
	99.99	100	100	100	100	100	100	100	100	100	100	100	100	100	100	100	100
	100.00	100	100	100	100	100	100	100	100	100	100	100	100	100	100	100	100

Table 26

PREDICTIVE VALUE OF POSITIVES (IN PERCENT)
SENSITIVITY= 50%

		SPECIFICITY (%)							(CONTINUED)	
		50.00	60.00	70.00	80.00	90.00	91.00	93.00	95.00	97.00	99.00
	1	0	0	0	0	0	0	0	0	0	0
	2	0	0	0	0	0	0	0	0	0	0
	3	0	0	0	0	0	0	0	0	0	0
PREVA-	4	0	0	0	0	0	0	0	0	0	0
LENCE	5	0	0	0	0	0	0	0	0	0	0
PER	10	0	0	0	0	0	0	0	0	0	0
100,000	20	0	0	0	0	0	0	0	0	0	1
	30	0	0	0	0	0	0	0	0	0	1
	40	0	0	0	0	0	0	0	0	1	2
	50	0	0	0	0	0	0	0	0	1	2
	100	0	0	0	0	0	1	1	1	2	5
	200	0	0	0	0	1	1	1	2	3	9
	300	0	0	0	1	1	2	2	3	5	13
	400	0	0	1	1	2	2	3	4	6	17
	500	1	1	1	1	2	3	3	5	8	20
	1000	1	1	2	2	5	5	7	9	14	34
	2000	2	2	3	5	9	10	13	17	25	51
	3000	3	4	5	7	13	15	18	24	34	61
	4000	4	5	6	9	17	19	23	29	41	68
	5000	5	6	8	12	21	23	27	34	47	72
	10000	10	12	16	22	36	38	44	53	65	85
	15000	15	18	23	31	47	50	56	64	75	90
	20000	20	24	29	38	56	58	64	71	81	93
	25000	25	29	36	45	63	65	70	77	85	94
	50000	50	56	62	71	83	85	88	91	94	98

Table 27

PREDICTIVE VALUE OF POSITIVES (IN PERCENT)
SENSITIVITY= 50%

		SPECIFICITY (%)									
		99.10	99.30	99.50	99.70	99.90	99.91	99.93	99.95	99.97	99.99	100.00
	1	0	0	0	0	0	1	1	1	2	5	100
	2	0	0	0	0	1	1	1	2	3	9	100
	3	0	0	0	0	1	2	2	3	5	13	100
PREVA-	4	0	0	0	1	2	2	3	4	6	17	100
LENCE	5	0	0	0	1	2	3	3	5	8	20	100
PER	10	1	1	1	2	5	5	7	9	14	33	100
100,000	20	1	1	2	3	9	10	13	17	25	50	100
	30	2	2	3	5	13	14	18	23	33	60	100
	40	2	3	4	6	17	18	22	29	40	67	100
	50	3	3	5	8	20	22	26	33	45	71	100
	100	5	7	9	14	33	36	42	50	63	83	100
	200	10	13	17	25	50	53	59	67	77	91	100
	300	14	18	23	33	60	63	68	75	83	94	100
	400	18	22	29	40	67	69	74	80	87	95	100
	500	22	26	33	46	72	74	78	83	89	96	100
	1000	36	42	50	63	83	85	88	91	94	98	100
	2000	53	59	67	77	91	92	94	95	97	99	100
	3000	63	69	76	84	94	94	96	97	98	99	100
	4000	70	75	81	87	95	96	97	98	99	100	100
	5000	75	79	84	90	96	97	97	98	99	100	100
	10000	86	89	92	95	98	98	99	99	99	100	100
	15000	91	93	95	97	99	99	99	99	100	100	100
	20000	93	95	96	98	99	99	99	100	100	100	100
	25000	95	96	97	98	99	99	100	100	100	100	100
	50000	98	99	99	99	100	100	100	100	100	100	100

Table 28

PREDICTIVE VALUE OF POSITIVES (IN PERCENT)
SENSITIVITY= 60%

SPECIFICITY (%)   (CONTINUED)

		50.00	60.00	70.00	80.00	90.00	91.00	93.00	95.00	97.00	99.00
PREVA-LENCE	1	0	0	0	0	0	0	0	0	0	0
	2	0	0	0	0	0	0	0	0	0	0
	3	0	0	0	0	0	0	0	0	0	0
	4	0	0	0	0	0	0	0	0	0	0
	5	0	0	0	0	0	0	0	0	0	0
PER 100,000	10	0	0	0	0	0	0	0	0	0	1
	20	0	0	0	0	0	0	0	0	0	1
	30	0	0	0	0	0	0	0	0	1	2
	40	0	0	0	0	0	0	0	0	1	2
	50	0	0	0	0	0	0	0	1	1	3
	100	0	0	0	0	1	1	1	1	2	6
	200	0	0	0	1	1	1	2	2	4	11
	300	0	0	1	1	2	2	3	3	6	15
	400	0	1	1	1	2	3	3	5	7	19
	500	1	1	1	1	3	3	4	6	9	23
	1000	1	1	2	3	6	6	8	11	17	38
	2000	2	3	4	6	11	12	15	20	29	55
	3000	4	4	6	8	16	17	21	27	38	65
	4000	5	6	8	11	20	22	26	33	45	71
	5000	6	7	10	14	24	26	31	39	51	76
	10000	12	14	18	25	4(	43	49	57	69	87
	15000	17	21	26	35	51	54	60	68	78	91
	20000	23	27	33	43	60	63	68	75	83	94
	25000	29	33	40	50	67	69	74	80	87	95
	50000	55	60	67	75	86	87	90	92	95	98

Table 29

PREDICTIVE VALUE OF POSITIVES (IN PERCENT)
SENSITIVITY= 60%

SPECIFICITY (%)

		99.10	99.30	99.50	99.70	99.90	99.91	99.93	99.95	99.97	99.99	100.00
PREVA-LENCE	1	0	0	0	0	1	1	1	1	2	6	100
	2	0	0	0	0	1	1	2	2	4	11	100
	3	0	0	0	1	2	2	3	3	6	15	100
	4	0	0	0	1	2	3	3	5	7	19	100
	5	0	0	1	1	3	3	4	6	9	23	100
PER 100,000	10	1	1	1	2	6	6	8	11	17	37	100
	20	1	2	2	4	11	12	15	19	29	55	100
	30	2	3	3	6	15	17	20	26	37	64	100
	40	3	3	5	7	19	21	26	32	44	71	100
	50	3	4	6	9	23	25	30	38	50	75	100
	100	6	8	11	17	38	40	46	55	67	86	100
	200	12	15	19	29	55	57	63	71	80	92	100
	300	17	21	27	38	64	67	72	78	86	95	100
	400	21	26	33	45	71	73	77	83	89	96	100
	500	25	30	38	50	75	77	81	86	91	97	100
	1000	40	46	55	67	86	87	90	92	95	98	100
	2000	58	64	71	80	92	93	95	96	98	99	100
	3000	67	73	79	86	95	95	96	97	98	99	100
	4000	74	78	83	89	96	97	97	98	99	100	100
	5000	78	82	86	91	97	97	98	98	99	100	100
	10000	88	90	93	96	99	99	99	99	100	100	100
	15000	92	94	95	97	99	99	99	100	100	100	100
	20000	94	96	97	98	99	99	100	100	100	100	100
	25000	96	97	98	99	100	100	100	100	100	100	100
	50000	99	99	99	100	100	100	100	100	100	100	100

Table 30

PREDICTIVE VALUE OF POSITIVES (IN PERCENT)
SENSITIVITY= 70%

SPECIFICITY (%) (CONTINUED)

		50.00	60.00	70.00	80.00	90.00	91.00	93.00	95.00	97.00	99.00
PREVA-LENCE	1	0	0	0	0	0	0	0	0	0	0
	2	0	0	0	0	0	0	0	0	0	0
	3	0	0	0	0	0	0	0	0	0	0
	4	0	0	0	0	0	0	0	0	0	0
	5	0	0	0	0	0	0	0	0	0	0
PER 100,000	10	0	0	0	0	0	0	0	0	0	1
	20	0	0	0	0	0	0	0	0	0	1
	30	0	0	0	0	0	0	0	0	1	2
	40	0	0	0	0	0	0	0	1	1	3
	50	0	0	0	0	0	0	0	1	1	3
	100	0	0	0	0	1	1	1	1	2	7
	200	0	0	0	1	1	2	2	3	4	12
	300	0	1	1	1	2	2	3	4	7	17
	400	1	1	1	1	3	3	4	5	9	22
	500	1	1	1	2	3	4	5	7	10	26
	1000	1	2	2	3	7	7	9	12	19	41
	2000	3	3	5	7	13	14	17	22	32	59
	3000	4	5	7	10	18	19	24	30	42	68
	4000	6	7	9	13	23	24	29	37	49	74
	5000	7	8	11	16	27	29	34	42	55	79
	10000	13	16	21	28	44	46	53	61	72	89
	15000	20	24	29	38	55	58	64	71	80	93
	20000	26	30	37	47	64	66	71	78	85	95
	25000	32	37	44	54	70	72	77	82	89	96
	50000	58	64	70	78	88	89	91	93	96	99

Table 31

PREDICTIVE VALUE OF POSITIVES (IN PERCENT)
SENSITIVITY= 70%

SPECIFICITY (%)

		99.10	99.30	99.50	99.70	99.90	99.91	99.93	99.95	99.97	99.99	100.00
PREVA-LENCE	1	0	0	0	0	1	1	1	1	2	7	100
	2	0	0	0	0	1	2	2	3	4	12	100
	3	0	0	0	1	2	2	3	4	7	17	100
	4	0	0	1	1	3	3	4	5	9	22	100
	5	0	0	1	1	3	4	5	7	10	26	100
PER 100,000	10	1	1	1	2	7	7	9	12	19	41	100
	20	2	2	3	4	12	13	17	22	32	58	100
	30	2	3	4	7	17	19	23	30	41	68	100
	40	3	4	5	9	22	24	29	36	48	74	100
	50	4	5	7	10	26	28	33	41	54	78	100
	100	7	9	12	19	41	44	50	58	70	88	100
	200	13	17	22	32	58	61	67	74	82	93	100
	300	19	23	30	41	68	70	75	81	88	95	100
	400	24	29	36	48	74	76	80	85	90	97	100
	500	28	33	41	54	78	80	83	88	92	97	100
	1000	44	50	59	70	88	89	91	93	96	99	100
	2000	61	67	74	83	93	94	95	97	98	99	100
	3000	71	76	81	88	96	96	97	98	99	100	100
	4000	76	81	85	91	97	97	98	98	99	100	100
	5000	80	84	88	92	97	98	98	99	99	100	100
	10000	90	92	94	96	99	99	99	99	100	100	100
	15000	93	95	96	98	99	99	99	100	100	100	100
	20000	95	96	97	98	99	99	100	100	100	100	100
	25000	96	97	98	99	100	100	100	100	100	100	100
	50000	99	99	99	100	100	100	100	100	100	100	100

Table 32

PREDICTIVE VALUE OF POSITIVES (IN PERCENT)
SENSITIVITY= 80%

SPECIFICITY (%) (CONTINUED)

		50.00	60.00	70.00	80.00	90.00	91.00	93.00	95.00	97.00	99.00
PREVA-LENCE	1	0	0	0	0	0	0	0	0	0	0
	2	0	0	0	0	0	0	0	0	0	0
	3	0	0	0	0	0	0	0	0	0	0
	4	0	0	0	0	0	0	0	0	0	0
	5	0	0	0	0	0	0	0	0	0	0
PER 100,000	10	0	0	0	0	0	0	0	0	0	1
	20	0	0	0	0	0	0	0	0	1	2
	30	0	0	0	0	0	0	0	0	1	2
	40	0	0	0	0	0	0	0	1	1	3
	50	0	0	0	0	0	0	1	1	1	4
	100	0	0	0	0	1	1	1	2	3	7
	200	0	0	1	1	2	2	2	3	5	14
	300	0	1	1	1	2	3	3	5	7	19
	400	1	1	1	2	3	3	4	6	10	24
	500	1	1	1	2	4	4	5	7	12	29
	1000	2	2	3	4	7	8	10	14	21	45
	2000	3	4	5	8	14	15	19	25	35	62
	3000	5	6	8	11	20	22	26	33	45	71
	4000	6	8	10	14	25	27	32	40	53	77
	5000	8	10	12	17	30	32	38	46	58	81
	10000	15	18	23	31	47	50	56	64	75	90
	15000	22	26	32	41	59	61	67	74	82	93
	20000	29	33	40	50	67	69	74	80	87	95
	25000	35	40	47	57	73	75	79	84	90	96
	50000	62	67	73	80	89	90	92	94	96	99

Table 33

PREDICTIVE VALUE OF POSITIVES (IN PERCENT)
SENSITIVITY= 80%

SPECIFICITY (%)

		99.10	99.30	99.50	99.70	99.90	99.91	99.93	99.95	99.97	99.99	100.00
PREVA-LENCE	1	0	0	0	0	1	1	1	2	3	7	100
	2	0	0	0	1	2	2	2	3	5	14	100
	3	0	0	0	1	2	3	3	5	7	19	100
	4	0	0	1	1	3	3	4	6	10	24	100
	5	0	1	1	1	4	4	5	7	12	29	100
PER 100,000	10	1	1	2	3	7	8	10	14	21	44	100
	20	2	2	3	5	14	15	19	24	35	62	100
	30	3	3	5	7	19	21	26	32	44	71	100
	40	3	4	6	10	24	26	31	39	52	76	100
	50	4	5	7	12	29	31	36	44	57	80	100
	100	8	10	14	21	44	47	53	62	73	89	100
	200	15	19	24	35	62	64	70	76	84	94	100
	300	21	26	32	45	71	73	77	83	89	96	100
	400	26	31	39	52	76	78	82	87	91	97	100
	500	31	36	45	57	80	82	85	89	93	98	100
	1000	47	54	62	73	89	90	92	94	96	99	100
	2000	64	7C	77	84	94	95	96	97	98	99	100
	3000	73	78	83	89	96	96	97	98	99	100	100
	4000	79	83	87	92	97	97	98	99	99	100	100
	5000	82	86	89	93	98	98	98	99	99	100	100
	10000	91	93	95	97	99	99	99	99	100	100	100
	15000	94	95	97	98	99	99	100	100	100	100	100
	20000	96	97	98	99	100	100	100	100	100	100	100
	25000	97	97	98	99	100	100	100	100	100	100	100
	50000	99	99	99	100	100	100	100	100	100	100	100

Table 34

PREDICTIVE VALUE OF POSITIVES (IN PERCENT)
SENSITIVITY= 85%

SPECIFICITY (%)   (CONTINUED)

PREVALENCE PER 100,000	50.00	60.00	70.00	80.00	90.00	91.00	93.00	95.00	97.00	99.00
1	0	0	0	0	0	0	0	0	0	0
2	0	0	0	0	0	0	0	0	0	0
3	0	0	0	0	0	0	0	0	0	0
4	0	0	0	0	0	0	0	0	0	0
5	0	0	0	0	0	0	0	0	0	0
10	0	0	0	0	0	0	0	0	0	1
20	0	0	0	0	0	0	0	0	1	2
30	0	0	0	0	0	0	0	1	1	2
40	0	0	0	0	0	0	0	1	1	3
50	0	0	0	0	0	0	1	1	1	4
100	0	0	0	0	1	1	1	2	3	8
200	0	0	1	1	2	2	2	3	5	15
300	1	1	1	1	2	3	4	5	8	20
400	1	1	1	2	3	4	5	6	10	25
500	1	1	1	2	4	5	6	8	12	30
1000	2	2	3	4	8	9	11	15	22	46
2000	3	4	5	8	15	16	20	26	37	63
3000	5	6	8	12	21	23	27	34	47	72
4000	7	8	11	15	26	28	34	41	54	78
5000	8	10	13	18	31	33	39	47	60	82
10000	16	19	24	32	49	51	57	65	76	90
15000	23	27	33	43	60	63	68	75	83	94
20000	30	35	41	52	68	70	75	81	88	96
25000	36	41	49	59	74	76	80	85	90	97
50000	63	68	74	81	89	90	92	94	97	99

Table 35

PREDICTIVE VALUE OF POSITIVES (IN PERCENT)
SENSITIVITY= 85%

SPECIFICITY (%)

PREVALENCE PER 100,000	99.10	99.30	99.50	99.70	99.90	99.91	99.93	99.95	99.97	99.99	100.00
1	0	0	0	0	1	1	1	2	3	8	100
2	0	0	0	1	2	2	2	3	5	15	100
3	0	0	1	1	2	3	4	5	8	20	100
4	0	0	1	1	3	4	5	6	10	25	100
5	0	1	1	1	4	5	6	8	12	30	100
10	1	1	2	3	8	9	11	15	22	46	100
20	2	2	3	5	15	16	20	25	36	63	100
30	3	4	5	8	20	22	27	34	46	72	100
40	4	5	6	10	25	27	33	40	53	77	100
50	5	6	8	12	30	32	38	46	59	81	100
100	9	11	15	22	46	49	55	63	74	89	100
200	16	20	25	36	63	65	71	77	85	94	100
300	22	27	34	46	72	74	79	84	89	96	100
400	27	33	41	53	77	79	83	87	92	97	100
500	32	38	46	59	81	83	86	90	93	98	100
1000	49	55	63	74	90	91	92	94	97	99	100
2000	66	71	78	85	95	95	96	97	98	99	100
3000	74	79	84	90	96	97	97	98	99	100	100
4000	80	83	88	92	97	98	98	99	99	100	100
5000	83	86	90	94	98	98	98	99	99	100	100
10000	91	93	95	97	99	99	99	99	100	100	100
15000	94	96	97	98	99	99	100	100	100	100	100
20000	96	97	98	99	100	100	100	100	100	100	100
25000	97	98	98	99	100	100	100	100	100	100	100
50000	99	99	99	100	100	100	100	100	100	100	100

Table 36

PREDICTIVE VALUE OF POSITIVES (IN PERCENT)
SENSITIVITY= 90%

					SPECIFICITY (%)				(CONTINUED)	
		50.00	60.00	70.00	80.00	90.00	91.00	93.00	95.00	97.00	99.00
PREVA-LENCE	1	0	0	0	0	0	0	0	0	0	0
	2	0	0	0	0	0	0	0	0	0	0
	3	0	0	0	0	0	0	0	0	0	0
	4	0	0	0	0	0	0	0	0	0	0
	5	0	0	0	0	0	0	0	0	0	0
PER 100,000	10	0	0	0	0	0	0	0	0	0	1
	20	0	0	0	0	0	0	0	0	1	2
	30	0	0	0	0	0	0	0	1	1	3
	40	0	0	0	0	0	0	1	1	1	3
	50	0	0	0	0	0	0	1	1	1	4
	100	0	0	0	0	1	1	1	2	3	8
	200	0	0	1	1	2	2	3	3	6	15
	300	1	1	1	1	3	3	4	5	8	21
	400	1	1	1	2	3	4	5	7	11	27
	500	1	1	1	2	4	5	6	8	13	31
	1000	2	2	3	4	8	9	11	15	23	48
	2000	4	4	6	8	16	17	21	27	38	65
	3000	5	7	8	12	22	24	28	36	48	74
	4000	7	9	11	16	27	29	35	43	56	79
	5000	9	11	14	19	32	34	40	49	61	83
	10000	17	20	25	33	50	53	59	67	77	91
	15000	24	28	35	44	61	64	69	76	84	94
	20000	31	36	43	53	69	71	76	82	88	96
	25000	37	43	50	60	75	77	81.	86	91	97
	50000	64	69	75	82	90	91	93	95	97	99

Table 37

PREDICTIVE VALUE OF POSITIVES (IN PERCENT)
SENSITIVITY= 90%

					SPECIFICITY (%)						
		99.10	99.30	99.50	99.70	99.90	99.91	99.93	99.95	99.97	99.99	100.00
PREVA-LENCE	1	0	0	0	0	1	1	1	2	3	8	100
	2	0	0	0	1	2	2	3	3	6	15	100
	3	0	0	1	1	3	3	4	5	8	21	100
	4	0	1	1	1	3	4	5	7	11	26	100
	5	0	1	1	1	4	5	6	8	13	31	100
PER 100,000	10	1	1	2	3	8	9	11	15	23	47	100
	20	2	3	3	6	15	17	20	26	37	64	100
	30	3	4	5	8	21	23	28	35	47	73	100
	40	4	5	7	11	26	29	34	42	55	78	100
	50	5	6	8	13	31	33	39	47	60	82	100
	100	9	11	15	23	47	50	56	64	75	90	100
	200	17	20	27	38	64	67	72	78	86	95	100
	300	23	28	35	47	73	75	79	84	90	96	100
	400	29	34	42	55	78	80	84	88	92	97	100
	500	33	39	47	60	82	83	87	90	94	98	100
	1000	50	56	65	75	90	91	93	95	97	99	100
	2000	67	72	79	86	95	95	96	97	98	99	100
	3000	76	80	85	90	97	97	98	98	99	100	100
	4000	81	84	88	93	97	98	98	99	99	100	100
	5000	84	87	90	94	98	98	99	99	99	100	100
	10000	92	93	95	97	99	99	99	100	100	100	100
	15000	95	96	97	98	99	99	100	100	100	100	100
	20000	96	97	98	99	100	100	100	100	100	100	100
	25000	97	98	98	99	100	100	100	100	100	100	100
	50000	99	99	99	100	100	100	100	100	100	100	100

185

Table 38

PREDICTIVE VALUE OF POSITIVES (IN PERCENT)
SENSITIVITY= 91%

SPECIFICITY (%)　　　　(CONTINUED)

		50.00	60.00	70.00	80.00	90.00	91.00	93.00	95.00	97.00	99.00
PREVA-LENCE	1	0	0	0	0	0	0	0	0	0	0
	2	0	0	0	0	0	0	0	0	0	0
	3	0	0	0	0	0	0	0	0	0	0
	4	0	0	0	0	0	0	0	0	0	0
	5	0	0	0	0	0	0	0	0	0	0
PER 100,000	10	0	0	0	0	0	0	0	0	0	1
	20	0	0	0	0	0	0	0	0	1	2
	30	0	0	0	0	0	0	0	1	1	3
	40	0	0	0	0	0	0	1	1	1	4
	50	0	0	0	0	0	1	1	1	1	4
	100	0	0	0	0	1	1	1	2	3	8
	200	0	0	1	1	2	2	3	4	6	15
	300	1	1	1	1	3	3	4	5	8	21
	400	1	1	1	2	4	4	5	7	11	27
	500	1	1	2	2	4	5	6	8	13	31
	1000	2	2	3	4	8	9	12	16	23	48
	2000	4	4	6	8	16	17	21	27	38	65
	3000	5	7	9	12	22	24	29	36	48	74
	4000	7	9	11	16	27	30	35	43	56	79
	5000	9	11	14	19	32	35	41	49	61	83
	10000	17	20	25	34	50	53	59	67	77	91
	15000	24	29	35	45	62	64	70	76	84	94
	20000	31	36	43	53	69	72	76	82	88	96
	25000	38	43	50	60	75	77	81	86	91	97
	50000	65	69	75	82	90	91	93	95	97	99

Table 39

PREDICTIVE VALUE OF POSITIVES (IN PERCENT)
SENSITIVITY= 91%

SPECIFICITY (%)

		99.10	99.30	99.50	99.70	99.90	99.91	99.93	99.95	99.97	99.99	100.00
PREVA-LENCE	1	0	0	0	0	1	1	1	2	3	8	100
	2	0	0	0	1	2	2	3	4	6	15	100
	3	0	0	1	1	3	3	4	5	8	21	100
	4	0	1	1	1	4	4	5	7	11	27	100
	5	1	1	1	1	4	5	6	8	13	31	100
PER 100,000	10	1	1	2	3	8	9	12	15	23	48	100
	20	2	3	4	6	15	17	21	27	38	65	100
	30	3	4	5	8	21	23	28	35	48	73	100
	40	4	5	7	11	27	29	34	42	55	78	100
	50	5	6	8	13	31	34	39	48	60	82	100
	100	9	12	15	23	48	50	57	65	75	90	100
	200	17	21	27	38	65	67	72	78	86	95	100
	300	23	28	35	48	73	75	80	85	90	96	100
	400	29	34	42	55	79	80	84	88	92	97	100
	500	34	40	48	60	82	84	87	90	94	98	100
	1000	51	57	65	75	90	91	93	95	97	99	100
	2000	67	73	79	86	95	95	96	97	98	99	100
	3000	76	80	85	90	97	97	98	98	99	100	100
	4000	81	84	88	93	97	98	98	99	99	100	100
	5000	84	87	91	94	98	98	99	99	99	100	100
	10000	92	94	95	97	99	99	99	100	100	100	100
	15000	95	96	97	98	99	99	100	100	100	100	100
	20000	96	97	98	99	100	100	100	100	100	100	100
	25000	97	98	98	99	100	100	100	100	100	100	100
	50000	99	99	99	100	100	100	100	100	100	100	100

Table 40

PREDICTIVE VALUE OF POSITIVES (IN PERCENT)
SENSITIVITY= 92%

SPECIFICITY (%)   (CONTINUED)

		50.00	60.00	70.00	80.00	90.00	91.00	93.00	95.00	97.00	99.00
	1	0	0	0	0	0	0	0	0	0	0
	2	0	0	0	0	0	0	0	0	0	0
	3	0	0	0	0	0	0	0	0	0	0
PREVA-	4	0	0	0	0	0	0	0	0	0	0
LENCE	5	0	0	0	0	0	0	0	0	0	0
PER	10	0	0	0	0	0	0	0	0	0	1
100,000	20	0	0	0	0	0	0	0	0	1	2
	30	0	0	0	0	0	0	0	1	1	3
	40	0	0	0	0	0	0	1	1	1	4
	50	0	0	0	0	0	1	1	1	2	4
	100	0	0	0	0	1	1	1	2	3	8
	200	0	0	1	1	2	2	3	4	6	16
	300	1	1	1	1	3	3	4	5	8	22
	400	1	1	1	2	4	4	5	7	11	27
	500	1	1	2	2	4	5	6	8	13	32
	1000	2	2	3	4	9	9	12	16	24	48
	2000	4	4	6	9	16	17	21	27	38	65
	3000	5	7	9	12	22	24	29	36	49	74
	4000	7	9	11	16	28	30	35	43	56	79
	5000	9	11	14	19	33	35	41	49	62	83
	10000	17	20	25	34	51	53	59	67	77	91
	15000	25	29	35	45	62	64	70	76	84	94
	20000	32	37	43	53	70	72	77	82	88	96
	25000	38	43	51	61	75	77	81	86	91	97
	50000	65	70	75	82	90	91	93	95	97	99

Table 41

PREDICTIVE VALUE OF POSITIVES (IN PERCENT)
SENSITIVITY= 92%

SPECIFICITY (%)

		99.10	99.30	99.50	99.70	99.90	99.91	99.93	99.95	99.97	99.99	100.00
	1	0	0	0	0	1	1	1	2	3	8	100
	2	0	0	0	1	2	2	3	4	6	16	100
	3	0	0	1	1	3	3	4	5	8	22	100
PREVA-	4	0	1	1	1	4	4	5	7	11	27	100
LENCE	5	1	1	1	2	4	5	6	8	13	31	100
PER	10	1	1	2	3	8	9	12	16	23	48	100
100,000	20	2	3	4	6	16	17	21	27	38	65	100
	30	3	4	5	8	22	23	28	36	48	73	100
	40	4	5	7	11	27	29	34	42	55	79	100
	50	5	6	8	13	32	34	40	48	61	82	100
	100	9	12	16	23	48	51	57	65	75	90	100
	200	17	21	27	38	65	67	72	79	86	95	100
	300	24	28	36	48	73	75	80	85	90	97	100
	400	29	35	42	55	79	80	84	88	92	97	100
	500	34	40	48	61	82	84	87	90	94	98	100
	1000	51	57	65	76	90	91	93	95	97	99	100
	2000	68	73	79	86	95	95	96	97	98	99	100
	3000	76	80	85	90	97	97	98	98	99	100	100
	4000	81	85	88	93	97	98	98	99	99	100	100
	5000	84	87	91	94	98	98	99	99	99	100	100
	10000	92	94	95	97	99	99	99	100	100	100	100
	15000	95	96	97	98	99	99	100	100	100	100	100
	20000	96	97	98	99	100	100	100	100	100	100	100
	25000	97	98	98	99	100	100	100	100	100	100	100
	50000	99	99	99	100	100	100	100	100	100	100	100

187

Table 42

PREDICTIVE VALUE OF POSITIVES (IN PERCENT)
SENSITIVITY= 93%

		SPECIFICITY (%)								(CONTINUED)	
		50.00	60.00	70.00	80.00	90.00	91.00	93.00	95.00	97.00	99.00
	1	0	0	0	0	0	0	0	0	0	0
	2	0	0	0	0	0	0	0	0	0	0
	3	0	0	0	0	0	0	0	0	0	0
PREVA-	4	0	0	0	0	0	0	0	0	0	0
LENCE	5	0	0	0	0	0	0	0	0	0	0
PER	10	0	0	0	0	0	0	0	0	0	1
100,000	20	0	0	0	0	0	0	0	0	1	2
	30	0	0	0	0	0	0	0	1	1	3
	40	0	0	0	0	0	0	1	1	1	4
	50	0	0	0	0	0	1	1	1	2	4
	100	0	0	0	0	1	1	1	2	3	9
	200	0	0	1	1	2	2	3	4	6	16
	300	1	1	1	1	3	3	4	5	9	22
	400	1	1	1	2	4	4	5	7	11	27
	500	1	1	2	2	4	5	6	9	13	32
	1000	2	2	3	4	9	9	12	16	24	48
	2000	4	5	6	9	16	17	21	28	39	65
	3000	5	7	9	13	22	24	29	37	49	74
	4000	7	9	11	16	28	30	36	44	56	79
	5000	9	11	14	20	33	35	41	49	62	83
	10000	17	21	26	34	51	53	60	67	78	91
	15000	25	29	35	45	62	65	70	77	85	94
	20000	32	37	44	54	70	72	77	82	89	96
	25000	38	44	51	61	76	77	82	86	91	97
	50000	65	70	76	82	90	91	93	95	97	99

Table 43

PREDICTIVE VALUE OF POSITIVES (IN PERCENT)
SENSITIVITY= 93%

		SPECIFICITY (%)									
		99.10	99.30	99.50	99.70	99.90	99.91	99.93	99.95	99.97	99.99	100.00
	1	0	0	0	0	1	1	1	2	3	9	100
	2	0	0	0	1	2	2	3	4	6	16	100
	3	0	0	1	1	3	3	4	5	9	22	100
PREVA-	4	0	1	1	1	4	4	5	7	11	27	100
LENCE	5	1	1	1	2	4	5	6	9	13	32	100
PER	10	1	1	2	3	9	9	12	16	24	48	100
100,000	20	2	3	4	6	16	17	21	27	38	65	100
	30	3	4	5	9	22	24	29	36	48	74	100
	40	4	5	7	11	27	29	35	43	55	79	100
	50	5	6	9	13	32	34	40	48	61	82	100
	100	9	12	16	24	48	51	57	65	76	90	100
	200	17	21	27	38	65	67	73	79	86	95	100
	300	24	29	36	48	74	76	80	85	90	97	100
	400	29	35	43	55	79	81	84	88	93	97	100
	500	34	40	48	61	82	84	87	90	94	98	100
	1000	51	57	65	76	90	91	93	95	97	99	100
	2000	68	73	79	86	95	95	96	97	98	99	100
	3000	76	80	85	91	97	97	98	98	99	100	100
	4000	81	85	89	93	97	98	98	99	99	100	100
	5000	84	87	91	94	98	98	99	99	99	100	100
	10000	92	94	95	97	99	99	99	100	100	100	100
	15000	95	96	97	98	99	99	100	100	100	100	100
	20000	96	97	98	99	100	100	100	100	100	100	100
	25000	97	98	98	99	100	100	100	100	100	100	100
	50000	99	99	99	100	100	100	100	100	100	100	100

Table 44

PREDICTIVE VALUE OF POSITIVES (IN PERCENT)
SENSITIVITY= 94%

SPECIFICITY (%)   (CONTINUED)

		50.00	60.00	70.00	80.00	90.00	91.00	93.00	95.00	97.00	99.00
	1	0	0	0	0	0	0	0	0	0	0
	2	0	0	0	0	0	0	0	0	0	0
	3	0	0	0	0	0	0	0	0	0	0
PREVA-	4	0	0	0	0	0	0	0	0	0	0
LENCE	5	0	0	0	0	0	0	0	0	0	0
PER	10	0	0	0	0	0	0	0	0	0	1
100,000	20	0	0	0	0	0	0	0	0	1	2
	30	0	0	0	0	0	0	0	1	1	3
	40	0	0	0	0	0	0	1	1	1	4
	50	0	0	0	0	0	1	1	1	2	4
	100	0	0	0	0	1	1	1	2	3	9
	200	0	0	1	1	2	2	3	4	6	16
	300	1	1	1	1	3	3	4	5	9	22
	400	1	1	1	2	4	4	5	7	11	27
	500	1	1	2	2	5	5	6	9	14	32
	1000	2	2	3	5	9	10	12	16	24	49
	2000	4	5	6	9	16	18	22	28	39	66
	3000	5	7	9	13	23	24	29	37	49	74
	4000	7	9	12	16	28	30	36	44	57	80
	5000	9	11	14	20	33	35	41	50	62	83
	10000	17	21	26	34	51	54	60	68	78	91
	15000	25	29	36	45	62	65	70	77	85	94
	20000	32	37	44	54	70	72	77	82	89	96
	25000	39	44	51	61	76	78	82	86	91	97
	50000	65	70	76	82	90	91	93	95	97	99

Table 45

PREDICTIVE VALUE OF POSITIVES (IN PERCENT)
SENSITIVITY= 94%

SPECIFICITY (%)

		99.10	99.30	99.50	99.70	99.90	99.91	99.93	99.95	99.97	99.99	100.00
	1	0	0	0	0	1	1	1	2	3	9	100
	2	0	0	0	1	2	2	3	4	6	16	100
	3	0	0	1	1	3	3	4	5	9	22	100
PREVA-	4	0	1	1	1	4	4	5	7	11	27	100
LENCE	5	1	1	1	2	4	5	6	9	14	32	100
PER	10	1	1	2	3	9	9	12	16	24	48	100
100,000	20	2	3	4	6	16	17	21	27	39	65	100
	30	3	4	5	9	22	24	29	36	48	74	100
	40	4	5	7	11	27	29	35	43	56	79	100
	50	5	6	9	14	32	34	40	48	61	82	100
	100	9	12	16	24	48	51	57	65	76	90	100
	200	17	21	27	39	65	68	73	79	86	95	100
	300	24	29	36	49	74	76	80	85	90	97	100
	400	30	35	43	56	79	81	84	88	93	97	100
	500	34	40	49	61	83	84	87	90	94	98	100
	1000	51	58	66	76	90	91	93	95	97	99	100
	2000	68	73	79	86	95	96	96	97	98	99	100
	3000	76	81	85	91	97	97	98	98	99	100	100
	4000	81	85	89	93	98	98	98	99	99	100	100
	5000	85	88	91	94	98	98	99	99	99	100	100
	10000	92	94	95	97	99	99	99	100	100	100	100
	15000	95	96	97	98	99	99	100	100	100	100	100
	20000	96	97	98	99	100	100	100	100	100	100	100
	25000	97	98	98	99	100	100	100	100	100	100	100
	50000	99	99	99	100	100	100	100	100	100	100	100

Table 46

PREDICTIVE VALUE OF POSITIVES (IN PERCENT)
SENSITIVITY= 95%

SPECIFICITY (%)   (CONTINUED)

		50.00	60.00	70.00	80.00	90.00	91.00	93.00	95.00	97.00	99.00
PREVA-LENCE	1	0	0	0	0	0	0	0	0	0	0
	2	0	0	0	0	0	0	0	0	0	0
	3	0	0	0	0	0	0	0	0	0	0
	4	0	0	0	0	0	0	0	0	0	0
	5	0	0	0	0	0	0	0	0	0	0
PER 100,000	10	0	0	0	0	0	0	0	0	0	1
	20	0	0	0	0	0	0	0	0	1	2
	30	0	0	0	0	0	0	0	1	1	3
	40	0	0	0	0	0	0	1	1	1	4
	50	0	0	0	0	0	1	1	1	2	5
	100	0	0	0	0	1	1	1	2	3	9
	200	0	0	1	1	2	2	3	4	6	16
	300	1	1	1	1	3	3	4	5	9	22
	400	1	1	1	2	4	4	5	7	11	28
	500	1	1	2	2	5	5	6	9	14	32
	1000	2	2	3	5	9	10	12	16	24	49
	2000	4	5	6	9	16	18	22	28	39	66
	3000	6	7	9	13	23	25	30	37	49	75
	4000	7	9	12	17	28	31	36	44	57	80
	5000	9	11	14	20	33	36	42	50	63	83
	10000	17	21	26	35	51	54	60	68	78	91
	15000	25	30	36	46	63	65	71	77	85	94
	20000	32	37	44	54	70	73	77	83	89	96
	25000	39	44	51	61	76	78	82	86	91	97
	50000	66	70	76	83	90	91	93	95	97	99

Table 47

PREDICTIVE VALUE OF POSITIVES (IN PERCENT)
SENSITIVITY= 95%

SPECIFICITY (%)

		99.10	99.30	99.50	99.70	99.90	99.91	99.93	99.95	99.97	99.99	100.00
PREVA-LENCE	1	0	0	0	0	1	1	1	2	3	9	100
	2	0	0	0	1	2	2	3	4	6	16	100
	3	0	0	1	1	3	3	4	5	9	22	100
	4	0	1	1	1	4	4	5	7	11	28	100
	5	1	1	1	2	5	5	6	9	14	32	100
PER 100,000	10	1	1	2	3	9	10	12	16	24	49	100
	20	2	3	4	6	16	17	21	28	39	65	100
	30	3	4	5	9	22	24	29	36	49	74	100
	40	4	5	7	11	28	30	35	43	56	79	100
	50	5	6	9	14	32	35	40	49	61	83	100
	100	10	12	16	24	49	51	58	66	76	90	100
	200	17	21	28	39	66	68	73	79	86	95	100
	300	24	29	36	49	74	76	80	85	90	97	100
	400	30	35	43	56	79	81	84	88	93	97	100
	500	35	41	49	61	83	84	87	91	94	98	100
	1000	52	58	66	76	91	91	93	95	97	99	100
	2000	68	73	79	87	95	96	97	97	98	99	100
	3000	77	81	85	91	97	97	98	98	99	100	100
	4000	81	85	89	93	98	98	98	99	99	100	100
	5000	85	88	91	94	98	98	99	99	99	100	100
	10000	92	94	95	97	99	99	99	100	100	100	100
	15000	95	96	97	98	99	99	100	100	100	100	100
	20000	96	97	98	99	100	100	100	100	100	100	100
	25000	97	98	98	99	100	100	100	100	100	100	100
	50000	99	99	99	100	100	100	100	100	100	100	100

Table 48

PREDICTIVE VALUE OF POSITIVES (IN PERCENT)
SENSITIVITY= 96%

SPECIFICITY (%)   (CONTINUED)

		50.00	60.00	70.00	80.00	90.00	91.00	93.00	95.00	97.00	99.00
	1	0	0	0	0	0	0	0	0	0	0
	2	0	0	0	0	0	0	0	0	0	0
	3	0	0	0	0	0	0	0	0	0	0
PREVA-	4	0	0	0	0	0	0	0	0	0	0
LENCE	5	0	0	0	0	0	0	0	0	0	0
PER	10	0	0	0	0	0	0	0	0	0	1
100,000	20	0	0	0	0	0	0	0	0	1	2
	30	0	0	0	0	0	0	0	1	1	3
	40	0	0	0	0	0	0	1	1	1	4
	50	0	0	0	0	0	1	1	1	2	5
	100	0	0	0	0	1	1	1	2	3	9
	200	0	0	1	1	2	2	3	4	6	16
	300	1	1	1	1	3	3	4	5	9	22
	400	1	1	1	2	4	4	5	7	11	28
	500	1	1	2	2	5	5	6	9	14	33
	1000	2	2	3	5	9	10	12	16	24	49
	2000	4	5	6	9	16	18	22	28	40	66
	3000	6	7	9	13	23	25	30	37	50	75
	4000	7	9	12	17	29	31	36	44	57	80
	5000	9	11	14	20	34	36	42	50	63	83
	10000	18	21	26	35	52	54	60	68	78	91
	15000	25	30	36	46	63	65	71	77	85	94
	20000	32	38	44	55	71	73	77	83	89	96
	25000	39	44	52	62	76	78	82	86	91	97
	50000	66	71	76	83	91	91	93	95	97	99

Table 49

PREDICTIVE VALUE OF POSITIVES (IN PERCENT)
SENSITIVITY= 96%

SPECIFICITY (%)

		99.10	99.30	99.50	99.70	99.90	99.91	99.93	99.95	99.97	99.99	100.00
	1	0	0	0	0	1	1	1	2	3	9	100
	2	0	0	0	1	2	2	3	4	6	16	100
	3	0	0	1	1	3	3	4	5	9	22	100
PREVA-	4	0	1	1	1	4	4	5	7	11	28	100
LENCE	5	1	1	1	2	5	5	6	9	14	32	100
PER	10	1	1	2	3	9	10	12	16	24	49	100
100,000	20	2	3	4	6	16	18	22	28	39	66	100
	30	3	4	5	9	22	24	29	37	49	74	100
	40	4	5	7	11	28	30	35	43	56	79	100
	50	5	6	9	14	32	35	41	49	62	83	100
	100	10	12	16	24	49	52	58	66	76	91	100
	200	18	22	28	39	66	68	73	79	87	95	100
	300	24	29	37	49	74	76	80	85	91	97	100
	400	30	36	44	56	79	81	85	89	93	97	100
	500	35	41	49	62	83	84	87	91	94	98	100
	1000	52	58	66	76	91	92	93	95	97	99	100
	2000	69	74	80	87	95	96	97	98	98	99	100
	3000	77	81	86	91	97	97	98	98	99	100	100
	4000	82	85	89	93	98	98	98	99	99	100	100
	5000	85	88	91	94	98	98	99	99	99	100	100
	10000	92	94	96	97	99	99	99	100	100	100	100
	15000	95	96	97	98	99	99	100	100	100	100	100
	20000	96	97	98	99	100	100	100	100	100	100	100
	25000	97	98	98	99	100	100	100	100	100	100	100
	50000	99	99	99	100	100	100	100	100	100	100	100

Table 50

PREDICTIVE VALUE OF POSITIVES (IN PERCENT)
SENSITIVITY= 97%

SPECIFICITY (%)　　　　　(CCNTINUED)

		50.00	60.00	70.00	80.00	90.00	91.00	93.00	95.00	97.00	99.00
PREVA-LENCE	1	0	0	0	0	0	0	0	0	0	0
	2	0	0	0	0	0	0	0	0	0	0
	3	0	0	0	0	0	0	0	0	0	0
	4	0	0	0	0	0	0	0	0	0	0
	5	0	0	0	0	0	0	0	0	0	0
PER 100,000	10	0	0	0	0	0	0	0	0	0	1
	20	0	0	0	0	0	0	0	0	1	2
	30	0	0	0	0	0	0	0	1	1	3
	40	0	0	0	0	0	0	1	1	1	4
	50	0	0	0	0	0	1	1	1	2	5
	100	0	0	0	0	1	1	1	2	3	9
	200	0	0	1	1	2	2	3	4	6	16
	300	1	1	1	1	3	3	4	6	9	23
	400	1	1	1	2	4	4	5	7	11	28
	500	1	1	2	2	5	5	7	9	14	33
	1000	2	2	3	5	9	10	12	16	25	49
	2000	4	5	6	9	17	18	22	28	40	66
	3000	6	7	9	13	23	25	30	38	50	75
	4000	7	9	12	17	29	31	37	45	57	80
	5000	9	11	15	20	34	36	42	51	63	84
	10000	18	21	26	35	52	54	61	68	78	92
	15000	26	30	36	46	63	66	71	77	85	94
	20000	33	38	45	55	71	73	78	83	89	96
	25000	39	45	52	62	76	78	82	87	92	97
	50000	66	71	76	83	91	92	93	95	97	99

Table 51

PREDICTIVE VALUE OF POSITIVES (IN PERCENT)
SENSITIVITY= 97%

SPECIFICITY (%)

		99.10	99.30	99.50	99.70	99.90	99.91	99.93	99.95	99.97	99.99	100.00
PREVA-LENCE	1	0	0	0	0	1	1	1	2	3	9	100
	2	0	0	0	1	2	2	3	4	6	16	100
	3	0	0	1	1	3	3	4	5	9	23	100
	4	0	1	1	1	4	4	5	7	11	28	100
	5	1	1	1	2	5	5	6	9	14	33	100
PER 100,000	10	1	1	2	3	9	10	12	16	24	49	100
	20	2	3	4	6	16	18	22	28	39	66	100
	30	3	4	6	9	23	24	29	37	49	74	100
	40	4	5	7	11	28	30	36	44	56	79	100
	50	5	6	9	14	33	35	41	49	62	83	100
	100	10	12	16	24	49	52	58	66	76	91	100
	200	18	22	28	39	66	68	74	80	87	95	100
	300	24	29	37	49	74	76	81	85	91	97	100
	400	30	36	44	56	80	81	85	89	93	97	100
	500	35	41	49	62	83	84	87	91	94	98	100
	1000	52	58	66	77	91	92	93	95	97	99	100
	2000	69	74	80	87	95	96	97	98	99	99	100
	3000	77	81	86	91	97	97	98	98	99	100	100
	4000	82	85	89	93	98	98	98	99	99	100	100
	5000	85	88	91	94	98	98	99	99	99	100	100
	10000	92	94	96	97	99	99	99	100	100	100	100
	15000	95	96	97	98	99	99	100	100	100	100	100
	20000	96	97	98	99	100	100	100	100	100	100	100
	25000	97	98	98	99	100	100	100	100	100	100	100
	50000	99	99	99	100	100	100	100	100	100	100	100

Table 52

PREDICTIVE VALUE OF POSITIVES (IN PERCENT)
SENSITIVITY= 98%

SPECIFICITY (%)　　　　　　　　　(CONTINUED)

		50.00	60.00	70.00	80.00	90.00	91.00	93.00	95.00	97.00	99.00
	1	0	0	0	0	0	0	0	0	0	0
	2	0	0	0	0	0	0	0	0	0	0
	3	0	0	0	0	0	0	0	0	0	0
PREVA-	4	0	0	0	0	0	0	0	0	0	0
LENCE	5	0	0	0	0	0	0	0	0	0	0
PER	10	0	0	0	0	0	0	0	0	0	1
100,000	20	0	0	0	0	0	0	0	0	1	2
	30	0	0	0	0	0	0	0	1	1	3
	40	0	0	0	0	0	0	1	1	1	4
	50	0	0	0	0	0	1	1	1	2	5
	100	0	0	0	0	1	1	1	2	3	9
	200	0	0	1	1	2	2	3	4	6	16
	300	1	1	1	1	3	3	4	6	9	23
	400	1	1	1	2	4	4	5	7	12	28
	500	1	1	2	2	5	5	7	9	14	33
	1000	2	2	3	5	9	10	12	17	25	50
	2000	4	5	6	9	17	18	22	29	40	67
	3000	6	7	9	13	23	25	30	38	50	75
	4000	8	9	12	17	29	31	37	45	58	80
	5000	9	11	15	21	34	36	42	51	63	84
	10000	18	21	27	35	52	55	61	69	78	92
	15000	26	30	37	46	63	66	71	78	85	95
	20000	33	38	45	55	71	73	78	83	89	96
	25000	40	45	52	62	77	78	82	87	92	97
	50000	66	71	77	83	91	92	93	95	97	99

Table 53

PREDICTIVE VALUE OF POSITIVES (IN PERCENT)
SENSITIVITY= 98%

SPECIFICITY (%)

		99.10	99.30	99.50	99.70	99.90	99.91	99.93	99.95	99.97	99.99	100.00
	1	0	0	0	0	1	1	1	2	3	9	100
	2	0	0	0	1	2	2	3	4	6	16	100
	3	0	0	1	1	3	3	4	6	9	23	100
PREVA-	4	0	1	1	1	4	4	5	7	12	28	100
LENCE	5	1	1	1	2	5	5	7	9	14	33	100
PER	10	1	1	2	3	9	10	12	16	25	49	100
100,000	20	2	3	4	6	16	18	22	28	40	66	100
	30	3	4	6	9	23	25	30	37	49	75	100
	40	4	5	7	12	28	30	36	44	57	80	100
	50	5	7	9	14	33	35	41	50	62	83	100
	100	10	12	16	25	50	52	58	66	77	91	100
	200	18	22	28	40	66	69	74	80	87	95	100
	300	25	30	37	50	75	77	81	86	91	97	100
	400	30	36	44	57	80	81	85	89	93	98	100
	500	35	41	50	62	83	85	88	91	94	98	100
	1000	52	59	66	77	91	92	93	95	97	99	100
	2000	69	74	80	87	95	96	97	98	99	100	100
	3000	77	81	86	91	97	97	98	98	99	100	100
	4000	82	85	89	93	98	98	98	99	99	100	100
	5000	85	88	91	95	98	98	99	99	99	100	100
	10000	92	94	96	97	99	99	99	100	100	100	100
	15000	95	96	97	98	99	99	100	100	100	100	100
	20000	96	97	98	99	100	100	100	100	100	100	100
	25000	97	98	98	99	100	100	100	100	100	100	100
	50000	99	99	99	100	100	100	100	100	100	100	100

Table 54

PREDICTIVE VALUE OF POSITIVES (IN PERCENT)
SENSITIVITY= 99%

		SPECIFICITY (%)								(CONTINUED)	
		50.00	60.00	70.00	80.00	90.00	91.00	93.00	95.00	97.00	99.00
PREVA-LENCE	1	0	C	0	0	0	0	0	0	0	0
	2	0	0	0	0	0	0	0	0	0	0
	3	0	0	0	0	0	C	0	0	0	0
	4	C	C	0	0	0	0	0	0	U	0
	5	0	0	0	0	0	C	0	0	0	0
PER 100,000	10	0	C	0	U	0	0	0	U	0	1
	20	0	0	0	0	0	0	0	0	1	2
	30	0	0	0	0	0	0	0	1	1	3
	40	0	0	0	0	0	C	1	1	1	4
	50	0	C	0	0	0	1	1	1	2	5
	100	C	C	C	0	1	1	1	2	3	9
	200	0	0	1	1	2	2	3	4	6	17
	300	1	1	1	1	3	3	4	6	9	23
	400	1	1	1	2	4	4	5	7	12	28
	500	1	1	2	2	5	5	7	9	14	33
	1000	2	2	3	5	9	10	13	17	25	50
	2000	4	5	6	9	17	18	22	29	40	67
	3000	6	7	9	13	23	25	30	38	51	75
	4000	8	9	12	17	29	31	37	45	58	80
	5000	9	12	15	21	34	37	43	51	63	84
	10000	18	22	27	35	52	55	61	69	79	92
	15000	26	30	37	47	64	66	71	78	85	95
	20000	33	38	45	55	71	73	78	83	89	96
	25000	40	45	52	62	77	79	82	87	92	97
	50000	66	71	77	83	91	92	93	95	97	99

Table 55

PREDICTIVE VALUE OF POSITIVES (IN PERCENT)
SENSITIVITY= 99%

		SPECIFICITY (%)										
		99.10	99.30	99.50	99.70	99.90	99.91	99.93	99.95	99.97	99.99	100.00
PREVA-LENCE	1	0	0	0	0	1	1	1	2	3	9	100
	2	0	0	0	1	2	2	3	4	6	17	100
	3	0	0	1	1	3	3	4	6	9	23	100
	4	0	1	1	1	4	4	5	7	12	28	100
	5	1	1	1	2	5	5	7	9	14	33	100
PER 100,000	10	1	1	2	3	9	10	12	17	25	50	100
	20	2	3	4	6	17	18	22	28	40	66	100
	30	3	4	6	9	23	25	30	37	50	75	100
	40	4	5	7	12	28	31	36	44	57	80	100
	50	5	7	9	14	33	35	41	50	62	83	100
	100	10	12	17	25	50	52	59	66	77	91	100
	200	18	22	28	40	66	69	74	80	87	95	100
	300	25	30	37	50	75	77	81	86	91	97	100
	400	31	36	44	57	80	82	85	89	93	98	100
	500	36	42	50	62	83	85	88	91	94	98	100
	1000	53	59	67	77	91	92	93	95	97	99	100
	2000	69	74	80	87	95	96	97	98	99	100	100
	3000	77	81	86	91	97	97	98	98	99	100	100
	4000	82	85	89	93	98	98	98	99	99	100	100
	5000	85	88	91	95	98	98	99	99	99	100	100
	10000	92	94	96	97	99	99	99	100	100	100	100
	15000	95	96	97	98	99	99	100	100	100	100	100
	20000	96	97	98	99	100	100	100	100	100	100	100
	25000	97	98	99	99	100	100	100	100	100	100	100
	50000	99	99	99	100	100	100	100	100	100	100	100

Table 56

PREDICTIVE VALUE OF POSITIVES (IN PERCENT)
SENSITIVITY=100%

SPECIFICITY (%)   (CONTINUED)

		50.00	60.00	70.00	80.00	90.00	91.00	93.00	95.00	97.00	99.00
	1	0	0	0	0	0	0	0	0	0	0
	2	0	0	0	0	0	0	0	0	0	0
	3	0	0	0	0	0	0	0	0	0	0
PREVA-	4	0	0	0	0	0	0	0	0	0	0
LENCE	5	0	0	0	0	0	0	0	0	0	0
PER	10	0	0	0	0	0	0	0	0	0	1
100,000	20	0	0	0	0	0	0	0	0	1	2
	30	0	0	0	0	0	0	0	1	1	3
	40	0	0	0	0	0	0	1	1	1	4
	50	0	0	0	0	0	1	1	1	2	5
	100	0	0	0	0	1	1	1	2	3	9
	200	0	0	1	1	2	2	3	4	6	17
	300	1	1	1	1	3	3	4	6	9	23
	400	1	1	1	2	4	4	5	7	12	29
	500	1	1	2	2	5	5	7	9	14	33
	1000	2	2	3	5	9	10	13	17	25	50
	2000	4	5	6	9	17	18	23	29	40	67
	3000	6	7	9	13	24	26	31	38	51	76
	4000	8	9	12	17	29	32	37	45	58	81
	5000	10	12	15	21	34	37	43	51	64	84
	10000	18	22	27	36	53	55	61	69	79	92
	15000	26	31	37	47	64	66	72	78	85	95
	20000	33	38	45	56	71	74	78	83	89	96
	25000	40	45	53	62	77	79	83	87	92	97
	50000	67	71	77	83	91	92	93	95	97	99

Table 57

PREDICTIVE VALUE OF POSITIVES (IN PERCENT)
SENSITIVITY=100%

SPECIFICITY (%)

		99.10	99.30	99.50	99.70	99.90	99.91	99.93	99.95	99.97	99.99	100.00
	1	0	0	0	0	1	1	1	2	3	9	100
	2	0	0	0	1	2	2	3	4	6	17	100
	3	0	0	1	1	3	3	4	6	9	23	100
PREVA-	4	0	1	1	1	4	4	5	7	12	29	100
LENCE	5	1	1	1	2	5	5	7	9	14	33	100
PER	10	1	1	2	3	9	10	12	17	25	50	100
100,000	20	2	3	4	6	17	18	22	29	40	67	100
	30	3	4	6	9	23	25	30	38	50	75	100
	40	4	5	7	12	29	31	36	44	57	80	100
	50	5	7	9	14	33	36	42	50	63	83	100
	100	10	13	17	25	50	53	59	67	77	91	100
	200	18	22	29	40	67	69	74	80	87	95	100
	300	25	30	38	50	75	77	81	86	91	97	100
	400	31	36	45	57	80	82	85	89	93	98	100
	500	36	42	50	63	83	85	88	91	94	98	100
	1000	53	59	67	77	91	92	94	95	97	99	100
	2000	69	74	80	87	95	96	97	98	99	100	100
	3000	77	82	86	91	97	97	98	98	99	100	100
	4000	82	86	89	93	98	98	98	99	99	100	100
	5000	85	88	91	95	98	98	99	99	99	100	100
	10000	93	94	96	97	99	99	99	100	100	100	100
	15000	95	96	97	98	99	99	100	100	100	100	100
	20000	97	97	98	99	100	100	100	100	100	100	100
	25000	97	98	99	99	100	100	100	100	100	100	100
	50000	99	99	100	100	100	100	100	100	100	100	100

Table 58

PREDICTIVE VALUE OF POSITIVES (IN PERCENT)
SPECIFICITY= 50.00%

		50	60	70	80	85	90	91	92	93	94	95	96	97	98	99	100
								SENSITIVITY (%)									
PREVA-LENCE	1	0	0	0	0	0	0	0	0	0	0	0	0	0	0	0	0
	2	0	0	0	0	0	0	0	0	0	0	0	0	0	0	0	0
	3	0	0	0	0	0	0	0	0	0	0	0	0	0	0	0	0
	4	0	0	0	0	0	0	0	0	0	0	0	0	0	0	0	0
	5	0	0	0	0	0	0	0	0	0	0	0	0	0	0	0	0
PER 100,000	10	0	0	0	0	0	0	0	0	0	0	0	0	0	0	0	0
	20	0	0	0	0	0	0	0	0	0	0	0	0	0	0	0	0
	30	0	0	0	0	0	0	0	0	0	0	0	0	0	0	0	0
	40	0	0	0	0	0	0	0	0	0	0	0	0	0	0	0	0
	50	0	0	0	0	0	0	0	0	0	0	0	0	0	0	0	0
	100	0	0	0	0	0	0	0	0	0	0	0	0	0	0	0	0
	200	0	0	0	0	0	0	0	0	0	0	0	0	0	0	0	0
	300	0	0	0	0	1	1	1	1	1	1	1	1	1	1	1	1
	400	0	0	1	1	1	1	1	1	1	1	1	1	1	1	1	1
	500	1	1	1	1	1	1	1	1	1	1	1	1	1	1	1	1
	1000	1	1	1	2	2	2	2	2	2	2	2	2	2	2	2	2
	2000	2	2	3	3	3	4	4	4	4	4	4	4	4	4	4	4
	3000	3	4	4	5	5	5	5	5	5	5	6	6	6	6	6	6
	4000	4	5	6	6	7	7	7	7	7	7	7	7	7	8	8	8
	5000	5	6	7	8	8	9	9	9	9	9	9	9	9	9	9	10
	10000	10	12	13	15	16	17	17	17	17	17	17	18	18	18	18	18
	15000	15	17	20	22	23	24	24	25	25	25	25	25	26	26	26	26
	20000	20	23	26	29	30	31	31	32	32	32	32	32	33	33	33	33
	25000	25	29	32	35	36	37	38	38	38	39	39	39	39	40	40	40
	50000	50	55	58	62	63	64	65	65	65	65	66	66	66	66	66	67

Table 59

PREDICTIVE VALUE OF POSITIVES (IN PERCENT)
SPECIFICITY= 60.00%

		50	60	70	80	85	90	91	92	93	94	95	96	97	98	99	100
								SENSITIVITY (%)									
PREVA-LENCE	1	0	0	0	0	0	0	0	0	0	0	0	0	0	0	0	0
	2	0	0	0	0	0	0	0	0	0	0	0	0	0	0	0	0
	3	0	0	0	0	0	0	0	0	0	0	0	0	0	0	0	0
	4	0	0	0	0	0	0	0	0	0	0	0	0	0	0	0	0
	5	0	0	0	0	0	0	0	0	0	0	0	0	0	0	0	0
PER 100,000	10	0	0	0	0	0	0	0	0	0	0	0	0	0	0	0	0
	20	0	0	0	0	0	0	0	0	0	0	0	0	0	0	0	0
	30	0	0	0	0	0	0	0	0	0	0	0	0	0	0	0	0
	40	0	0	0	0	0	0	0	0	0	0	0	0	0	0	0	0
	50	0	0	0	0	0	0	0	0	0	0	0	0	0	0	0	0
	100	0	0	0	0	0	0	0	0	0	0	0	0	0	0	0	0
	200	0	0	0	0	0	0	0	0	0	0	0	0	0	0	0	0
	300	0	0	1	1	1	1	1	1	1	1	1	1	1	1	1	1
	400	0	1	1	1	1	1	1	1	1	1	1	1	1	1	1	1
	500	1	1	1	1	1	1	1	1	1	1	1	1	1	1	1	1
	1000	1	1	2	2	2	2	2	2	2	2	2	2	2	2	2	2
	2000	2	3	3	4	4	4	4	4	5	5	5	5	5	5	5	5
	3000	4	4	5	6	6	7	7	7	7	7	7	7	7	7	7	7
	4000	5	6	7	8	8	9	9	9	9	9	9	9	9	9	9	9
	5000	6	7	8	10	10	11	11	11	11	11	11	11	11	11	12	12
	10000	12	14	16	18	19	20	20	20	21	21	21	21	21	21	22	22
	15000	18	21	24	26	27	28	29	29	29	29	30	30	30	30	30	31
	20000	24	27	30	33	35	36	36	37	37	37	37	38	38	38	38	38
	25000	29	33	37	40	41	43	43	43	44	44	44	44	45	45	45	45
	50000	56	60	64	67	68	69	69	70	70	70	70	71	71	71	71	71

Table 60

PREDICTIVE VALUE OF POSITIVES (IN PERCENT)
SPECIFICITY= 70.00%

								SENSITIVITY (%)								
		50	60	70	80	85	90	91	92	93	94	95	96	97	98	99	100
	1	0	0	0	0	0	0	0	0	0	0	0	0	0	0	0	0
	2	0	0	0	0	0	0	0	0	0	0	0	0	0	0	0	0
	3	0	0	0	0	0	0	0	0	0	0	0	0	0	0	0	0
PREVA-	4	0	0	0	0	0	0	0	0	0	0	0	0	0	0	0	0
LENCE	5	0	0	0	0	0	0	0	0	0	0	0	0	0	0	0	0
PER	10	0	0	0	0	0	0	0	0	0	0	0	0	0	0	0	0
100,000	20	0	0	0	0	0	0	0	0	0	0	0	0	0	0	0	0
	30	0	0	0	0	0	0	0	0	0	0	0	0	0	0	0	0
	40	0	0	0	0	0	0	0	0	0	0	0	0	0	0	0	0
	50	0	0	0	0	0	0	0	0	0	0	0	0	0	0	0	0
	100	0	0	0	0	0	0	0	0	0	0	0	0	0	0	0	0
	200	0	0	0	1	1	1	1	1	1	1	1	1	1	1	1	1
	300	0	1	1	1	1	1	1	1	1	1	1	1	1	1	1	1
	400	1	1	1	1	1	1	1	1	1	1	1	1	1	1	1	1
	500	1	1	1	1	1	1	2	2	2	2	2	2	2	2	2	2
	1000	2	2	2	3	3	3	3	3	3	3	3	3	3	3	3	3
	2000	3	4	5	5	5	6	6	6	6	6	6	6	6	6	6	6
	3000	5	6	7	8	8	8	9	9	9	9	9	9	9	9	9	9
	4000	6	8	9	10	11	11	11	11	11	12	12	12	12	12	12	12
	5000	8	10	11	12	13	14	14	14	14	14	14	14	15	15	15	15
	10000	16	18	21	23	24	25	25	25	26	26	26	26	26	27	27	27
	15000	23	26	29	32	33	35	35	35	35	36	36	36	36	37	37	37
	20000	29	33	37	40	41	43	43	43	44	44	44	44	45	45	45	45
	25000	36	40	44	47	49	50	50	51	51	51	51	52	52	52	52	53
	50000	62	67	70	73	74	75	75	75	76	76	76	76	76	77	77	77

Table 61

PREDICTIVE VALUE OF POSITIVES (IN PERCENT)
SPECIFICITY= 80.00%

								SENSITIVITY (%)								
		50	60	70	80	85	90	91	92	93	94	95	96	97	98	99	100
	1	0	0	0	0	0	0	0	0	0	0	0	0	0	0	0	0
	2	0	0	0	0	0	0	0	0	0	0	0	0	0	0	0	0
	3	0	0	0	0	0	0	0	0	0	0	0	0	0	0	0	0
PREVA-	4	0	0	0	0	0	0	0	0	0	0	0	0	0	0	0	0
LENCE	5	0	0	0	0	0	0	0	0	0	0	0	0	0	0	0	0
PER	10	0	0	0	0	0	0	0	0	0	0	0	0	0	0	0	0
100,000	20	0	0	0	0	0	0	0	0	0	0	0	0	0	0	0	0
	30	0	0	0	0	0	0	0	0	0	0	0	0	0	0	0	0
	40	0	0	0	0	0	0	0	0	0	0	0	0	0	0	0	0
	50	0	0	0	0	0	0	0	0	0	0	0	0	0	0	0	0
	100	0	0	0	0	0	0	0	0	0	0	0	0	0	0	0	0
	200	0	1	1	1	1	1	1	1	1	1	1	1	1	1	1	1
	300	1	1	1	1	1	1	1	1	1	1	1	1	1	1	1	1
	400	1	1	1	2	2	2	2	2	2	2	2	2	2	2	2	2
	500	1	1	2	2	2	2	2	2	2	2	2	2	2	2	2	2
	1000	2	3	3	4	4	4	4	4	4	5	5	5	5	5	5	5
	2000	5	6	7	8	8	8	8	9	9	9	9	9	9	9	9	9
	3000	7	8	10	11	12	12	12	12	13	13	13	13	13	13	13	13
	4000	9	11,	13	14	15	16	16	16	16	16	17	17	17	17	17	17
	5000	12	14	16	17	18	19	19	19	20	20	20	20	20	21	21	21
	10000	22	25	28	31	32	33	34	34	34	34	35	35	35	35	35	36
	15000	31	35	38	41	43	44	45	45	45	45	46	46	46	46	47	47
	20000	38	43	47	50	52	53	53	53	54	54	54	55	55	55	55	56
	25000	45	50	54	57	59	60	60	61	61	61	61	62	62	62	62	62
	50000	71	75	78	80	81	82	82	82	82	82	83	83	83	83	83	83

Table 62

PREDICTIVE VALUE OF POSITIVES (IN PERCENT)
SPECIFICITY= 90.00%

		SENSITIVITY (%)															
		50	60	70	80	85	90	91	92	93	94	95	96	97	98	99	100
PREVA-LENCE	1	0	0	0	0	0	0	0	0	0	0	0	0	0	0	0	0
	2	0	0	0	0	0	0	0	0	0	0	0	0	0	0	0	0
	3	0	0	0	0	0	0	0	0	0	0	0	0	0	0	0	0
	4	0	0	0	0	0	0	0	0	0	0	0	0	0	0	0	0
	5	0	0	0	0	0	0	0	0	0	0	0	0	0	0	0	0
PER 100,000	10	0	0	0	0	0	0	0	0	0	0	0	0	0	0	0	0
	20	0	0	0	0	0	0	0	0	0	0	0	0	0	0	0	0
	30	0	0	0	0	0	0	0	0	0	0	0	0	0	0	0	0
	40	0	0	0	0	0	0	0	0	0	0	0	0	0	0	0	0
	50	0	0	0	0	0	0	0	0	0	0	0	0	0	0	0	0
	100	0	1	1	1	1	1	1	1	1	1	1	1	1	1	1	1
	200	1	1	1	2	2	2	2	2	2	2	2	2	2	2	2	2
	300	1	2	2	2	2	3	3	3	3	3	3	3	3	3	3	3
	400	2	2	3	3	3	3	4	4	4	4	4	4	4	4	4	4
	500	2	3	3	4.	4	4	4	4	4	5	5	5	5	5	5	5
	1000	5	6	7	7	8	8	8	9	9	9	9	9	9	9	9	9
	2000	9	11	13	14	15	16	16	16	16	16	16	16	17	17	17	17
	3000	13	16	18	20	21	22	22	22	22	23	23	23	23	23	23	24
	4000	17	20	23	25	26	27	27	28	28	28	28	29	29	29	29	29
	5000	21	24	27	30	31	32	32	33	33	33	33	34	34	34	34	34
	10000	36	40	44	47	49	50	50	51	51	51	51	52	52	52	52	53
	15000	47	51	55	59	60	61	62	62	62	62	63	63	63	63	64	64
	20000	56	60	64	67	68	69	69	70	70	70	70	71	71	71	71	71
	25000	63	67	70	73	74	75	75	75	76	76	76	76	76	77	77	77
	50000	83	86	88	89	89	90	90	90	90	90	90	91	91	91	91	91

Table 63

PREDICTIVE VALUE OF POSITIVES (IN PERCENT)
SPECIFICITY= 91.00%

		SENSITIVITY (%)															
		50	60	70	80	85	90	91	92	93	94	95	96	97	98	99	100
PREVA-LENCE	1	0	0	0	0	0	0	0	0	0	0	0	0	0	0	0	0
	2	0	0	0	0	0	0	0	0	0	0	0	0	0	0	0	0
	3	0	0	0	0	0	0	0	0	0	0	0	0	0	0	0	0
	4	0	0	0	0	0	0	0	0	0	0	0	0	0	0	0	0
	5	0	0	0	0	0	0	0	0	0	0	0	0	0	0	0	0
PER 100,000	10	0	0	0	0	0	0	0	0	0	0	0	0	0	0	0	0
	20	0	0	0	0	0	0	0	0	0	0	0	0	0	0	0	0
	30	0	0	0	0	0	0	0	0	0	0	0	0	0	0	0	0
	40	0	0	0	0	0	0	0	0	0	0	0	0	0	0	0	0
	50	0	0	0	0	0	0	1	1	1	1	1	1	1	1	1	1
	100	1	1	1	1	1	1	1	1	1	1	1	1	1	1	1	1
	200	1	1	2	2	2	2	2	2	2	2	2	2	2	2	2	2
	300	2	2	2	3	3	3	3	3	3	3	3	3	3	3	3	3
	400	2	3	3	3	4	4	4	4	4	4	4	4	4	4	4	4
	500	3	3	4	4	5	5	5	5	5	5	5	5	5	5	5	5
	1000	5	6	7	8	9	9	9	9	9	10	10	10	10	10	10	10
	2000	10	12	14	15	16	17	17	17	17	18	18	18	18	18	18	18
	3000	15	17	19	22	23	24	24	24	24	24	25	25	25	25	25	26
	4000	19	22	24	27	28	29	30	30	30	30	31	31	31	31	31	32
	5000	23	26	29	32	33	34	35	35	35	35	36	36	36	36	37	37
	10000	38	43	46	50	51	53	53	53	53	54	54	54	54	55	55	55
	15000	50	54	58	61	63	64	64	64	65	65	65	65	66	66	66	66
	20000	58	63	66	69	70	71	72	72	72	72	73	73	73	73	73	74
	25000	65	69	72	75	76	77	77	77	77	78	78	78	78	78	79	79
	50000	85	87	89	90	90	91	91	91	91	91	91	91	92	92	92	92

Table 64

PREDICTIVE VALUE OF POSITIVES (IN PERCENT)
SPECIFICITY= 93.00%

| | | \multicolumn{16}{c}{SENSITIVITY (%)} | | | | | | | | | | | | | | |
		50	60	70	80	85	90	91	92	93	94	95	96	97	98	99	100
PREVA-LENCE	1	0	0	0	0	0	0	0	0	0	0	0	0	0	0	0	0
	2	0	0	0	0	0	0	0	0	0	0	0	0	0	0	0	0
	3	0	0	0	0	0	0	0	0	0	0	0	0	0	0	0	0
	4	0	0	0	0	0	0	0	0	0	0	0	0	0	0	0	0
	5	0	0	0	0	0	0	0	0	0	0	0	0	0	0	0	0
PER 100,000	10	0	0	0	0	0	0	0	0	0	0	0	0	0	0	0	0
	20	0	0	0	0	0	0	0	0	0	0	0	0	0	0	0	0
	30	0	0	0	0	0	0	0	0	0	0	0	0	0	0	0	0
	40	0	0	0	0	0	1	1	1	1	1	1	1	1	1	1	1
	50	0	0	0	1	1	1	1	1	1	1	1	1	1	1	1	1
	100	1	1	1	1	1	1	1	1	1	1	1	1	1	1	1	1
	200	1	2	2	2	2	3	3	3	3	3	3	3	3	3	3	3
	300	2	3	3	3	4	4	4	4	4	4	4	4	4	4	4	4
	400	3	3	4	4	5	5	5	5	5	5	5	5	5	5	5	5
	500	3	4	5	5	6	6	6	6	6	6	6	6	7	7	7	7
	1000	7	8	9	10	11	11	12	12	12	12	12	12	12	12	13	13
	2000	13	15	17	19	20	21	21	21	21	22	22	22	22	22	22	23
	3000	18	21	24	26	27	28	29	29	29	29	30	30	30	30	30	31
	4000	23	26	29	32	34	35	35	35	36	36	36	36	37	37	37	37
	5000	27	31	34	38	39	40	41	41	41	41	42	42	42	42	43	43
	10000	44	49	53	56	57	59	59	59	60	60	60	60	61	61	61	61
	15000	56	60	64	67	68	69	70	70	70	70	71	71	71	71	71	72
	20000	64	68	71	74	75	76	76	77	77	77	77	77	78	78	78	78
	25000	70	74	77	79	80	81	81	81	82	82	82	82	82	82	82	83
	50000	88	90	91	92	92	93	93	93	93	93	93	93	93	93	93	93

Table 65

PREDICTIVE VALUE OF POSITIVES (IN PERCENT)
SPECIFICITY= 95.00%

| | | \multicolumn{16}{c}{SENSITIVITY (%)} | | | | | | | | | | | | | | |
		50	60	70	80	85	90	91	92	93	94	95	96	97	98	99	100
PREVA-LENCE	1	0	0	0	0	0	0	0	0	0	0	0	0	0	0	0	0
	2	0	0	0	0	0	0	0	0	0	0	0	0	0	0	0	0
	3	0	0	0	0	0	0	0	0	0	0	0	0	0	0	0	0
	4	0	0	0	0	0	0	0	0	0	0	0	0	0	0	0	0
	5	0	0	0	0	0	0	0	0	0	0	0	0	0	0	0	0
PER 100,000	10	0	0	0	0	0	0	0	0	0	0	0	0	0	0	0	0
	20	0	0	0	0	0	0	0	0	0	0	0	0	0	0	0	0
	30	0	0	0	0	1	1	1	1	1	1	1	1	1	1	1	1
	40	0	0	1	1	1	1	1	1	1	1	1	1	1	1	1	1
	50	0	1	1	1	1	1	1	1	1	1	1	1	1	1	1	1
	100	1	1	1	2	2	2	2	2	2	2	2	2	2	2	2	2
	200	2	2	3	3	3	4	4	4	4	4	4	4	4	4	4	4
	300	3	3	4	5	5	5	5	5	5	5	5	5	6	6	6	6
	400	4	5	5	6	6	7	7	7	7	7	7	7	7	7	7	7
	500	5	6	7	7	8	8	8	8	9	9	9	9	9	9	9	9
	1000	9	11	12	14	15	15	16	16	16	16	16	16	16	17	17	17
	2000	17	20	22	25	26	27	27	27	28	28	28	28	28	29	29	29
	3000	24	27	30	33	34	36	36	36	37	37	37	37	38	38	38	38
	4000	29	33	37	40	41	43	43	43	44	44	44	44	45	45	45	45
	5000	34	39	42	46	47	49	49	49	49	50	50	50	51	51	51	51
	10000	53	57	61	64	65	67	67	67	67	68	68	68	68	69	69	69
	15000	64	68	71	74	75	76	76	76	77	77	77	77	77	78	78	78
	20000	71	75	78	80	81	82	82	82	82	82	83	83	83	83	83	83
	25000	77	80	82	84	85	86	86	86	86	86	86	86	87	87	87	87
	50000	91	92	93	94	94	95	95	95	95	95	95	95	95	95	95	95

Table 66

PREDICTIVE VALUE OF POSITIVES (IN PERCENT)
SPECIFICITY= 97.00%

							SENSITIVITY (%)									
		50	60	70	80	85	90	91	92	93	94	95	96	97	98	99	100
	1	0	0	0	0	0	0	0	0	0	0	0	0	0	0	0	0
	2	0	0	0	0	0	0	0	0	0	0	0	0	0	0	0	0
	3	0	0	0	0	0	0	0	0	0	0	0	0	0	0	0	0
PREVA-	4	0	0	0	0	0	0	0	0	0	0	0	0	0	0	0	0
LENCE	5	0	0	0	0	0	0	0	0	0	0	0	0	0	0	0	0
PER	10	0	0	0	0	0	0	0	0	0	0	0	0	0	0	0	0
100,000	20	0	0	0	1	1	1	1	1	1	1	1	1	1	1	1	1
	30	0	1	1	1	1	1	1	1	1	1	1	1	1	1	1	1
	40	1	1	1	1	1	1	1	1	1	1	1	1	1	1	1	1
	50	1	1	1	1	1	1	1	2	2	2	2	2	2	2	2	2
	100	2	2	2	3	3	3	3	3	3	3	3	3	3	3	3	3
	200	3	4	4	5	5	6	6	6	6	6	6	6	6	6	6	6
	300	5	6	7	7	8	8	8	8	9	9	9	9	9	9	9	9
	400	6	7	9	10	10	11	11	11	11	11	11	11	11	12	12	12
	500	8	9	10	12	12	13	13	13	13	14	14	14	14	14	14	14
	1000	14	17	19	21	22	23	23	24	24	24	24	24	25	25	25	25
	2000	25	29	32	35	37	38	38	38	39	39	39	40	40	40	40	40
	3000	34	38	42	45	47	48	48	49	49	49	49	50	50	50	51	51
	4000	41	45	49	53	54	56	56	56	56	57	57	57	57	58	58	58
	5000	47	51	55	58	60	61	61	62	62	62	63	63	63	63	63	64
	10000	65	69	72	75	76	77	77	77	78	78	78	78	78	78	79	79
	15000	75	78	80	82	83	84	84	84	85	85	85	85	85	85	85	85
	20000	81	83	85	87	88	88	88	88	89	89	89	89	89	89	89	89
	25000	85	87	89	90	90	91	91	91	91	91	91	91	92	92	92	92
	50000	94	95	96	96	97	97	97	97	97	97	97	97	97	97	97	97

Table 67

PREDICTIVE VALUE OF POSITIVES (IN PERCENT)
SPECIFICITY= 99.00%

							SENSITIVITY (%)									
		50	60	70	80	85	90	91	92	93	94	95	96	97	98	99	100
	1	0	0	0	0	0	0	0	0	0	0	0	0	0	0	0	0
	2	0	0	0	0	0	0	0	0	0	0	0	0	0	0	0	0
	3	0	0	0	0	0	0	0	0	0	0	0	0	0	0	0	0
PREVA-	4	0	0	0	0	0	0	0	0	0	0	0	0	0	0	0	0
LENCE	5	0	0	0	0	0	0	0	0	0	0	0	0	0	0	0	0
PER	10	0	1	1	1	1	1	1	1	1	1	1	1	1	1	1	1
100,000	20	1	1	1	2	2	2	2	2	2	2	2	2	2	2	2	2
	30	1	2	2	2	2	3	3	3	3	3	3	3	3	3	3	3
	40	2	2	3	3	3	3	4	4	4	4	4	4	4	4	4	4
	50	2	3	3	4	4	4	4	4	4	4	5	5	5	5	5	5
	100	5	6	7	7	8	8	8	8	9	9	9	9	9	9	9	9
	200	9	11	12	14	15	15	15	16	16	16	16	16	16	16	17	17
	300	13	15	17	19	20	21	21	22	22	22	22	22	23	23	23	23
	400	17	19	22	24	25	27	27	27	27	27	28	28	28	28	28	29
	500	20	23	26	29	30	31	31	32	32	32	32	33	33	33	33	33
	1000	34	38	41	45	46	48	48	48	48	49	49	49	49	50	50	50
	2000	51	55	59	62	63	65	65	65	65	66	66	66	66	67	67	67
	3000	61	65	68	71	72	74	74	74	74	74	75	75	75	75	75	76
	4000	68	71	74	77	78	79	79	79	79	80	80	80	80	80	80	81
	5000	72	76	79	81	82	83	83	83	83	83	83	83	84	84	84	84
	10000	85	87	89	90	90	91	91	91	91	91	91	91	92	92	92	92
	15000	90	91	93	93	94	94	94	94	94	94	94	94	94	95	95	95
	20000	93	94	95	95	96	96	96	96	96	96	96	96	96	96	96	96
	25000	94	95	96	96	97	97	97	97	97	97	97	97	97	97	97	97
	50000	98	98	99	99	99	99	99	99	99	99	99	99	99	99	99	99

Table 68

PREDICTIVE VALUE OF POSITIVES (IN PERCENT)
SPECIFICITY= 99.10%

								SENSITIVITY (%)									
		50	60	70	80	85	90	91	92	93	94	95	96	97	98	99	100
	1	0	0	0	0	0	0	0	0	0	0	0	0	0	0	0	0
	2	0	0	0	0	0	0	0	0	0	0	0	0	0	0	0	0
	3	0	0	0	0	0	0	0	0	0	0	0	0	0	0	0	0
PREVA-	4	0	0	0	0	0	0	0	0	0	0	0	0	0	0	0	0
LENCE	5	0	0	0	0	0	0	1	1	1	1	1	1	1	1	1	1
PER	10	1	1	1	1	1	1	1	1	1	1	1	1	1	1	1	1
100,000	20	1	1	2	2	2	2	2	2	2	2	2	2	2	2	2	2
	30	2	2	2	3	3	3	3	3	3	3	3	3	3	3	3	3
	40	2	3	3	3	4	4	4	4	4	4	4	4	4	4	4	4
	50	3	3	4	4	5	5	5	5	5	5	5	5	5	5	5	5
	100	5	6	7	8	9	9	9	9	9	9	10	10	10	10	10	10
	200	10	12	13	15	16	17	17	17	17	17	17	18	18	18	18	18
	300	14	17	19	21	22	23	23	24	24	24	24	24	24	25	25	25
	400	18	21	24	26	27	29	29	29	29	30	30	30	30	30	31	31
	500	22	25	28	31	32	33	34	34	34	34	35	35	35	35	36	36
	1000	36	40	44	47	49	50	51	51	51	51	52	52	52	52	53	53
	2000	53	58	61	64	66	67	67	68	68	68	68	69	69	69	69	69
	3000	63	67	71	73	74	76	76	76	76	76	77	77	77	77	77	77
	4000	70	74	76	79	80	81	81	81	81	81	81	82	82	82	82	82
	5000	75	78	80	82	83	84	84	84	84	85	85	85	85	85	85	85
	10000	86	88	90	91	91	92	92	92	92	92	92	92	92	92	92	93
	15000	91	92	93	94	94	95	95	95	95	95	95	95	95	95	95	95
	20000	93	94	95	96	96	96	96	96	96	96	96	96	96	96	96	97
	25000	95	96	96	97	97	97	97	97	97	97	97	97	97	97	97	97
	50000	98	99	99	99	99	99	99	99	99	99	99	99	99	99	99	99

Table 69

PREDICTIVE VALUE OF POSITIVES (IN PERCENT)
SPECIFICITY= 99.30%

								SENSITIVITY (%)									
		50	60	70	80	85	90	91	92	93	94	95	96	97	98	99	100
	1	0	0	0	0	0	0	0	0	0	0	0	0	0	0	0	0
	2	0	0	0	0	0	0	0	0	0	0	0	0	0	0	0	0
	3	0	0	0	0	0	0	0	0	0	0	0	0	0	0	0	0
PREVA-	4	0	0	0	0	0	1	1	1	1	1	1	1	1	1	1	1
LENCE	5	0	0	0	1	1	1	1	1	1	1	1	1	1	1	1	1
PER	10	1	1	1	1	1	1	1	1	1	1	1	1	1	1	1	1
100,000	20	1	2	2	2	2	3	3	3	3	3	3	3	3	3	3	3
	30	2	3	3	3	4	4	4	4	4	4	4	4	4	4	4	4
	40	3	3	4	4	5	5	5	5	5	5	5	5	5	5	5	5
	50	3	4	5	5	6	6	6	6	6	6	6	6	6	7	7	7
	100	7	8	9	10	11	11	12	12	12	12	12	12	12	12	12	13
	200	13	15	17	19	20	20	21	21	21	21	21	22	22	22	22	22
	300	18	21	23	26	27	28	28	28	29	29	29	29	29	30	30	30
	400	22	26	29	31	33	34	34	35	35	35	35	36	36	36	36	36
	500	26	30	33	36	38	39	40	40	40	40	41	41	41	41	42	42
	1000	42	46	50	54	55	56	57	57	57	58	58	58	58	59	59	59
	2000	59	64	67	70	71	72	73	73	73	73	73	74	74	74	74	74
	3000	69	73	76	78	79	80	80	80	80	81	81	81	81	81	81	82
	4000	75	78	81	83	83	84	84	85	85	85	85	85	85	85	85	86
	5000	79	82	84	86	86	87	87	87	87	88	88	88	88	88	88	88
	10000	89	90	92	93	93	93	94	94	94	94	94	94	94	94	94	94
	15000	93	94	95	95	96	96	96	96	96	96	96	96	96	96	96	96
	20000	95	96	96	97	97	97	97	97	97	97	97	97	97	97	97	97
	25000	96	97	97	97	98	98	98	98	98	98	98	98	98	98	98	98
	50000	99	99	99	99	99	99	99	99	99	99	99	99	99	99	99	99

Table 70

PREDICTIVE VALUE OF POSITIVES (IN PERCENT)
SPECIFICITY= 99.50%

							SENSITIVITY (%)									
		50	60	70	80	85	90	91	92	93	94	95	96	97	98	99	100
	1	0	0	0	0	0	0	0	0	0	0	0	0	0	0	0	0
	2	0	0	0	0	0	0	0	0	0	0	0	0	0	0	0	0
	3	0	0	0	0	1	1	1	1	1	1	1	1	1	1	1	1
PREVA–	4	0	0	1	1	1	1	1	1	1	1	1	1	1	1	1	1
LENCE	5	0	1	1	1	1	1	1	1	1	1	1	1	1	1	1	1
PER	10	1	1	1	2	2	2	2	2	2	2	2	2	2	2	2	2
100,000	20	2	2	3	3	3	3	4	4	4	4	4	4	4	4	4	4
	30	3	3	4	5	5	5	5	5	5	5	5	5	6	6	6	6
	40	4	5	5	6	6	7	7	7	7	7	7	7	7	7	7	7
	50	5	6	7	7	8	8	8	8	9	9	9	9	9	9	9	9
	100	9	11	12	14	15	15	15	16	16	16	16	16	16	16	17	17
	200	17	19	22	24	25	27	27	27	27	27	28	28	28	28	28	29
	300	23	27	30	32	34	35	35	36	36	36	36	37	37	37	37	38
	400	29	33	36	39	41	42	42	42	43	43	43	44	44	44	44	45
	500	33	38	41	45	46	47	48	48	48	49	49	49	49	50	50	50
	1000	50	55	59	62	63	65	65	65	65	66	66	66	66	66	67	67
	2000	67	71	74	77	78	79	79	79	79	79	79	80	80	80	80	80
	3000	76	79	81	83	84	85	85	85	85	85	85	86	86	86	86	86
	4000	81	83	85	87	88	88	88	88	89	89	89	89	89	89	89	89
	5000	84	86	88	89	90	90	91	91	91	91	91	91	91	91	91	91
	10000	92	93	94	95	95	95	95	95	95	95	95	96	96	96	96	96
	15000	95	95	96	97	97	97	97	97	97	97	97	97	97	97	97	97
	20000	96	97	97	98	98	98	98	98	98	98	98	98	98	98	98	98
	25000	97	98	98	98	98	98	98	98	98	98	98	98	98	98	99	99
	50000	99	99	99	99	99	99	99	99	99	99	99	99	99	99	99	100

Table 71

PREDICTIVE VALUE OF POSITIVES (IN PERCENT)
SPECIFICITY= 99.70%

							SENSITIVITY (%)									
		50	60	70	80	85	90	91	92	93	94	95	96	97	98	99	100
	1	0	0	0	0	0	0	0	0	0	0	0	0	0	0	0	0
	2	0	0	0	1	1	1	1	1	1	1	1	1	1	1	1	1
	3	0	1	1	1	1	1	1	1	1	1	1	1	1	1	1	1
PREVA–	4	1	1	1	1	1	1	1	1	1	1	1	1	1	1	1	1
LENCE	5	1	1	1	1	1	1	1	2	2	2	2	2	2	2	2	2
PER	10	2	2	2	3	3	3	3	3	3	3	3	3	3	3	3	3
100,000	20	3	4	4	5	5	6	6	6	6	6	6	6	6	6	6	6
	30	5	6	7	7	8	8	8	8	9	9	9	9	9	9	9	9
	40	6	7	9	10	10	11	11	11	11	11	11	11	11	12	12	12
	50	8	9	10	12	12	13	13	13	13	14	14	14	14	14	14	14
	100	14	17	19	21	22	23	23	23	24	24	24	24	24	25	25	25
	200	25	29	32	35	36	38	38	38	38	39	39	39	39	40	40	40
	300	33	38	41	45	46	47	48	48	48	49	49	49	49	50	50	50
	400	40	45	48	52	53	55	55	55	55	56	56	56	56	57	57	57
	500	46	50	54	57	59	60	60	61	61	61	61	62	62	62	62	63
	1000	63	67	70	73	74	75	75	76	76	76	76	76	77	77	77	77
	2000	77	80	83	84	85	86	86	86	86	86	87	87	87	87	87	87
	3000	84	86	88	89	90	90	90	90	91	91	91	91	91	91	91	91
	4000	87	89	91	92	92	93	93	93	93	93	93	93	93	93	93	93
	5000	90	91	92	93	94	94	94	94	94	94	94	94	94	95	95	95
	10000	95	96	96	97	97	97	97	97	97	97	97	97	97	97	97	97
	15000	97	97	98	98	98	98	98	98	98	98	98	98	98	98	98	98
	20000	98	98	98	99	99	99	99	99	99	99	99	99	99	99	99	99
	25000	98	99	99	99	99	99	99	99	99	99	99	99	99	99	99	99
	50000	99	100	100	100	100	100	100	100	100	100	100	100	100	100	100	100

Table 72

PREDICTIVE VALUE OF POSITIVES (IN PERCENT)
SPECIFICITY= 99.90%

		SENSITIVITY (%)														
		50	60	70	80	85	90	91	92	93	94	95	96	97	98	99	100
PREVA-LENCE	1	0	1	1	1	1	1	1	1	1	1	1	1	1	1	1	1
	2	1	1	1	2	2	2	2	2	2	2	2	2	2	2	2	2
	3	1	2	2	2	2	3	3	3	3	3	3	3	3	3	3	3
	4	2	2	3	3	3	3	4	4	4	4	4	4	4	4	4	4
	5	2	3	3	4	4	4	4	4	4	4	5	5	5	5	5	5
PER 100,000	10	5	6	7	7	8	8	8	8	9	9	9	9	9	9	9	9
	20	9	11	12	14	15	15	15	16	16	16	16	16	16	16	17	17
	30	13	15	17	19	20	21	21	22	22	22	22	22	23	23	23	23
	40	17	19	22	24	25	26	27	27	27	27	28	28	28	28	28	29
	50	20	23	26	29	30	31	31	32	32	32	32	32	33	33	33	33
	100	33	38	41	44	46	47	48	48	48	48	49	49	49	50	50	50
	200	50	55	58	62	63	64	65	65	65	65	66	66	66	66	66	67
	300	60	64	68	71	72	73	73	73	74	74	74	74	74	75	75	75
	400	67	71	74	76	77	78	79	79	79	79	79	79	79	80	80	80
	500	72	75	78	80	81	82	82	82	82	82	83	83	83	83	83	83
	1000	83	86	88	89	90	90	90	90	90	90	91	91	91	91	91	91
	2000	91	92	93	94	95	95	95	95	95	95	95	95	95	95	95	95
	3000	94	95	96	96	96	97	97	97	97	97	97	97	97	97	97	97
	4000	95	96	97	97	97	97	97	97	97	98	98	98	98	98	98	98
	5000	96	97	97	98	98	98	98	98	98	98	98	98	98	98	98	98
	10000	98	99	99	99	99	99	99	99	99	99	99	99	99	99	99	99
	15000	99	99	99	99	99	99	99	99	99	99	99	99	99	99	99	99
	20000	99	99	99	100	100	100	100	100	100	100	100	100	100	100	100	100
	25000	99	100	100	100	100	100	100	100	100	100	100	100	100	100	100	100
	50000	100	100	100	100	100	100	100	100	100	100	100	100	100	100	100	100

Table 73

PREDICTIVE VALUE OF POSITIVES (IN PERCENT)
SPECIFICITY= 99.91%

		SENSITIVITY (%)														
		50	60	70	80	85	90	91	92	93	94	95	96	97	98	99	100
PREVA-LENCE	1	1	1	1	1	1	1	1	1	1	1	1	1	1	1	1	1
	2	1	1	2	2	2	2	2	2	2	2	2	2	2	2	2	2
	3	2	2	2	3	3	3	3	3	3	3	3	3	3	3	3	3
	4	2	3	3	3	4	4	4	4	4	4	4	4	4	4	4	4
	5	3	3	4	4	5	5	5	5	5	5	5	5	5	5	5	5
PER 100,000	10	5	6	7	8	9	9	9	9	9	9	10	10	10	10	10	10
	20	10	12	13	15	16	17	17	17	17	17	17	18	18	18	18	18
	30	14	17	19	21	22	23	23	23	24	24	24	24	24	25	25	25
	40	18	21	24	26	27	29	29	29	29	29	30	30	30	30	31	31
	50	22	25	28	31	32	33	34	34	34	34	35	35	35	35	35	36
	100	36	40	44	47	49	50	50	51	51	51	51	52	52	52	52	53
	200	53	57	61	64	65	67	67	67	67	68	68	68	68	69	69	69
	300	63	67	70	73	74	75	75	75	76	76	76	76	76	77	77	77
	400	69	73	76	78	79	80	80	80	81	81	81	81	81	81	82	82
	500	74	77	80	82	83	83	84	84	84	84	84	84	84	85	85	85
	1000	85	87	89	90	91	91	91	91	91	91	91	92	92	92	92	92
	2000	92	93	94	95	95	95	95	95	95	96	96	96	96	96	96	96
	3000	94	95	96	96	97	97	97	97	97	97	97	97	97	97	97	97
	4000	96	97	97	97	98	98	98	98	98	98	98	98	98	98	98	98
	5000	97	97	98	98	98	98	98	98	98	98	98	98	98	98	98	98
	10000	98	99	99	99	99	99	99	99	99	99	99	99	99	99	99	99
	15000	99	99	99	99	99	99	99	99	99	99	99	99	99	99	99	99
	20000	99	99	99	100	100	100	100	100	100	100	100	100	100	100	100	100
	25000	99	100	100	100	100	100	100	100	100	100	100	100	100	100	100	100
	50000	100	100	100	100	100	100	100	100	100	100	100	100	100	100	100	100

Table 74

PREDICTIVE VALUE OF POSITIVES (IN PERCENT)
SPECIFICITY= 99.92%

								SENSITIVITY (%)								
		50	60	70	80	85	90	91	92	93	94	95	96	97	98	99	100
PREVA-LENCE	1	1	1	1	1	1	1	1	1	1	1	1	1	1	1	1	1
	2	1	1	2	2	2	2	2	2	2	2	2	2	2	2	2	2
	3	2	2	3	3	3	3	3	3	3	3	3	3	4	4	4	4
	4	2	3	3	4	4	4	4	4	4	4	5	5	5	5	5	5
	5	3	4	4	5	5	5	5	5	5	6	6	6	6	6	6	6
PER 100,000	10	6	7	8	9	10	10	10	10	10	11	11	11	11	11	11	11
	20	11	13	15	17	18	18	19	19	19	19	19	20	20	20	20	20
	30	16	18	21	23	24	25	25	26	26	26	26	26	27	27	27	27
	40	20	23	26	29	30	31	31	32	32	32	32	32	33	33	33	33
	50	24	27	30	33	35	36	36	37	37	37	37	38	38	38	38	38
	100	38	43	47	50	52	53	53	54	54	54	54	55	55	55	55	56
	200	56	60	64	67	68	69	70	70	70	70	70	71	71	71	71	71
	300	65	69	72	75	76	77	77	78	78	78	78	78	78	79	79	79
	400	72	75	78	80	81	82	82	82	82	83	83	83	83	83	83	83
	500	76	79	81	83	84	85	85	85	85	86	86	86	86	86	86	86
	1000	86	88	90	91	91	92	92	92	92	92	92	92	92	93	93	93
	2000	93	94	95	95	96	96	96	96	96	96	96	96	96	96	96	96
	3000	95	96	96	97	97	97	97	97	97	97	97	97	97	97	97	97
	4000	96	97	97	98	98	98	98	98	98	98	98	98	98	98	98	98
	5000	97	98	98	98	98	98	98	98	98	98	98	98	98	98	98	99
	10000	99	99	99	99	99	99	99	99	99	99	99	99	99	99	99	99
	15000	99	99	99	99	99	99	100	100	100	100	100	100	100	100	100	100
	20000	99	99	100	100	100	100	100	100	100	100	100	100	100	100	100	100
	25000	100	100	100	100	100	100	100	100	100	100	100	100	100	100	100	100
	50000	100	100	100	100	100	100	100	100	100	100	100	100	100	100	100	100

Table 75

PREDICTIVE VALUE OF POSITIVES (IN PERCENT)
SPECIFICITY= 99.93%

								SENSITIVITY (%)								
		50	60	70	80	85	90	91	92	93	94	95	96	97	98	99	100
PREVA-LENCE	1	1	1	1	1	1	1	1	1	1	1	1	1	1	1	1	1
	2	1	2	2	2	2	3	3	3	3	3	3	3	3	3	3	3
	3	2	3	3	3	4	4	4	4	4	4	4	4	4	4	4	4
	4	3	3	4	4	5	5	5	5	5	5	5	5	5	5	5	5
	5	3	4	5	5	6	6	6	6	6	6	6	6	6	7	7	7
PER 100,000	10	7	8	9	10	11	11	12	12	12	12	12	12	12	12	12	12
	20	13	15	17	19	20	20	21	21	21	21	21	22	22	22	22	22
	30	18	20	23	26	27	28	28	28	29	29	29	29	29	30	30	30
	40	22	26	29	31	33	34	34	34	35	35	35	35	36	36	36	36
	50	26	30	33	36	38	39	39	40	40	40	40	41	41	41	41	42
	100	42	46	50	53	55	56	57	57	57	57	58	58	58	58	59	59
	200	59	63	67	70	71	72	72	72	73	73	73	74	74	74	74	74
	300	68	72	75	77	79	79	80	80	80	80	80	80	81	81	81	81
	400	74	77	80	82	83	84	84	84	84	84	84	85	85	85	85	85
	500	78	81	83	85	86	87	87	87	87	87	87	87	87	88	88	88
	1000	88	90	91	92	92	93	93	93	93	93	93	93	93	93	93	94
	2000	94	95	95	96	96	96	96	96	96	96	97	97	97	97	97	97
	3000	96	96	97	97	97	98	98	98	98	98	98	98	98	98	98	98
	4000	97	97	98	98	98	98	98	98	98	98	98	98	98	98	98	98
	5000	97	98	98	98	98	99	99	99	99	99	99	99	99	99	99	99
	10000	99	99	99	99	99	99	99	99	99	99	99	99	99	99	99	99
	15000	99	99	99	100	100	100	100	100	100	100	100	100	100	100	100	100
	20000	99	100	100	100	100	100	100	100	100	100	100	100	100	100	100	100
	25000	100	100	100	100	100	100	100	100	100	100	100	100	100	100	100	100
	50000	100	100	100	100	100	100	100	100	100	100	100	100	100	100	100	100

Table 76

PREDICTIVE VALUE OF POSITIVES (IN PERCENT)
SPECIFICITY= 99.94%

		50	60	70	80	85	90	91	92	93	94	95	96	97	98	99	100
								SENSITIVITY (%)									
	1	1	1	1	1	1	1	1	2	2	2	2	2	2	2	2	2
	2	2	2	2	3	3	3	3	3	3	3	3	3	3	3	3	3
	3	2	3	3	4	4	4	4	4	4	4	5	5	5	5	5	5
PREVA-	4	3	4	4	5	5	6	6	6	6	6	6	6	6	6	6	6
LENCE	5	4	5	6	6	7	7	7	7	7	7	7	7	7	8	8	8
PER	10	8	9	10	12	12	13	13	13	13	14	14	14	14	14	14	14
100,000	20	14	17	19	21	22	23	23	23	24	24	24	24	24	25	25	25
	30	20	23	26	29	30	31	31	32	32	32	32	32	33	33	33	33
	40	25	29	32	35	36	38	38	38	38	39	39	39	39	40	40	40
	50	29	33	37	40	41	43	43	43	44	44	44	44	45	45	45	45
	100	45	50	54	57	59	60	60	61	61	61	61	62	62	62	62	63
	200	63	67	70	73	74	75	75	75	76	76	76	76	76	77	77	77
	300	71	75	78	80	81	82	82	82	82	82	83	83	83	83	83	83
	400	77	80	82	84	85	86	86	86	86	86	86	87	87	87	87	87
	500	81	83	85	87	88	88	88	89	89	89	89	89	89	89	89	89
	1000	89	91	92	93	93	94	94	94	94	94	94	94	94	94	94	94
	2000	94	95	96	96	97	97	97	97	97	97	97	97	97	97	97	97
	3000	96	97	97	98	98	98	98	98	98	98	98	98	98	98	98	98
	4000	97	98	98	98	98	98	98	98	98	98	99	99	99	99	99	99
	5000	98	98	98	99	99	99	99	99	99	99	99	99	99	99	99	99
	10000	99	99	99	99	99	99	99	99	99	99	99	99	99	99	99	99
	15000	99	99	100	100	100	100	100	100	100	100	100	100	100	100	100	100
	20000	100	100	100	100	100	100	100	100	100	100	100	100	100	100	100	100
	25000	100	100	100	100	100	100	100	100	100	100	100	100	100	100	100	100
	50000	100	100	100	100	100	100	100	100	100	100	100	100	100	100	100	100

Table 77

PREDICTIVE VALUE OF POSITIVES (IN PERCENT)
SPECIFICITY= 99.95%

		50	60	70	80	85	90	91	92	93	94	95	96	97	98	99	100
								SENSITIVITY (%)									
	1	1	1	1	2	2	2	2	2	2	2	2	2	2	2	2	2
	2	2	2	3	3	3	3	4	4	4	4	4	4	4	4	4	4
	3	3	3	4	5	5	5	5	5	5	5	5	5	5	6	6	6
PREVA-	4	4	5	5	6	6	7	7	7	7	7	7	7	7	7	7	7
LENCE	5	5	6	7	7	8	8	8	8	9	9	9	9	9	9	9	9
PER	10	9	11	12	14	15	15	15	16	16	16	16	16	16	16	17	17
100,000	20	17	19	22	24	25	26	27	27	27	27	28	28	28	28	28	29
	30	23	26	30	32	34	35	35	36	36	36	36	37	37	37	37	38
	40	29	32	36	39	40	42	42	42	43	43	43	43	44	44	44	44
	50	33	38	41	44	46	47	48	48	48	48	49	49	49	50	50	50
	100	50	55	58	62	63	64	65	65	65	65	66	66	66	66	66	67
	200	67	71	74	76	77	78	78	79	79	79	79	79	80	80	80	80
	300	75	78	81	83	84	84	85	85	85	85	85	85	85	86	86	86
	400	80	83	85	87	87	88	88	88	88	88	88	89	89	89	89	89
	500	83	86	88	89	90	90	90	90	90	90	91	91	91	91	91	91
	1000	91	92	93	94	94	95	95	95	95	95	95	95	95	95	95	95
	2000	95	96	97	97	97	97	97	97	97	97	97	98	98	98	98	98
	3000	97	97	98	98	98	98	98	98	98	98	98	98	98	98	98	98
	4000	98	98	98	99	99	99	99	99	99	99	99	99	99	99	99	99
	5000	98	98	99	99	99	99	99	99	99	99	99	99	99	99	99	99
	10000	99	99	99	99	99	100	100	100	100	100	100	100	100	100	100	100
	15000	99	100	100	100	100	100	100	100	100	100	100	100	100	100	100	100
	20000	100	100	100	100	100	100	100	100	100	100	100	100	100	100	100	100
	25000	100	100	100	100	100	100	100	100	100	100	100	100	100	100	100	100
	50000	100	100	100	100	100	100	100	100	100	100	100	100	100	100	100	100

Table 78

PREDICTIVE VALUE OF POSITIVES (IN PERCENT)
SPECIFICITY= 99.96%

		SENSITIVITY (%)														
		50	60	70	80	85	90	91	92	93	94	95	96	97	98	99	100
	1	1	1	2	2	2	2	2	2	2	2	2	2	2	2	2	2
	2	2	3	3	4	4	4	4	4	4	4	5	5	5	5	5	5
	3	4	4	5	6	6	6	6	6	7	7	7	7	7	7	7	7
PREVA-	4	5	6	7	7	8	8	8	8	9	9	9	9	9	9	9	9
LENCE	5	6	7	8	9	10	10	10	10	10	11	11	11	11	11	11	11
PER	10	11	13	15	17	18	18	19	19	19	19	19	19	20	20	20	20
100,000	20	20	23	26	29	30	31	31	32	32	32	32	32	33	33	33	33
	30	27	31	34	38	39	40	41	41	41	41	42	42	42	42	43	43
	40	33	38	41	44	46	47	48	48	48	48	49	49	49	49	50	50
	50	38	43	47	50	52	53	53	53	54	54	54	55	55	55	55	56
	100	56	60	64	67	68	69	69	70	70	70	70	71	71	71	71	71
	200	71	75	78	80	81	82	82	82	82	82	83	83	83	83	83	83
	300	79	82	84	86	86	87	87	87	87	88	88	88	88	88	88	88
	400	83	86	88	89	90	90	90	90	90	90	91	91	91	91	91	91
	500	86	88	90	91	91	92	92	92	92	92	92	92	92	92	93	93
	1000	93	94	95	95	96	96	96	96	96	96	96	96	96	96	96	96
	2000	96	97	97	98	98	98	98	98	98	98	98	98	98	98	98	98
	3000	97	98	98	98	99	99	99	99	99	99	99	99	99	99	99	.99
	4000	98	98	99	99	99	99	99	99	99	99	99	99	99	99	99	99
	5000	99	99	99	99	99	99	99	99	99	99	99	99	99	99	99	99
	10000	99	99	99	100	100	100	100	100	100	100	100	100	100	100	100	100
	15000	100	100	100	100	100	100	100	100	100	100	100	100	100	100	100	100
	20000	100	100	100	100	100	100	100	100	100	100	100	100	100	100	100	100
	25000	100	100	100	100	100	100	100	100	100	100	100	100	100	100	100	100
	50000	100	100	100	100	100	100	100	100	100	100	100	100	100	100	100	100

Table 79

PREDICTIVE VALUE OF POSITIVES (IN PERCENT)
SPECIFICITY= 99.97%

		SENSITIVITY (%)														
		50	60	70	80	85	90	91	92	93	94	95	96	97	98	99	100
	1	2	2	2	3	3	3	3	3	3	3	3	3	3	3	3	3
	2	3	4	4	5	5	6	6	6	6	6	6	6	6	6	6	6
	3	5	6	7	7	8	8	8	8	9	9	9	9	9	9	9	9
PREVA-	4	6	7	9	10	10	11	11	11	11	11	11	11	11	11	12	12
LENCE	5	8	9	10	12	12	13	13	13	13	13	14	14	14	14	14	14
PER	10	14	17	19	21	22	23	23	23	24	24	24	24	24	25	25	25
100,000	20	25	29	32	35	36	37	38	38	38	39	39	39	39	40	40	40
	30	33	37	41	44	46	47	48	48	48	48	49	49	49	49	50	50
	40	40	44	48	52	53	55	55	55	55	56	56	56	56	57	57	57
	50	45	50	54	57	59	60	60	61	61	61	61	62	62	62	62	63
	100	63	67	70	73	74	75	75	75	76	76	76	76	76	77	77	77
	200	77	80	82	84	85	86	86	86	86	86	86	87	87	87	87	87
	300	83	86	88	89	89	90	90	90	90	90	90	91	91	91	91	91
	400	87	89	90	91	92	92	92	92	93	93	93	93	93	93	93	93
	500	89	91	92	93	93	94	94	94	94	94	94	94	94	94	94	94
	1000	94	95	96	96	97	97	97	97	97	97	97	97	97	97	97	97
	2000	97	98	98	98	98	98	98	98	98	98	98	98	99	99	99	99.
	3000	98	98	99	99	99	99	99	99	99	99	99	99	99	99	99	99
	4000	99	99	99	99	99	99	99	99	99	99	99	99	99	99	99	99
	5000	99	99	99	99	99	99	99	99	99	99	99	99	99	99	99	99
	10000	99	100	100	100	100	100	100	100	100	100	100	100	100	100	100	100
	15000	100	100	100	100	100	100	100	100	100	100	100	100	100	100	100	100
	20000	100	100	100	100	100	100	100	100	100	100	100	100	100	100	100	100
	25000	100	100	100	100	100	100	100	100	100	100	100	100	100	100	100	100
	50000	100	100	100	100	100	100	100	100	100	100	100	100	100	100	100	100

Table 80

PREDICTIVE VALUE OF POSITIVES (IN PERCENT)
SPECIFICITY= 99.98%

		50	60	70	80	85	90	91	92	93	94	95	96	97	98	99	100
								SENSITIVITY (%)									
PREVA-LENCE	1	2	3	3	4	4	4	4	4	4	4	5	5	5	5	5	5
	2	5	6	7	7	8	8	8	8	9	9	9	9	9	9	9	9
	3	7	8	10	11	11	12	12	12	12	12	12	13	13	13	13	13
	4	9	11	12	14	15	15	15	16	16	16	16	16	16	16	17	17
	5	11	13	15	17	18	18	19	19	19	19	19	19	20	20	20	20
PER 100,000	10	20	23	26	29	30	31	31	32	32	32	32	32	33	33	33	33
	20	33	37	41	44	46	47	48	48	48	48	49	49	49	49	50	50
	30	43	47	51	55	56	57	58	58	58	59	59	59	59	60	60	60
	40	50	55	58	62	63	64	65	65	65	65	66	66	66	66	66	67
	50	56	60	64	67	68	69	69	70	70	70	70	71	71	71	71	71
	100	71	75	78	80	81	82	82	82	82	82	83	83	83	83	83	83
	200	83	86	88	89	89	90	90	90	90	90	90	91	91	91	91	91
	300	88	90	91	92	93	93	93	93	93	93	93	94	94	94	94	94
	400	91	92	93	94	94	95	95	95	95	95	95	95	95	95	95	95
	500	93	94	95	95	96	96	96	96	96	96	96	96	96	96	96	96
	1000	96	97	97	98	98	98	98	98	98	98	98	98	98	98	98	98
	2000	98	98	99	99	99	99	99	99	99	99	99	99	99	99	99	99
	3000	99	99	99	99	99	99	99	99	99	99	99	99	99	99	99	99
	4000	99	99	99	99	99	99	99	99	99	99	99	100	100	100	100	100
	5000	99	99	99	100	100	100	100	100	100	100	100	100	100	100	100	100
	10000	100	100	100	100	100	100	100	100	100	100	100	100	100	100	100	100
	15000	100	100	100	100	100	100	100	100	100	100	100	100	100	100	100	100
	20000	100	100	100	100	100	100	100	100	100	100	100	100	100	100	100	100
	25000	100	100	100	100	100	100	100	100	100	100	100	100	100	100	100	100
	50000	100	100	100	100	100	100	100	100	100	100	100	100	100	100	100	100

Table 81

PREDICTIVE VALUE OF POSITIVES (IN PERCENT)
SPECIFICITY= 99.99%

		50	60	70	80	85	90	91	92	93	94	95	96	97	98	99	100
								SENSITIVITY (%)									
PREVA-LENCE	1	5	6	7	7	8	8	8	8	9	9	9	9	9	9	9	9
	2	9	11	12	14	15	15	15	16	16	16	16	16	16	16	17	17
	3	13	15	17	19	20	21	21	22	22	22	22	22	23	23	23	23
	4	17	19	22	24	25	26	27	27	27	27	28	28	28	28	28	29
	5	20	23	26	29	30	31	31	31	32	32	32	32	33	33	33	33
PER 100,000	10	33	37	41	44	46	47	48	48	48	48	49	49	49	49	50	50
	20	50	55	58	62	63	64	65	65	65	65	65	66	66	66	66	67
	30	60	64	68	71	72	73	73	73	74	74	74	74	74	75	75	75
	40	67	71	74	76	77	78	78	79	79	79	79	79	79	80	80	80
	50	71	75	78	80	81	82	82	82	82	82	83	83	83	83	83	83
	100	83	86	88	89	89	90	90	90	90	90	90	91	91	91	91	91
	200	91	92	93	94	94	95	95	95	95	95	95	95	95	95	95	95
	300	94	95	95	96	96	96	96	97	97	97	97	97	97	97	97	97
	400	95	96	97	97	97	97	97	97	97	97	97	97	97	98	98	98
	500	96	97	97	98	98	98	98	98	98	98	98	98	98	98	98	98
	1000	98	98	99	99	99	99	99	99	99	99	99	99	99	99	99	99
	2000	99	99	99	99	99	99	99	99	99	99	99	99	99	100	100	100
	3000	99	99	100	100	100	100	100	100	100	100	100	100	100	100	100	100
	4000	100	100	100	100	100	100	100	100	100	100	100	100	100	100	100	100
	5000	100	100	100	100	100	100	100	100	100	100	100	100	100	100	100	100
	10000	100	100	100	100	100	100	100	100	100	100	100	100	100	100	100	100
	15000	100	100	100	100	100	100	100	100	100	100	100	100	100	100	100	100
	20000	100	100	100	100	100	100	100	100	100	100	100	100	100	100	100	100
	25000	100	100	100	100	100	100	100	100	100	100	100	100	100	100	100	100
	50000	100	100	100	100	100	100	100	100	100	100	100	100	100	100	100	100

Table 82

PREDICTIVE VALUE OF POSITIVES (IN PERCENT)
SPECIFICITY=100.00%

SENSITIVITY (%)

		50	60	70	80	85	90	91	92	93	94	95	96	97	98	99	100
	1	100	100	100	100	100	100	100	100	100	100	100	100	100	100	100	100
	2	100	100	100	100	100	100	100	100	100	100	100	100	100	100	100	100
	3	100	100	100	100	100	100	100	100	100	100	100	100	100	100	100	100
PREVA-	4	100	100	100	100	100	100	100	100	100	100	100	100	100	100	100	100
LENCE	5	100	100	100	100	100	100	100	100	100	100	100	100	100	100	100	100
PER	10	100	100	100	100	100	100	100	100	100	100	100	100	100	100	100	100
100,000	20	100	100	100	100	100	100	100	100	100	100	100	100	100	100	100	100
	30	100	100	100	100	100	100	100	100	100	100	100	100	100	100	100	100
	40	100	100	100	100	100	100	100	100	100	100	100	100	100	100	100	100
	50	100	100	100	100	100	100	100	100	100	100	100	100	100	100	100	100
	100	100	100	100	100	100	100	100	100	100	100	100	100	100	100	100	100
	200	100	100	100	100	100	100	100	100	100	100	100	100	100	100	100	100
	300	100	100	100	100	100	100	100	100	100	100	100	100	100	100	100	100
	400	100	100	100	100	100	100	100	100	100	100	100	100	100	100	100	100
	500	100	100	100	100	100	100	100	100	100	100	100	100	100	100	100	100
	1000	100	100	100	100	100	100	100	100	100	100	100	100	100	100	100	100
	2000	100	100	100	100	100	100	100	100	100	100	100	100	100	100	100	100
	3000	100	100	100	100	100	100	100	100	100	100	100	100	100	100	100	100
	4000	100	100	100	100	100	100	100	100	100	100	100	100	100	100	100	100
	5000	100	100	100	100	100	100	100	100	100	100	100	100	100	100	100	100
	10000	100	100	100	100	100	100	100	100	100	100	100	100	100	100	100	100
	15000	100	100	100	100	100	100	100	100	100	100	100	100	100	100	100	100
	20000	100	100	100	100	100	100	100	100	100	100	100	100	100	100	100	100
	25000	100	100	100	100	100	100	100	100	100	100	100	100	100	100	100	100
	50000	100	100	100	100	100	100	100	100	100	100	100	100	100	100	100	100

PREDICTIVE VALUE OF A NEGATIVE TEST BASED ON
TEST SENSITIVITY, SPECIFICITY, AND DISEASE PREVALENCE*

Three relationships are possible between sensitivity and specificity for any test. The sensitivity may be greater than the specificity, the sensitivity may be equal to the specificity, or the sensitivity may be less than the specificity. Let us review what happens to the predictive value of a negative test under each of these circumstances in the face of fixed as well as increasing disease prevalence:

At a given prevalence, an incremental increase in sensitivity results in a greater increase in the predictive value of a negative test than the same incremental increase in specificity. As prevalence increases, the predictive value of a negative test decreases regardless of the relationship between sensitivity and specificity.

Table 83

PREDICTIVE VALUE OF NEGATIVES (IN PERCENT)
PREVALENCE=   1 PER 100,000

SENSITIVITY (%)

		50	60	70	80	85	90	91	92	93	94	95	96	97	98	99	100
	50.00	100	100	100	100	100	100	100	100	100	100	100	100	100	100	100	100
	60.00	100	100	100	100	100	100	100	100	100	100	100	100	100	100	100	100
	70.00	100	100	100	100	100	100	100	100	100	100	100	100	100	100	100	100
SPECI-	80.00	100	100	100	100	100	100	100	100	100	100	100	100	100	100	100	100
FICITY	90.00	100	100	100	100	100	100	100	100	100	100	100	100	100	100	100	100
(%)	91.00	100	100	100	100	100	100	100	100	100	100	100	100	100	100	100	100
	93.00	100	100	100	100	100	100	100	100	100	100	100	100	100	100	100	100
	95.00	100	100	100	100	100	100	100	100	100	100	100	100	100	100	100	100
	97.00	100	100	100	100	100	100	100	100	100	100	100	100	100	100	100	100
	99.00	100	100	100	100	100	100	100	100	100	100	100	100	100	100	100	100
	99.10	100	100	100	100	100	100	100	100	100	100	100	100	100	100	100	100
	99.30	100	100	100	100	100	100	100	100	100	100	100	100	100	100	100	100
	99.50	100	100	100	100	100	100	100	100	100	100	100	100	100	100	100	100
	99.70	100	100	100	100	100	100	100	100	100	100	100	100	100	100	100	100
	99.90	100	100	100	100	100	100	100	100	100	100	100	100	100	100	100	100
	99.91	100	100	100	100	100	100	100	100	100	100	100	100	100	100	100	100
	99.92	100	100	100	100	100	100	100	100	100	100	100	100	100	100	100	100
	99.93	100	100	100	100	100	100	100	100	100	100	100	100	100	100	100	100
	99.94	100	100	100	100	100	100	100	100	100	100	100	100	100	100	100	100
	99.95	100	100	100	100	100	100	100	100	100	100	100	100	100	100	100	100
	99.96	100	100	100	100	100	100	100	100	100	100	100	100	100	100	100	100
	99.97	100	100	100	100	100	100	100	100	100	100	100	100	100	100	100	100
	99.98	100	100	100	100	100	100	100	100	100	100	100	100	100	100	100	100
	99.99	100	100	100	100	100	100	100	100	100	100	100	100	100	100	100	100
	100.00	100	100	100	100	100	100	100	100	100	100	100	100	100	100	100	100

Table 84

PREDICTIVE VALUE OF NEGATIVES (IN PERCENT)
PREVALENCE=   2 PER 100,000

SENSITIVITY (%)

		50	60	70	80	85	90	91	92	93	94	95	96	97	98	99	100
	50.00	100	100	100	100	100	100	100	100	100	100	100	100	100	100	100	100
	60.00	100	100	100	100	100	100	100	100	100	100	100	100	100	100	100	100
	70.00	100	100	100	100	100	100	100	100	100	100	100	100	100	100	100	100
SPECI-	80.00	100	100	100	100	100	100	100	100	100	100	100	100	100	100	100	100
FICITY	90.00	100	100	100	100	100	100	100	100	100	100	100	100	100	100	100	100
(%)	91.00	100	100	100	100	100	100	100	100	100	100	100	100	100	100	100	100
	93.00	100	100	100	100	100	100	100	100	100	100	100	100	100	100	100	100
	95.00	100	100	100	100	100	100	100	100	100	100	100	100	100	100	100	100
	97.00	100	100	100	100	100	100	100	100	100	100	100	100	100	100	100	100
	99.00	100	100	100	100	100	100	100	100	100	100	100	100	100	100	100	100
	99.10	100	100	100	100	100	100	100	100	100	100	100	100	100	100	100	100
	99.30	100	100	100	100	100	100	100	100	100	100	100	100	100	100	100	100
	99.50	100	100	100	100	100	100	100	100	100	100	100	100	100	100	100	100
	99.70	100	100	100	100	100	100	100	100	100	100	100	100	100	100	100	100
	99.90	100	100	100	100	100	100	100	100	100	100	100	100	100	100	100	100
	99.91	100	100	100	100	100	100	100	100	100	100	100	100	100	100	100	100
	99.92	100	100	100	100	100	100	100	100	100	100	100	100	100	100	100	100
	99.93	100	100	100	100	100	100	100	100	100	100	100	100	100	100	100	100
	99.94	100	100	100	100	100	100	100	100	100	100	100	100	100	100	100	100
	99.95	100	100	100	100	100	100	100	100	100	100	100	100	100	100	100	100
	99.96	100	100	100	100	100	100	100	100	100	100	100	100	100	100	100	100
	99.97	100	100	100	100	100	100	100	100	100	100	100	100	100	100	100	100
	99.98	100	100	100	100	100	100	100	100	100	100	100	100	100	100	100	100
	99.99	100	100	100	100	100	100	100	100	100	100	100	100	100	100	100	100
	100.00	100	100	100	100	100	100	100	100	100	100	100	100	100	100	100	100

Table 85

PREDICTIVE VALUE OF NEGATIVES (IN PERCENT)
PREVALENCE=   3 PER 100,000

								SENSITIVITY (%)								
		50	60	70	80	85	90	91	92	93	94	95	96	97	98	99	100
	50.00	100	100	100	100	100	100	100	100	100	100	100	100	100	100	100	100
	60.00	100	100	100	100	100	100	100	100	100	100	100	100	100	100	100	100
	70.00	100	100	100	100	100	100	100	100	100	100	100	100	100	100	100	100
SPECI-	80.00	100	100	100	100	100	100	100	100	100	100	100	100	100	100	100	100
FICITY	90.00	100	100	100	100	100	100	100	100	100	100	100	100	100	100	100	100
(%)	91.00	100	100	100	100	100	100	100	100	100	100	100	100	100	100	100	100
	93.00	100	100	100	100	100	100	100	100	100	100	100	100	100	100	100	100
	95.00	100	100	100	100	100	100	100	100	100	100	100	100	100	100	100	100
	97.00	100	100	100	100	100	100	100	100	100	100	100	100	100	100	100	100
	99.00	100	100	100	100	100	100	100	100	100	100	100	100	100	100	100	100
	99.10	100	100	100	100	100	100	100	100	100	100	100	100	100	100	100	100
	99.30	100	100	100	100	100	100	100	100	100	100	100	100	100	100	100	100
	99.50	100	100	100	100	100	100	100	100	100	100	100	100	100	100	100	100
	99.70	100	100	100	100	100	100	100	100	100	100	100	100	100	100	100	100
	99.90	100	100	100	100	100	100	100	100	100	100	100	100	100	100	100	100
	99.91	100	100	100	100	100	100	100	100	100	100	100	100	100	100	100	100
	99.92	100	100	100	100	100	100	100	100	100	100	100	100	100	100	100	100
	99.93	100	100	100	100	100	100	100	100	100	100	100	100	100	100	100	100
	99.94	100	100	100	100	100	100	100	100	100	100	100	100	100	100	100	100
	99.95	100	100	100	100	100	100	100	100	100	100	100	100	100	100	100	100
	99.96	100	100	100	100	100	100	100	100	100	100	100	100	100	100	100	100
	99.97	100	100	100	100	100	100	100	100	100	100	100	100	100	100	100	100
	99.98	100	100	100	100	100	100	100	100	100	100	100	100	100	100	100	100
	99.99	100	100	100	100	100	100	100	100	100	100	100	100	100	100	100	100
	100.00	100	100	100	100	100	100	100	100	100	100	100	100	100	100	100	100

Table 86

PREDICTIVE VALUE OF NEGATIVES (IN PERCENT)
PREVALENCE=   4 PER 100,000

								SENSITIVITY (%)								
		50	60	70	80	85	90	91	92	93	94	95	96	97	98	99	100
	50.00	100	100	100	100	100	100	100	100	100	100	100	100	100	100	100	100
	60.00	100	100	100	100	100	100	100	100	100	100	100	100	100	100	100	100
	70.00	100	100	100	100	100	100	100	100	100	100	100	100	100	100	100	100
SPECI-	80.00	100	100	100	100	100	100	100	100	100	100	100	100	100	100	100	100
FICITY	90.00	100	100	100	100	100	100	100	100	100	100	100	100	100	100	100	100
(%)	91.00	100	100	100	100	100	100	100	100	100	100	100	100	100	100	100	100
	93.00	100	100	100	100	100	100	100	100	100	100	100	100	100	100	100	100
	95.00	100	100	100	100	100	100	100	100	100	100	100	100	100	100	100	100
	97.00	100	100	100	100	100	100	100	100	100	100	100	100	100	100	100	100
	99.00	100	100	100	100	100	100	100	100	100	100	100	100	100	100	100	100
	99.10	100	100	100	100	100	100	100	100	100	100	100	100	100	100	100	100
	99.30	100	100	100	100	100	100	100	100	100	100	100	100	100	100	100	100
	99.50	100	100	100	100	100	100	100	100	100	100	100	100	100	100	100	100
	99.70	100	100	100	100	100	100	100	100	100	100	100	100	100	100	100	100
	99.90	100	100	100	100	100	100	100	100	100	100	100	100	100	100	100	100
	99.91	100	100	100	100	100	100	100	100	100	100	100	100	100	100	100	100
	99.92	100	100	100	100	100	100	100	100	100	100	100	100	100	100	100	100
	99.93	100	100	100	100	100	100	100	100	100	100	100	100	100	100	100	100
	99.94	100	100	100	100	100	100	100	100	100	100	100	100	100	100	100	100
	99.95	100	100	100	100	100	100	100	100	100	100	100	100	100	100	100	100
	99.96	100	100	100	100	100	100	100	100	100	100	100	100	100	100	100	100
	99.97	100	100	100	100	100	100	100	100	100	100	100	100	100	100	100	100
	99.98	100	100	100	100	100	100	100	100	100	100	100	100	100	100	100	100
	99.99	100	100	100	100	100	100	100	100	100	100	100	100	100	100	100	100
	100.00	100	100	100	100	100	100	100	100	100	100	100	100	100	100	100	100

Table 87

PREDICTIVE VALUE OF NEGATIVES (IN PERCENT)
PREVALENCE=   5 PER 100,000

SENSITIVITY (%)

		50	60	70	80	85	90	91	92	93	94	95	96	97	98	99	100
	50.00	100	100	100	100	100	100	100	100	100	100	100	100	100	100	100	100
	60.00	100	100	100	100	100	100	100	100	100	100	100	100	100	100	100	100
	70.00	100	100	100	100	100	100	100	100	100	100	100	100	100	100	100	100
SPECI-	80.00	100	100	100	100	100	100	100	100	100	100	100	100	100	100	100	100
FICITY	90.00	100	100	100	100	100	100	100	100	100	100	100	100	100	100	100	100
(%)	91.00	100	100	100	100	100	100	100	100	100	100	100	100	100	100	100	100
	93.00	100	100	100	100	100	100	100	100	100	100	100	100	100	100	100	100
	95.00	100	100	100	100	100	100	100	100	100	100	100	100	100	100	100	100
	97.00	100	100	100	100	100	100	100	100	100	100	100	100	100	100	100	100
	99.00	100	100	100	100	100	100	100	100	100	100	100	100	100	100	100	100
	99.10	100	100	100	100	100	100	100	100	100	100	100	100	100	100	100	100
	99.30	100	100	100	100	100	100	100	100	100	100	100	100	100	100	100	100
	99.50	100	100	100	100	100	100	100	100	100	100	100	100	100	100	100	100
	99.70	100	100	100	100	100	100	100	100	100	100	100	100	100	100	100	100
	99.90	100	100	100	100	100	100	100	100	100	100	100	100	100	100	100	100
	99.91	100	100	100	100	100	100	100	100	100	100	100	100	100	100	100	100
	99.92	100	100	100	100	100	100	100	100	100	100	100	100	100	100	100	100
	99.93	100	100	100	100	100	100	100	100	100	100	100	100	100	100	100	100
	99.94	100	100	100	100	100	100	100	100	100	100	100	100	100	100	100	100
	99.95	100	100	100	100	100	100	100	100	100	100	100	100	100	100	100	100
	99.96	100	100	100	100	100	100	100	100	100	100	100	100	100	100	100	100
	99.97	100	100	100	100	100	100	100	100	100	100	100	100	100	100	100	100
	99.98	100	100	100	100	100	100	100	100	100	100	100	100	100	100	100	100
	99.99	100	100	100	100	100	100	100	100	100	100	100	100	100	100	100	100
	100.00	100	100	100	100	100	100	100	100	100	100	100	100	100	100	100	100

Table 88

PREDICTIVE VALUE OF NEGATIVES (IN PERCENT)
PREVALENCE=   10 PER 100,000

SENSITIVITY (%)

		50	60	70	80	85	90	91	92	93	94	95	96	97	98	99	100
	50.00	100	100	100	100	100	100	100	100	100	100	100	100	100	100	100	100
	60.00	100	100	100	100	100	100	100	100	100	100	100	100	100	100	100	100
	70.00	100	100	100	100	100	100	100	100	100	100	100	100	100	100	100	100
SPECI-	80.00	100	100	100	100	100	100	100	100	100	100	100	100	100	100	100	100
FICITY	90.00	100	100	100	100	100	100	100	100	100	100	100	100	100	100	100	100
(%)	91.00	100	100	100	100	100	100	100	100	100	100	100	100	100	100	100	100
	93.00	100	100	100	100	100	100	100	100	100	100	100	100	100	100	100	100
	95.00	100	100	100	100	100	100	100	100	100	100	100	100	100	100	100	100
	97.00	100	100	100	100	100	100	100	100	100	100	100	100	100	100	100	100
	99.00	100	100	100	100	100	100	100	100	100	100	100	100	100	100	100	100
	99.10	100	100	100	100	100	100	100	100	100	100	100	100	100	100	100	100
	99.30	100	100	100	100	100	100	100	100	100	100	100	100	100	100	100	100
	99.50	100	100	100	100	100	100	100	100	100	100	100	100	100	100	100	100
	99.70	100	100	100	100	100	100	100	100	100	100	100	100	100	100	100	100
	99.90	100	100	100	100	100	100	100	100	100	100	100	100	100	100	100	100
	99.91	100	100	100	100	100	100	100	100	100	100	100	100	100	100	100	100
	99.92	100	100	100	100	100	100	100	100	100	100	100	100	100	100	100	100
	99.93	100	100	100	100	100	100	100	100	100	100	100	100	100	100	100	100
	99.94	100	100	100	100	100	100	100	100	100	100	100	100	100	100	100	100
	99.95	100	100	100	100	100	100	100	100	100	100	100	100	100	100	100	100
	99.96	100	100	100	100	100	100	100	100	100	100	100	100	100	100	100	100
	99.97	100	100	100	100	100	100	100	100	100	100	100	100	100	100	100	100
	99.98	100	100	100	100	100	100	100	100	100	100	100	100	100	100	100	100
	99.99	100	100	100	100	100	100	100	100	100	100	100	100	100	100	100	100
	100.00	100	100	100	100	100	100	100	100	100	100	100	100	100	100	100	100

Table 89

PREDICTIVE VALUE OF NEGATIVES (IN PERCENT)
PREVALENCE=   20 PER 100,000

SENSITIVITY (%)

		50	60	70	80	85	90	91	92	93	94	95	96	97	98	99	100
	50.00	100	100	100	100	100	100	100	100	100	100	100	100	100	100	100	100
	60.00	100	100	100	100	100	100	100	100	100	100	100	100	100	100	100	100
	70.00	100	100	100	100	100	100	100	100	100	100	100	100	100	100	100	100
SPECI-	80.00	100	100	100	100	100	100	100	100	100	100	100	100	100	100	100	100
FICITY	90.00	100	100	100	100	100	100	100	100	100	100	100	100	100	100	100	100
(%)	91.00	100	100	100	100	100	100	100	100	100	100	100	100	100	100	100	100
	93.00	100	100	100	100	100	100	100	100	100	100	100	100	100	100	100	100
	95.00	100	100	100	100	100	100	100	100	100	100	100	100	100	100	100	100
	97.00	100	100	100	100	100	100	100	100	100	100	100	100	100	100	100	100
	99.00	100	100	100	100	100	100	100	100	100	100	100	100	100	100	100	100
	99.10	100	100	100	100	100	100	100	100	100	100	100	100	100	100	100	100
	99.30	100	100	100	100	100	100	100	100	100	100	100	100	100	100	100	100
	99.50	100	100	100	100	100	100	100	100	100	100	100	100	100	100	100	100
	99.70	100	100	100	100	100	100	100	100	100	100	100	100	100	100	100	100
	99.90	100	100	100	100	100	100	100	100	100	100	100	100	100	100	100	100
	99.91	100	100	100	100	100	100	100	100	100	100	100	100	100	100	100	100
	99.92	100	100	100	100	100	100	100	100	100	100	100	100	100	100	100	100
	99.93	100	100	100	100	100	100	100	100	100	100	100	100	100	100	100	100
	99.94	100	100	100	100	100	100	100	100	100	100	100	100	100	100	100	100
	99.95	100	100	100	100	100	100	100	100	100	100	100	100	100	100	100	100
	99.96	100	100	100	100	100	100	100	100	100	100	100	100	100	100	100	100
	99.97	100	100	100	100	100	100	100	100	100	100	100	100	100	100	100	100
	99.98	100	100	100	100	100	100	100	100	100	100	100	100	100	100	100	100
	99.99	100	100	100	100	100	100	100	100	100	100	100	100	100	100	100	100
	100.00	100	100	100	100	100	100	100	100	100	100	100	100	100	100	100	100

Table 90

PREDICTIVE VALUE OF NEGATIVES (IN PERCENT)
PREVALENCE=   30 PER 100,000

SENSITIVITY (%)

		50	60	70	80	85	90	91	92	93	94	95	96	97	98	99	100
	50.00	100	100	100	100	100	100	100	100	100	100	100	100	100	100	100	100
	60.00	100	100	100	100	100	100	100	100	100	100	100	100	100	100	100	100
	70.00	100	100	100	100	100	100	100	100	100	100	100	100	100	100	100	100
SPECI-	80.00	100	100	100	100	100	100	100	100	100	100	100	100	100	100	100	100
FICITY	90.00	100	100	100	100	100	100	100	100	100	100	100	100	100	100	100	100
(%)	91.00	100	100	100	100	100	100	100	100	100	100	100	100	100	100	100	100
	93.00	100	100	100	100	100	100	100	100	100	100	100	100	100	100	100	100
	95.00	100	100	100	100	100	100	100	100	100	100	100	100	100	100	100	100
	97.00	100	100	100	100	100	100	100	100	100	100	100	100	100	100	100	100
	99.00	100	100	100	100	100	100	100	100	100	100	100	100	100	100	100	100
	99.10	100	100	100	100	100	100	100	100	100	100	100	100	100	100	100	100
	99.30	100	100	100	100	100	100	100	100	100	100	100	100	100	100	100	100
	99.50	100	100	100	100	100	100	100	100	100	100	100	100	100	100	100	100
	99.70	100	100	100	100	100	100	100	100	100	100	100	100	100	100	100	100
	99.90	100	100	100	100	100	100	100	100	100	100	100	100	100	100	100	100
	99.91	100	100	100	100	100	100	100	100	100	100	100	100	100	100	100	100
	99.92	100	100	100	100	100	100	100	100	100	100	100	100	100	100	100	100
	99.93	100	100	100	100	100	100	100	100	100	100	100	100	100	100	100	100
	99.94	100	100	100	100	100	100	100	100	100	100	100	100	100	100	100	100
	99.95	100	100	100	100	100	100	100	100	100	100	100	100	100	100	100	100
	99.96	100	100	100	100	100	100	100	100	100	100	100	100	100	100	100	100
	99.97	100	100	100	100	100	100	100	100	100	100	100	100	100	100	100	100
	99.98	100	100	100	100	100	100	100	100	100	100	100	100	100	100	100	100
	99.99	100	100	100	100	100	100	100	100	100	100	100	100	100	100	100	100
	100.00	100	100	100	100	100	100	100	100	100	100	100	100	100	100	100	100

Table 91

PREDICTIVE VALUE OF NEGATIVES (IN PERCENT)
PREVALENCE=   40 PER 100,000

		SENSITIVITY (%)														
		50	60	70	80	85	90	91	92	93	94	95	96	97	98	99	100
	50.00	100	100	100	100	100	100	100	100	100	100	100	100	100	100	100	100
	60.00	100	100	100	100	100	100	100	100	100	100	100	100	100	100	100	100
	70.00	100	100	100	100	100	100	100	100	100	100	100	100	100	100	100	100
SPECI-	80.00	100	100	100	100	100	100	100	100	100	100	100	100	100	100	100	100
FICITY	90.00	100	100	100	100	100	100	100	100	100	100	100	100	100	100	100	100
(%)	91.00	100	100	100	100	100	100	100	100	100	100	100	100	100	100	100	100
	93.00	100	100	100	100	100	100	100	100	100	100	100	100	100	100	100	100
	95.00	100	100	100	100	100	100	100	100	100	100	100	100	100	100	100	100
	97.00	100	100	100	100	100	100	100	100	100	100	100	100	100	100	100	100
	99.00	100	100	100	100	100	100	100	100	100	100	100	100	100	100	100	100
	99.10	100	100	100	100	100	100	100	100	100	100	100	100	100	100	100	100
	99.30	100	100	100	100	100	100	100	100	100	100	100	100	100	100	100	100
	99.50	100	100	100	100	100	100	100	100	100	100	100	100	100	100	100	100
	99.70	100	100	100	100	100	100	100	100	100	100	100	100	100	100	100	100
	99.90	100	100	100	100	100	100	100	100	100	100	100	100	100	100	100	100
	99.91	100	100	100	100	100	100	100	100	100	100	100	100	100	100	100	100
	99.92	100	100	100	100	100	100	100	100	100	100	100	100	100	100	100	100
	99.93	100	100	100	100	100	100	100	100	100	100	100	100	100	100	100	100
	99.94	100	100	100	100	100	100	100	100	100	100	100	100	100	100	100	100
	99.95	100	100	100	100	100	100	100	100	100	100	100	100	100	100	100	100
	99.96	100	100	100	100	100	100	100	100	100	100	100	100	100	100	100	100
	99.97	100	100	100	100	100	100	100	100	100	100	100	100	100	100	100	100
	99.98	100	100	100	100	100	100	100	100	100	100	100	100	100	100	100	100
	99.99	100	100	100	100	100	100	100	100	100	100	100	100	100	100	100	100
	100.00	100	100	100	100	100	100	100	100	100	100	100	100	100	100	100	100

Table 92

PREDICTIVE VALUE OF NEGATIVES (IN PERCENT)
PREVALENCE=   50 PER 100,000

		SENSITIVITY (%)														
		50	60	70	80	85	90	91	92	93	94	95	96	97	98	99	100
	50.00	100	100	100	100	100	100	100	100	100	100	100	100	100	100	100	100
	60.00	100	100	100	100	100	100	100	100	100	100	100	100	100	100	100	100
	70.00	100	100	100	100	100	100	100	100	100	100	100	100	100	100	100	100
SPECI-	80.00	100	100	100	100	100	100	100	100	100	100	100	100	100	100	100	100
FICITY	90.00	100	100	100	100	100	100	100	100	100	100	100	100	100	100	100	100
(%)	91.00	100	100	100	100	100	100	100	100	100	100	100	100	100	100	100	100
	93.00	100	100	100	100	100	100	100	100	100	100	100	100	100	100	100	100
	95.00	100	100	100	100	100	100	100	100	100	100	100	100	100	100	100	100
	97.00	100	100	100	100	100	100	100	100	100	100	100	100	100	100	100	100
	99.00	100	100	100	100	100	100	100	100	100	100	100	100	100	100	100	100
	99.10	100	100	100	100	100	100	100	100	100	100	100	100	100	100	100	100
	99.30	100	100	100	100	100	100	100	100	100	100	100	100	100	100	100	100
	99.50	100	100	100	100	100	100	100	100	100	100	100	100	100	100	100	100
	99.70	100	100	100	100	100	100	100	100	100	100	100	100	100	100	100	100
	99.90	100	100	100	100	100	100	100	100	100	100	100	100	100	100	100	100
	99.91	100	100	100	100	100	100	100	100	100	100	100	100	100	100	100	100
	99.92	100	100	100	100	100	100	100	100	100	100	100	100	100	100	100	100
	99.93	100	100	100	100	100	100	100	100	100	100	100	100	100	100	100	100
	99.94	100	100	100	100	100	100	100	100	100	100	100	100	100	100	100	100
	99.95	100	100	100	100	100	100	100	100	100	100	100	100	100	100	100	100
	99.96	100	100	100	100	100	100	100	100	100	100	100	100	100	100	100	100
	99.97	100	100	100	100	100	100	100	100	100	100	100	100	100	100	100	100
	99.98	100	100	100	100	100	100	100	100	100	100	100	100	100	100	100	100
	99.99	100	100	100	100	100	100	100	100	100	100	100	100	100	100	100	100
	100.00	100	100	100	100	100	100	100	100	100	100	100	100	100	100	100	100

Table 93

PREDICTIVE VALUE OF NEGATIVES (IN PERCENT)
PREVALENCE= 100 PER 100,000

SENSITIVITY (%)

		50	60	70	80	85	90	91	92	93	94	95	96	97	98	99	100
	50.00	100	100	100	100	100	100	100	100	100	100	100	100	100	100	100	100
	60.00	100	100	100	100	100	100	100	100	100	100	100	100	100	100	100	100
	70.00	100	100	100	100	100	100	100	100	100	100	100	100	100	100	100	100
SPECI-	80.00	100	100	100	100	100	100	100	100	100	100	100	100	100	100	100	100
FICITY	90.00	100	100	100	100	100	100	100	100	100	100	100	100	100	100	100	100
(%)	91.00	100	100	100	100	100	100	100	100	100	100	100	100	100	100	100	100
	93.00	100	100	100	100	100	100	100	100	100	100	100	100	100	100	100	100
	95.00	100	100	100	100	100	100	100	100	100	100	100	100	100	100	100	100
	97.00	100	100	100	100	100	100	100	100	100	100	100	100	100	100	100	100
	99.00	100	100	100	100	100	100	100	100	100	100	100	100	100	100	100	100
	99.10	100	100	100	100	100	100	100	100	100	100	100	100	100	100	100	100
	99.30	100	100	100	100	100	100	100	100	100	100	100	100	100	100	100	100
	99.50	100	100	100	100	100	100	100	100	100	100	100	100	100	100	100	100
	99.70	100	100	100	100	100	100	100	100	100	100	100	100	100	100	100	100
	99.90	100	100	100	100	100	100	100	100	100	100	100	100	100	100	100	100
	99.91	100	100	100	100	100	100	100	100	100	100	100	100	100	100	100	100
	99.92	100	100	100	100	100	100	100	100	100	100	100	100	100	100	100	100
	99.93	100	100	100	100	100	100	100	100	100	100	100	100	100	100	100	100
	99.94	100	100	100	100	100	100	100	100	100	100	100	100	100	100	100	100
	99.95	100	100	100	100	100	100	100	100	100	100	100	100	100	100	100	100
	99.96	100	100	100	100	100	100	100	100	100	100	100	100	100	100	100	100
	99.97	100	100	100	100	100	100	100	100	100	100	100	100	100	100	100	100
	99.98	100	100	100	100	100	100	100	100	100	100	100	100	100	100	100	100
	99.99	100	100	100	100	100	100	100	100	100	100	100	100	100	100	100	100
	100.00	100	100	100	100	100	100	100	100	100	100	100	100	100	100	100	100

Table 94

PREDICTIVE VALUE OF NEGATIVES (IN PERCENT)
PREVALENCE= 200 PER 100,000

SENSITIVITY (%)

		50	60	70	80	85	90	91	92	93	94	95	96	97	98	99	100
	50.00	100	100	100	100	100	100	100	100	100	100	100	100	100	100	100	100
	60.00	100	100	100	100	100	100	100	100	100	100	100	100	100	100	100	100
	70.00	100	100	100	100	100	100	100	100	100	100	100	100	100	100	100	100
SPECI-	80.00	100	100	100	100	100	100	100	100	100	100	100	100	100	100	100	100
FICITY	90.00	100	100	100	100	100	100	100	100	100	100	100	100	100	100	100	100
(%)	91.00	100	100	100	100	100	100	100	100	100	100	100	100	100	100	100	100
	93.00	100	100	100	100	100	100	100	100	100	100	100	100	100	100	100	100
	95.00	100	100	100	100	100	100	100	100	100	100	100	100	100	100	100	100
	97.00	100	100	100	100	100	100	100	100	100	100	100	100	100	100	100	100
	99.00	100	100	100	100	100	100	100	100	100	100	100	100	100	100	100	100
	99.10	100	100	100	100	100	100	100	100	100	100	100	100	100	100	100	100
	99.30	100	100	100	100	100	100	100	100	100	100	100	100	100	100	100	100
	99.50	100	100	100	100	100	100	100	100	100	100	100	100	100	100	100	100
	99.70	100	100	100	100	100	100	100	100	100	100	100	100	100	100	100	100
	99.90	100	100	100	100	100	100	100	100	100	100	100	100	100	100	100	100
	99.91	100	100	100	100	100	100	100	100	100	100	100	100	100	100	100	100
	99.92	100	100	100	100	100	100	100	100	100	100	100	100	100	100	100	100
	99.93	100	100	100	100	100	100	100	100	100	100	100	100	100	100	100	100
	99.94	100	100	100	100	100	100	100	100	100	100	100	100	100	100	100	100
	99.95	100	100	100	100	100	100	100	100	100	100	100	100	100	100	100	100
	99.96	100	100	100	100	100	100	100	100	100	100	100	100	100	100	100	100
	99.97	100	100	100	100	100	100	100	100	100	100	100	100	100	100	100	100
	99.98	100	100	100	100	100	100	100	100	100	100	100	100	100	100	100	100
	99.99	100	100	100	100	100	100	100	100	100	100	100	100	100	100	100	100
	100.00	100	100	100	100	100	100	100	100	100	100	100	100	100	100	100	100

Table 95

SENSITIVITY (%)

	50	60	70	80	85	90	91	92	93	94	95	96	97	98	99	100
50.00	100	100	100	100	100	100	100	100	100	100	100	100	100	100	100	100
60.00	100	100	100	100	100	100	100	100	100	100	100	100	100	100	100	100
70.00	100	100	100	100	100	100	100	100	100	100	100	100	100	100	100	100
SPECI- 80.00	100	100	100	100	100	100	100	100	100	100	100	100	100	100	100	100
FICITY 90.00	100	100	100	100	100	100	100	100	100	100	100	100	100	100	100	100
(%) 91.00	100	100	100	100	100	100	100	100	100	100	100	100	100	100	100	100
93.00	100	100	100	100	100	100	100	100	100	100	100	100	100	100	100	100
95.00	100	100	100	100	100	100	100	100	100	100	100	100	100	100	100	100
97.00	100	100	100	100	100	100	100	100	100	100	100	100	100	100	100	100
99.00	100	100	100	100	100	100	100	100	100	100	100	100	100	100	100	100
99.10	100	100	100	100	100	100	100	100	100	100	100	100	100	100	100	100
99.30	100	100	100	100	100	100	100	100	100	100	100	100	100	100	100	100
99.50	100	100	100	100	100	100	100	100	100	100	100	100	100	100	100	100
99.70	100	100	100	100	100	100	100	100	100	100	100	100	100	100	100	100
99.90	100	100	100	100	100	100	100	100	100	100	100	100	100	100	100	100
99.91	100	100	100	100	100	100	100	100	100	100	100	100	100	100	100	100
99.92	100	100	100	100	100	100	100	100	100	100	100	100	100	100	100	100
99.93	100	100	100	100	100	100	100	100	100	100	100	100	100	100	100	100
99.94	100	100	100	100	100	100	100	100	100	100	100	100	100	100	100	100
99.95	100	100	100	100	100	100	100	100	100	100	100	100	100	100	100	100
99.96	100	100	100	100	100	100	100	100	100	100	100	100	100	100	100	100
99.97	100	100	100	100	100	100	100	100	100	100	100	100	100	100	100	100
99.98	100	100	100	100	100	100	100	100	100	100	100	100	100	100	100	100
99.99	100	100	100	100	100	100	100	100	100	100	100	100	100	100	100	100
100.00	100	100	100	100	100	100	100	100	100	100	100	100	100	100	100	100

Table 96

SENSITIVITY (%)

	50	60	70	80	85	90	91	92	93	94	95	96	97	98	99	100
50.00	100	100	100	100	100	100	100	100	100	100	100	100	100	100	100	100
60.00	100	100	100	100	100	100	100	100	100	100	100	100	100	100	100	100
70.00	100	100	100	100	100	100	100	100	100	100	100	100	100	100	100	100
SPECI- 80.00	100	100	100	100	100	100	100	100	100	100	100	100	100	100	100	100
FICITY 90.00	100	100	100	100	100	100	100	100	100	100	100	100	100	100	100	100
(%) 91.00	100	100	100	100	100	100	100	100	100	100	100	100	100	100	100	100
93.00	100	100	100	100	100	100	100	100	100	100	100	100	100	100	100	100
95.00	100	100	100	100	100	100	100	100	100	100	100	100	100	100	100	100
97.00	100	100	100	100	100	100	100	100	100	100	100	100	100	100	100	100
99.00	100	100	100	100	100	100	100	100	100	100	100	100	100	100	100	100
99.10	100	100	100	100	100	100	100	100	100	100	100	100	100	100	100	100
99.30	100	100	100	100	100	100	100	100	100	100	100	100	100	100	100	100
99.50	100	100	100	100	100	100	100	100	100	100	100	100	100	100	100	100
99.70	100	100	100	100	100	100	100	100	100	100	100	100	100	100	100	100
99.90	100	100	100	100	100	100	100	100	100	100	100	100	100	100	100	100
99.91	100	100	100	100	100	100	100	100	100	100	100	100	100	100	100	100
99.92	100	100	100	100	100	100	100	100	100	100	100	100	100	100	100	100
99.93	100	100	100	100	100	100	100	100	100	100	100	100	100	100	100	100
99.94	100	100	100	100	100	100	100	100	100	100	100	100	100	100	100	100
99.95	100	100	100	100	100	100	100	100	100	100	100	100	100	100	100	100
99.96	100	100	100	100	100	100	100	100	100	100	100	100	100	100	100	100
99.97	100	100	100	100	100	100	100	100	100	100	100	100	100	100	100	100
99.98	100	100	100	100	100	100	100	100	100	100	100	100	100	100	100	100
99.99	100	100	100	100	100	100	100	100	100	100	100	100	100	100	100	100
100.00	100	100	100	100	100	100	100	100	100	100	100	100	100	100	100	100

Table 97

PREDICTIVE VALUE OF NEGATIVES (IN PERCENT)
PREVALENCE= 500 PER 100,000

		\multicolumn{16}{c}{SENSITIVITY (%)}														
		50	60	70	80	85	90	91	92	93	94	95	96	97	98	99	100
	50.00	100	100	100	100	100	100	100	100	100	100	100	100	100	100	100	100
	60.00	100	100	100	100	100	100	100	100	100	100	100	100	100	100	100	100
	70.00	100	100	100	100	100	100	100	100	100	100	100	100	100	100	100	100
SPECI-	80.00	100	100	100	100	100	100	100	100	100	100	100	100	100	100	100	100
FICITY	90.00	100	100	100	100	100	100	100	100	100	100	100	100	100	100	100	100
(%)	91.00	100	100	100	100	100	100	100	100	100	100	100	100	100	100	100	100
	93.00	100	100	100	100	100	100	100	100	100	100	100	100	100	100	100	100
	95.00	100	100	100	100	100	100	100	100	100	100	100	100	100	100	100	100
	97.00	100	100	100	100	100	100	100	100	100	100	100	100	100	100	100	100
	99.00	100	100	100	100	100	100	100	100	100	100	100	100	100	100	100	100
	99.10	100	100	100	100	100	100	100	100	100	100	100	100	100	100	100	100
	99.30	100	100	100	100	100	100	100	100	100	100	100	100	100	100	100	100
	99.50	100	100	100	100	100	100	100	100	100	100	100	100	100	100	100	100
	99.70	100	100	100	100	100	100	100	100	100	100	100	100	100	100	100	100
	99.90	100	100	100	100	100	100	100	100	100	100	100	100	100	100	100	100
	99.91	100	100	100	100	100	100	100	100	100	100	100	100	100	100	100	100
	99.92	100	100	100	100	100	100	100	100	100	100	100	100	100	100	100	100
	99.93	100	100	100	100	100	100	100	100	100	100	100	100	100	100	100	100
	99.94	100	100	100	100	100	100	100	100	100	100	100	100	100	100	100	100
	99.95	100	100	100	100	100	100	100	100	100	100	100	100	100	100	100	100
	99.96	100	100	100	100	100	100	100	100	100	100	100	100	100	100	100	100
	99.97	100	100	100	100	100	100	100	100	100	100	100	100	100	100	100	100
	99.98	100	100	100	100	100	100	100	100	100	100	100	100	100	100	100	100
	99.99	100	100	100	100	100	100	100	100	100	100	100	100	100	100	100	100
	100.00	100	100	100	100	100	100	100	100	100	100	100	100	100	100	100	100

Table 98

PREDICTIVE VALUE OF NEGATIVES (IN PERCENT)
PREVALENCE= 1000 PER 100,000

		\multicolumn{16}{c}{SENSITIVITY (%)}														
		50	60	70	80	85	90	91	92	93	94	95	96	97	98	99	100
	50.00	99	99	99	100	100	100	100	100	100	100	100	100	100	100	100	100
	60.00	99	99	99	100	100	100	100	100	100	100	100	100	100	100	100	100
	70.00	99	99	100	100	100	100	100	100	100	100	100	100	100	100	100	100
SPECI-	80.00	99	99	100	100	100	100	100	100	100	100	100	100	100	100	100	100
FICITY	90.00	99	100	100	100	100	100	100	100	100	100	100	100	100	100	100	100
(%)	91.00	99	100	100	100	100	100	100	100	100	100	100	100	100	100	100	100
	93.00	99	100	100	100	100	100	100	100	100	100	100	100	100	100	100	100
	95.00	99	100	100	100	100	100	100	100	100	100	100	100	100	100	100	100
	97.00	99	100	100	100	100	100	100	100	100	100	100	100	100	100	100	100
	99.00	99	100	100	100	100	100	100	100	100	100	100	100	100	100	100	100
	99.10	99	100	100	100	100	100	100	100	100	100	100	100	100	100	100	100
	99.30	99	100	100	100	100	100	100	100	100	100	100	100	100	100	100	100
	99.50	99	100	100	100	100	100	100	100	100	100	100	100	100	100	100	100
	99.70	99	100	100	100	100	100	100	100	100	100	100	100	100	100	100	100
	99.90	99	100	100	100	100	100	100	100	100	100	100	100	100	100	100	100
	99.91	99	100	100	100	100	100	100	100	100	100	100	100	100	100	100	100
	99.92	99	100	100	100	100	100	100	100	100	100	100	100	100	100	100	100
	99.93	99	100	100	100	100	100	100	100	100	100	100	100	100	100	100	100
	99.94	99	100	100	100	100	100	100	100	100	100	100	100	100	100	100	100
	99.95	99	100	100	100	100	100	100	100	100	100	100	100	100	100	100	100
	99.96	99	100	100	100	100	100	100	100	100	100	100	100	100	100	100	100
	99.97	99	100	100	100	100	100	100	100	100	100	100	100	100	100	100	100
	99.98	99	100	100	100	100	100	100	100	100	100	100	100	100	100	100	100
	99.99	99	100	100	100	100	100	100	100	100	100	100	100	100	100	100	100
	100.00	99	100	100	100	100	100	100	100	100	100	100	100	100	100	100	100

Table 99

PREDICTIVE VALUE OF NEGATIVES (IN PERCENT)
PREVALENCE= 2000 PER 100,000

		SENSITIVITY (%)														
		50	60	70	80	85	90	91	92	93	94	95	96	97	98	99	100
SPECI-FICITY (%)	50.00	98	98	99	99	99	100	100	100	100	100	100	100	100	100	100	100
	60.00	98	99	99	99	99	100	100	100	100	100	100	100	100	100	100	100
	70.00	99	99	99	99	100	100	100	100	100	100	100	100	100	100	100	100
	80.00	99	99	99	99	100	100	100	100	100	100	100	100	100	100	100	100
	90.00	99	99	99	100	100	100	100	100	100	100	100	100	100	100	100	100
	91.00	99	99	99	100	100	100	100	100	100	100	100	100	100	100	100	100
	93.00	99	99	99	100	100	100	100	100	100	100	100	100	100	100	100	100
	95.00	99	99	99	100	100	100	100	100	100	100	100	100	100	100	100	100
	97.00	99	99	99	100	100	100	100	100	100	100	100	100	100	100	100	100
	99.00	99	99	99	100	100	100	100	100	100	100	100	100	100	100	100	100
	99.10	99	99	99	100	100	100	100	100	100	100	100	100	100	100	100	100
	99.30	99	99	99	100	100	100	100	100	100	100	100	100	100	100	100	100
	99.50	99	99	99	100	100	100	100	100	100	100	100	100	100	100	100	100
	99.70	99	99	99	100	100	100	100	100	100	100	100	100	100	100	100	100
	99.90	99	99	99	100	100	100	100	100	100	100	100	100	100	100	100	100
	99.91	99	99	99	100	100	100	100	100	100	100	100	100	100	100	100	100
	99.92	99	99	99	100	100	100	100	100	100	100	100	100	100	100	100	100
	99.93	99	99	99	100	100	100	100	100	100	100	100	100	100	100	100	100
	99.94	99	99	99	100	100	100	100	100	100	100	100	100	100	100	100	100
	99.95	99	99	99	100	100	100	100	100	100	100	100	100	100	100	100	100
	99.96	99	99	99	100	100	100	100	100	100	100	100	100	100	100	100	100
	99.97	99	99	99	100	100	100	100	100	100	100	100	100	100	100	100	100
	99.98	99	99	99	100	100	100	100	100	100	100	100	100	100	100	100	100
	99.99	99	99	99	100	100	100	100	100	100	100	100	100	100	100	100	100
	100.00	99	99	99	100	100	100	100	100	100	100	100	100	100	100	100	100

Table 100

PREDICTIVE VALUE OF NEGATIVES (IN PERCENT)
PREVALENCE= 3000 PER 100,000

		SENSITIVITY (%)														
		50	60	70	80	85	90	91	92	93	94	95	96	97	98	99	100
SPECI-FICITY (%)	50.00	57	98	98	99	99	99	99	100	100	100	100	100	100	100	100	100
	60.00	97	98	98	99	99	99	100	100	100	100	100	100	100	100	100	100
	70.00	98	98	99	99	99	100	100	100	100	100	100	100	100	100	100	100
	80.00	98	98	99	99	99	100	100	100	100	100	100	100	100	100	100	100
	90.00	98	99	99	99	99	100	100	100	100	100	100	100	100	100	100	100
	91.00	98	99	99	99	99	100	100	100	100	100	100	100	100	100	100	100
	93.00	98	99	99	99	100	100	100	100	100	100	100	100	100	100	100	100
	95.00	98	99	99	99	100	100	100	100	100	100	100	100	100	100	100	100
	97.00	98	99	99	99	100	100	100	100	100	100	100	100	100	100	100	100
	99.00	98	99	99	99	100	100	100	100	100	100	100	100	100	100	100	100
	99.10	98	99	99	99	100	100	100	100	100	100	100	100	100	100	100	100
	99.30	98	99	99	99	100	100	100	100	100	100	100	100	100	100	100	100
	99.50	98	99	99	99	100	100	100	100	100	100	100	100	100	100	100	100
	99.70	98	99	99	99	100	100	100	100	100	100	100	100	100	100	100	100
	99.90	98	99	99	99	100	100	100	100	100	100	100	100	100	100	100	100
	99.91	98	99	99	99	100	100	100	100	100	100	100	100	100	100	100	100
	99.92	98	99	99	99	100	100	100	100	100	100	100	100	100	100	100	100
	99.93	98	99	99	99	100	100	100	100	100	100	100	100	100	100	100	100
	99.94	98	99	99	99	100	100	100	100	100	100	100	100	100	100	100	100
	99.95	98	99	99	99	100	100	100	100	100	100	100	100	100	100	100	100
	99.96	98	99	99	99	100	100	100	100	100	100	100	100	100	100	100	100
	99.97	98	99	99	99	100	100	100	100	100	100	100	100	100	100	100	100
	99.98	98	99	99	99	100	100	100	100	100	100	100	100	100	100	100	100
	99.99	98	99	99	99	100	100	100	100	100	100	100	100	100	100	100	100
	100.00	98	99	99	99	100	100	100	100	100	100	100	100	100	100	100	100

Table 101

PREDICTIVE VALUE OF NEGATIVES (IN PERCENT)
PREVALENCE= 4000 PER 100,000

		50	60	70	80	85	90	91	92	93	94	95	96	97	98	99	100
							SENSITIVITY (%)										
	50.00	96	97	98	98	99	99	99	99	99	100	100	100	100	100	100	100
	60.00	97	97	98	99	99	99	99	99	100	100	100	100	100	100	100	100
	70.00	97	98	98	99	99	99	99	100	100	100	100	100	100	100	100	100
SPECI-	80.00	97	98	98	99	99	99	100	100	100	100	100	100	100	100	100	100
FICITY	90.00	98	98	99	99	99	100	100	100	100	100	100	100	100	100	100	100
(%)	91.00	98	98	99	99	99	100	100	100	100	100	100	100	100	100	100	100
	93.00	98	98	99	99	99	100	100	100	100	100	100	100	100	100	100	100
	95.00	98	98	99	99	99	100	100	100	100	100	100	100	100	100	100	100
	97.00	98	98	99	99	99	100	100	100	100	100	100	100	100	100	100	100
	99.00	98	98	99	99	99	100	100	100	100	100	100	100	100	100	100	100
	99.10	98	98	99	99	99	100	100	100	100	100	100	100	100	100	100	100
	99.30	98	98	99	99	99	100	100	100	100	100	100	100	100	100	100	100
	99.50	98	98	99	99	99	100	100	100	100	100	100	100	100	100	100	100
	99.70	98	98	99	99	99	100	100	100	100	100	100	100	100	100	100	100
	99.90	98	98	99	99	99	100	100	100	100	100	100	100	100	100	100	100
	99.91	98	98	99	99	99	100	100	100	100	100	100	100	100	100	100	100
	99.92	98	98	99	99	99	100	100	100	100	100	100	100	100	100	100	100
	99.93	98	98	99	99	99	100	100	100	100	100	100	100	100	100	100	100
	99.94	98	98	99	99	99	100	100	100	100	100	100	100	100	100	100	100
	99.95	98	98	99	99	99	100	100	100	100	100	100	100	100	100	100	100
	99.96	98	98	99	99	99	100	100	100	100	100	100	100	100	100	100	100
	99.97	98	98	99	99	99	100	100	100	100	100	100	100	100	100	100	100
	99.98	98	98	99	99	99	100	100	100	100	100	100	100	100	100	100	100
	99.99	98	98	99	99	99	100	100	100	100	100	100	100	100	100	100	100
	100.00	98	98	99	99	99	100	100	100	100	100	100	100	100	100	100	100

Table 102

PREDICTIVE VALUE OF NEGATIVES (IN PERCENT)
PREVALENCE= 5000 PER 100,000

		50	60	70	80	85	90	91	92	93	94	95	96	97	98	99	100
							SENSITIVITY (%)										
	50.00	95	96	97	98	98	99	99	99	99	99	99	100	100	100	100	100
	60.00	96	97	97	98	99	99	99	99	99	99	100	100	100	100	100	100
	70.00	96	97	98	99	99	99	99	99	99	100	100	100	100	100	100	100
SPECI-	80.00	97	97	98	99	99	99	99	99	100	100	100	100	100	100	100	100
FICITY	90.00	97	98	98	99	99	99	99	100	100	100	100	100	100	100	100	100
(%)	91.00	97	98	98	99	99	99	99	100	100	100	100	100	100	100	100	100
	93.00	97	98	98	99	99	99	99	100	100	100	100	100	100	100	100	100
	95.00	97	98	98	99	99	99	100	100	100	100	100	100	100	100	100	100
	97.00	97	98	98	99	99	99	100	100	100	100	100	100	100	100	100	100
	99.00	97	98	98	99	99	99	100	100	100	100	100	100	100	100	100	100
	99.10	97	98	98	99	99	99	100	100	100	100	100	100	100	100	100	100
	99.30	97	98	98	99	99	99	100	100	100	100	100	100	100	100	100	100
	99.50	97	98	98	99	99	99	100	100	100	100	100	100	100	100	100	100
	99.70	97	98	98	99	99	99	100	100	100	100	100	100	100	100	100	100
	99.90	97	98	98	99	99	99	100	100	100	100	100	100	100	100	100	100
	99.91	97	98	98	99	99	99	100	100	100	100	100	100	100	100	100	100
	99.92	97	98	98	99	99	99	100	100	100	100	100	100	100	100	100	100
	99.93	97	98	98	99	99	99	100	100	100	100	100	100	100	100	100	100
	99.94	97	98	98	99	99	99	100	100	100	100	100	100	100	100	100	100
	99.95	97	98	98	99	99	99	100	100	100	100	100	100	100	100	100	100
	99.96	97	98	98	99	99	99	100	100	100	100	100	100	100	100	100	100
	99.97	97	98	98	99	99	99	100	100	100	100	100	100	100	100	100	100
	99.98	97	98	98	99	99	99	100	100	100	100	100	100	100	100	100	100
	99.99	97	98	98	99	99	99	100	100	100	100	100	100	100	100	100	100
	100.00	97	98	98	99	99	99	100	100	100	100	100	100	100	100	100	100

Table 103

PREDICTIVE VALUE OF NEGATIVES (IN PERCENT)
PREVALENCE=10000 PER 100,000

		SENSITIVITY (%)														
		50	60	70	80	85	90	91	92	93	94	95	96	97	98	99	100
	50.00	90	92	94	96	97	98	98	98	98	99	99	99	99	100	100	100
	60.00	92	93	95	96	97	98	98	99	99	99	99	99	99	100	100	100
	70.00	93	94	95	97	98	98	99	99	99	99	99	99	100	100	100	100
SPECI-	80.00	94	95	96	97	98	99	99	99	99	99	99	99	100	100	100	100
FICITY	90.00	94	95	96	98	98	99	99	99	99	99	99	100	100	100	100	100
(%)	91.00	94	95	96	98	98	99	99	99	99	99	99	100	100	100	100	100
	93.00	94	95	97	98	98	99	99	99	99	99	99	100	100	100	100	100
	95.00	94	96	97	98	98	99	99	99	99	99	99	100	100	100	100	100
	97.00	95	96	97	98	98	99	99	99	99	99	99	100	100	100	100	100
	99.00	95	96	97	98	98	99	99	99	99	99	99	100	100	100	100	100
	99.10	95	96	97	98	98	99	99	99	99	99	99	100	100	100	100	100
	99.30	95	96	97	98	98	99	99	99	99	99	99	100	100	100	100	100
	99.50	95	96	97	98	98	99	99	99	99	99	99	100	100	100	100	100
	99.70	95	96	97	98	98	99	99	99	99	99	99	100	100	100	100	100
	99.90	95	96	97	98	98	99	99	99	99	99	99	100	100	100	100	100
	99.91	95	96	97	98	98	99	99	99	99	99	99	100	100	100	100	100
	99.92	95	96	97	98	98	99	99	99	99	99	99	100	100	100	100	100
	99.93	95	96	97	98	98	99	99	99	99	99	99	100	100	100	100	100
	99.94	95	96	97	98	98	99	99	99	99	99	99	100	100	100	100	100
	99.95	95	96	97	98	98	99	99	99	99	99	99	100	100	100	100	100
	99.96	95	96	97	98	98	99	99	99	99	99	99	100	100	100	100	100
	99.97	95	96	97	98	98	99	99	99	99	99	99	100	100	100	100	100
	99.98	95	96	97	98	98	99	99	99	99	99	99	100	100	100	100	100
	99.99	95	96	97	98	98	99	99	99	99	99	99	100	100	100	100	100
	100.00	95	96	97	98	98	99	99	99	99	99	99	100	100	100	100	100

Table 104

PREDICTIVE VALUE OF NEGATIVES (IN PERCENT)
PREVALENCE=15000 PER 100,000

		SENSITIVITY (%)														
		50	60	70	80	85	90	91	92	93	94	95	96	97	98	99	100
	50.00	85	88	90	93	95	97	97	97	98	98	98	99	99	99	100	100
	60.00	87	89	92	94	96	97	97	98	98	98	99	99	99	99	100	100
	70.00	89	91	93	95	96	98	98	98	98	99	99	99	99	99	100	100
SPECI-	80.00	90	92	94	96	97	98	98	98	98	99	99	99	99	100	100	100
FICITY	90.00	91	93	94	96	97	98	98	98	99	99	99	99	99	100	100	100
(%)	91.00	91	93	95	96	97	98	98	98	99	99	99	99	99	100	100	100
	93.00	91	93	95	96	97	98	98	99	99	99	99	99	99	100	100	100
	95.00	92	93	95	96	97	98	98	99	99	99	99	99	99	100	100	100
	97.00	92	93	95	96	97	98	98	99	99	99	99	99	99	100	100	100
	99.00	92	93	95	97	97	98	98	99	99	99	99	99	99	100	100	100
	99.10	92	93	95	97	97	98	98	99	99	99	99	99	99	100	100	100
	99.30	92	93	95	97	97	98	98	99	99	99	99	99	99	100	100	100
	99.50	92	93	95	97	97	98	98	99	99	99	99	99	99	100	100	100
	99.70	92	93	95	97	97	98	98	99	99	99	99	99	99	100	100	100
	99.90	92	93	95	97	97	98	98	99	99	99	99	99	99	100	100	100
	99.91	92	93	95	97	97	98	98	99	99	99	99	99	99	100	100	100
	99.92	92	93	95	97	97	98	98	99	99	99	99	99	99	100	100	100
	99.93	92	93	95	97	97	98	98	99	99	99	99	99	99	100	100	100
	99.94	92	93	95	97	97	98	98	99	99	99	99	99	99	100	100	100
	99.95	92	93	95	97	97	98	98	99	99	99	99	99	99	100	100	100
	99.96	92	93	95	97	97	98	98	99	99	99	99	99	99	100	100	100
	99.97	92	93	95	97	97	98	98	99	99	99	99	99	99	100	100	100
	99.98	92	93	95	97	97	98	98	99	99	99	99	99	99	100	100	100
	99.99	92	93	95	97	97	98	98	99	99	99	99	99	99	100	100	100
	100.00	92	93	95	97	97	98	98	99	99	99	99	99	99	100	100	100

Table 105

PREDICTIVE VALUE OF NEGATIVES (IN PERCENT)
PREVALENCE=20000 PER 100,000

		SENSITIVITY (%)															
		50	60	70	80	85	90	91	92	93	94	95	96	97	98	99	100
	50.00	80	83	87	91	93	95	96	96	97	97	98	98	99	99	100	100
	60.00	83	86	89	92	94	96	96	97	97	98	98	98	99	99	100	100
	70.00	85	88	90	93	95	97	97	97	98	98	98	99	99	99	100	100
SPECI-	80.00	86	89	91	94	96	97	97	98	98	98	98	99	99	99	100	100
FICITY	90.00	88	90	92	95	96	97	98	98	98	98	99	99	99	99	100	100
(%)	91.00	88	90	92	95	96	97	98	98	98	98	99	99	99	99	100	100
	93.00	88	90	93	95	96	97	98	98	98	98	99	99	99	99	100	100
	95.00	88	90	93	95	96	97	98	98	98	98	99	99	99	99	100	100
	97.00	89	91	93	95	96	97	98	98	98	98	99	99	99	99	100	100
	99.00	89	91	93	95	96	98	98	98	98	99	99	99	99	99	100	100
	99.10	89	91	93	95	96	98	98	98	98	99	99	99	99	99	100	100
	99.30	89	91	93	95	96	98	98	98	98	99	99	99	99	99	100	100
	99.50	89	91	93	95	96	98	98	98	98	99	99	99	99	100	100	100
	99.70	89	91	93	95	96	98	98	98	98	99	99	99	99	100	100	100
	99.90	89	91	93	95	96	98	98	98	98	99	99	99	99	100	100	100
	99.91	89	91	93	95	96	98	98	98	98	99	99	99	99	100	100	100
	99.92	89	91	93	95	96	98	98	98	98	99	99	99	99	100	100	100
	99.93	89	91	93	95	96	98	98	98	98	99	99	99	99	100	100	100
	99.94	89	91	93	95	96	98	98	98	98	99	99	99	99	100	100	100
	99.95	89	91	93	95	96	98	98	98	98	99	99	99	99	100	100	100
	99.96	89	91	93	95	96	98	98	98	98	99	99	99	99	100	100	100
	99.97	89	91	93	95	96	98	98	98	98	99	99	99	99	100	100	100
	99.98	89	91	93	95	96	98	98	98	98	99	99	99	99	100	100	100
	99.99	89	91	93	95	96	98	98	98	98	99	99	99	99	100	100	100
	100.00	89	91	93	95	96	98	98	98	98	99	99	99	99	100	100	100

Table 106

PREDICTIVE VALUE OF NEGATIVES (IN PERCENT)
PREVALENCE=25000 PER 100,000

		SENSITIVITY (%)															
		50	60	70	80	85	90	91	92	93	94	95	96	97	98	99	100
	50.00	75	79	83	88	91	94	94	95	96	96	97	97	98	99	99	100
	60.00	78	82	86	90	92	95	95	96	96	97	97	98	98	99	99	100
	70.00	81	84	88	91	93	95	96	96	97	97	98	98	99	99	100	100
SPECI-	80.00	83	86	89	92	94	96	96	97	97	98	98	98	99	99	100	100
FICITY	90.00	84	87	90	93	95	96	97	97	97	98	98	99	99	99	100	100
(%)	91.00	85	87	90	93	95	96	97	97	98	98	98	99	99	99	100	100
	93.00	85	87	90	93	95	97	97	97	98	98	98	99	99	99	100	100
	95.00	85	88	90	93	95	97	97	97	98	98	98	99	99	99	100	100
	97.00	85	88	91	94	95	97	97	97	98	98	98	99	99	99	100	100
	99.00	86	88	91	94	95	97	97	97	98	98	98	99	99	99	100	100
	99.10	86	88	91	94	95	97	97	97	98	98	98	99	99	99	100	100
	99.30	86	88	91	94	95	97	97	97	98	98	98	99	99	99	100	100
	99.50	86	88	91	94	95	97	97	97	98	98	98	99	99	99	100	100
	99.70	86	88	91	94	95	97	97	97	98	98	98	99	99	99	100	100
	99.90	86	88	91	94	95	97	97	97	98	98	98	99	99	99	100	100
	99.91	86	88	91	94	95	97	97	97	98	98	98	99	99	99	100	100
	99.92	86	88	91	94	95	97	97	97	98	98	98	99	99	99	100	100
	99.93	86	88	91	94	95	97	97	97	98	98	98	99	99	99	100	100
	99.94	86	88	91	94	95	97	97	97	98	98	98	99	99	99	100	100
	99.95	86	88	91	94	95	97	97	97	98	98	98	99	99	99	100	100
	99.96	86	88	91	94	95	97	97	97	98	98	98	99	99	99	100	100
	99.97	86	88	91	94	95	97	97	97	98	98	98	99	99	99	100	100
	99.98	86	88	91	94	95	97	97	97	98	98	98	99	99	99	100	100
	99.99	86	88	91	94	95	97	97	97	98	98	98	99	99	99	100	100
	100.00	86	88	91	94	95	97	97	97	98	98	98	99	99	99	100	100

Table 107

PREDICTIVE VALUE OF NEGATIVES (IN PERCENT)
PREVALENCE=50000 PER 100,000

		50	60	70	80	85	90	91	92	93	94	95	96	97	98	99	100
							SENSITIVITY (%)										
	50.00	50	56	63	71	77	83	85	86	88	89	91	93	94	96	98	100
	60.00	55	60	67	75	80	86	87	88	90	91	92	94	95	97	98	100
	70.00	58	64	70	78	82	88	89	90	91	92	93	95	96	97	99	100
SPECI-	80.00	62	67	73	80	84	89	90	91	92	93	94	95	96	98	99	100
FICITY	90.00	64	69	75	82	86	90	91	92	93	94	95	96	97	98	99	100
(%)	91.00	65	69	75	82	86	90	91	92	93	94	95	96	97	98	99	100
	93.00	65	70	76	82	86	90	91	92	93	94	95	96	97	98	99	100
	95.00	66	70	76	83	86	90	91	92	93	94	95	96	97	98	99	100
	97.00	66	71	76	83	87	91	92	92	93	94	95	96	97	98	99	100
	99.00	66	71	77	83	87	91	92	93	93	94	95	96	97	98	99	100
	99.10	66	71	77	83	87	91	92	93	93	94	95	96	97	98	99	100
	99.30	67	71	77	83	87	91	92	93	93	94	95	96	97	98	99	100
	99.50	67	71	77	83	87	91	92	93	93	94	95	96	97	98	99	100
	99.70	67	71	77	83	87	91	92	93	93	94	95	96	97	98	99	100
	99.90	67	71	77	83	87	91	92	93	93	94	95	96	97	98	99	100
	99.91	67	71	77	83	87	91	92	93	93	94	95	96	97	98	99	100
	99.92	67	71	77	83	87	91	92	93	93	94	95	96	97	98	99	100
	99.93	67	71	77	83	87	91	92	93	93	94	95	96	97	98	99	100
	99.94	67	71	77	83	87	91	92	93	93	94	95	96	97	98	99	100
	99.95	67	71	77	83	87	91	92	93	93	94	95	96	97	98	99	100
	99.96	67	71	77	83	87	91	92	93	93	94	95	96	97	98	99	100
	99.97	67	71	77	83	87	91	92	93	93	94	95	96	97	98	99	100
	99.98	67	71	77	83	87	91	92	93	93	94	95	96	97	98	99	100
	99.99	67	71	77	83	87	91	92	93	93	94	95	96	97	98	99	100
	100.00	67	71	77	83	87	91	92	93	93	94	95	96	97	98	99	100

EFFICIENCY OF A LABORATORY TEST BASED ON TEST SENSITIVITY, SPECIFICITY, AND DISEASE PREVALENCE*

Three relationships are possible between sensitivity and specificity for any test. The sensitivity may be greater than the specificity, the sensitivity may be equal to the specificity, or the sensitivity may be less than the specificity. Let us review what happens to the efficiency of a laboratory test under each of these circumstances in the face of fixed as well as increasing disease prevalence:

At a given prevalence (up to 50%) an incremental increase in specificity results in a great increase in the efficiency of a test than the same incremental increase in sensitivity. As prevalence increases, the efficiency of a test increases only if sensitivity is greater than specificity. When sensitivity is less than specificity, the efficiency of a test decreases with increasing prevalence. When sensitivity equals specificity, test efficiency is independent of prevalence and equal to sensitivity (or specificity). The value of test efficiency in all other cases falls between the value of test sensitivity and specificity, regardless of the relationship between sensitivity and specificity and disease prevalence.

* © 1972 by Robert S. Galen, M.D., M.P.H. Galen Tables of the predictive value of clinical laboratory tests: 72-386841.

Table 108

EFFICIENCY OF TEST (IN PERCENT)
PREVALENCE=   1 PER 100,000

SENSITIVITY (%)

		50	60	70	80	85	90	91	92	93	94	95	96	97	98	99	100
	50.00	50	50	50	50	50	50	50	50	50	50	50	50	50	50	50	50
	60.00	60	60	60	60	60	60	60	60	60	60	60	60	60	60	60	60
	70.00	70	70	70	70	70	70	70	70	70	70	70	70	70	70	70	70
SPECI-	80.00	80	80	80	80	80	80	80	80	80	80	80	80	80	80	80	80
FICITY	90.00	90	90	90	90	90	90	90	90	90	90	90	90	90	90	90	90
	91.00	91	91	91	91	91	91	91	91	91	91	91	91	91	91	91	91
(%)	93.00	93	93	93	93	93	93	93	93	93	93	93	93	93	93	93	93
	95.00	95	95	95	95	95	95	95	95	95	95	95	95	95	95	95	95
	97.00	97	97	97	97	97	97	97	97	97	97	97	97	97	97	97	97
	99.00	99	99	99	99	99	99	99	99	99	99	99	99	99	99	99	99
	99.10	99	99	99	99	99	99	99	99	99	99	99	99	99	99	99	99
	99.30	99	99	99	99	99	99	99	99	99	99	99	99	99	99	99	99
	99.50	99	99	99	99	99	99	99	99	99	99	99	99	99	99	99	100
	99.70	100	100	100	100	100	100	100	100	100	100	100	100	100	100	100	100
	99.90	100	100	100	100	100	100	100	100	100	100	100	100	100	100	100	100
	99.91	100	100	100	100	100	100	100	100	100	100	100	100	100	100	100	100
	99.92	100	100	100	100	100	100	100	100	100	100	100	100	100	100	100	100
	99.93	100	100	100	100	100	100	100	100	100	100	100	100	100	100	100	100
	99.94	100	100	100	100	100	100	100	100	100	100	100	100	100	100	100	100
	99.95	100	100	100	100	100	100	100	100	100	100	100	100	100	100	100	100
	99.96	100	100	100	100	100	100	100	100	100	100	100	100	100	100	100	100
	99.97	100	100	100	100	100	100	100	100	100	100	100	100	100	100	100	100
	99.98	100	100	100	100	100	100	100	100	100	100	100	100	100	100	100	100
	99.99	100	100	100	100	100	100	100	100	100	100	100	100	100	100	100	100
	100.00	100	100	100	100	100	100	100	100	100	100	100	100	100	100	100	100

Table 109

EFFICIENCY OF TEST (IN PERCENT)
PREVALENCE=   2 PER 100,000

SENSITIVITY (%)

		50	60	70	80	85	90	91	92	93	94	95	96	97	98	99	100
	50.00	50	50	50	50	50	50	50	50	50	50	50	50	50	50	50	50
	60.00	60	60	60	60	60	60	60	60	60	60	60	60	60	60	60	60
	70.00	70	70	70	70	70	70	70	70	70	70	70	70	70	70	70	70
SPECI-	80.00	80	80	80	80	80	80	80	80	80	80	80	80	80	80	80	80
FICITY	90.00	90	90	90	90	90	90	90	90	90	90	90	90	90	90	90	90
(%)	91.00	91	91	91	91	91	91	91	91	91	91	91	91	91	91	91	91
	93.00	93	93	93	93	93	93	93	93	93	93	93	93	93	93	93	93
	95.00	95	95	95	95	95	95	95	95	95	95	95	95	95	95	95	95
	97.00	97	97	97	97	97	97	97	97	97	97	97	97	97	97	97	97
	99.00	99	99	99	99	99	99	99	99	99	99	99	99	99	99	99	99
	99.10	99	99	99	99	99	99	99	99	99	99	99	99	99	99	99	99
	99.30	99	99	99	99	99	99	99	99	99	99	99	99	99	99	99	99
	99.50	99	99	99	99	99	99	99	99	99	99	99	99	99	99	99	100
	99.70	100	100	100	100	100	100	100	100	100	100	100	100	100	100	100	100
	99.90	100	100	100	100	100	100	100	100	100	100	100	100	100	100	100	100
	99.91	100	100	100	100	100	100	100	100	100	100	100	100	100	100	100	100
	99.92	100	100	100	100	100	100	100	100	100	100	100	100	100	100	100	100
	99.93	100	100	100	100	100	100	100	100	100	100	100	100	100	100	100	100
	99.94	100	100	100	100	100	100	100	100	100	100	100	100	100	100	100	100
	99.95	100	100	100	100	100	100	100	100	100	100	100	100	100	100	100	100
	99.96	100	100	100	100	100	100	100	100	100	100	100	100	100	100	100	100
	99.97	100	100	100	100	100	100	100	100	100	100	100	100	100	100	100	100
	99.98	100	100	100	100	100	100	100	100	100	100	100	100	100	100	100	100
	99.99	100	100	100	100	100	100	100	100	100	100	100	100	100	100	100	100
	100.00	100	100	100	100	100	100	100	100	100	100	100	100	100	100	100	100

Table 110

EFFICIENCY OF TEST (IN PERCENT)
PREVALENCE=   3 PER 100,000

SENSITIVITY (%)

SPECIFICITY (%)	50	60	70	80	85	90	91	92	93	94	95	96	97	98	99	100
50.00	50	50	50	50	50	50	50	50	50	50	50	50	50	50	50	50
60.00	60	60	60	60	60	60	60	60	60	60	60	60	60	60	60	60
70.00	70	70	70	70	70	70	70	70	70	70	70	70	70	70	70	70
80.00	80	80	80	80	80	80	80	80	80	80	80	80	80	80	80	80
90.00	90	90	90	90	90	90	90	90	90	90	90	90	90	90	90	90
91.00	91	91	91	91	91	91	91	91	91	91	91	91	91	91	91	91
93.00	93	93	93	93	93	93	93	93	93	93	93	93	93	93	93	93
95.00	95	95	95	95	95	95	95	95	95	95	95	95	95	95	95	95
97.00	97	97	97	97	97	97	97	97	97	97	97	97	97	97	97	97
99.00	99	99	99	99	99	99	99	99	99	99	99	99	99	99	99	99
99.10	99	99	99	99	99	99	99	99	99	99	99	99	99	99	99	99
99.30	99	99	99	99	99	99	99	99	99	99	99	99	99	99	99	99
99.50	99	99	99	99	99	99	99	99	99	99	99	99	99	99	99	100
99.70	100	100	100	100	100	100	100	100	100	100	100	100	100	100	100	100
99.90	100	100	100	100	100	100	100	100	100	100	100	100	100	100	100	100
99.91	100	100	100	100	100	100	100	100	100	100	100	100	100	100	100	100
99.92	100	100	100	100	100	100	100	100	100	100	100	100	100	100	100	100
99.93	100	100	100	100	100	100	100	100	100	100	100	100	100	100	100	100
99.94	100	100	100	100	100	100	100	100	100	100	100	100	100	100	100	100
99.95	100	100	100	100	100	100	100	100	100	100	100	100	100	100	100	100
99.96	100	100	100	100	100	100	100	100	100	100	100	100	100	100	100	100
99.97	100	100	100	100	100	100	100	100	100	100	100	100	100	100	100	100
99.98	100	100	100	100	100	100	100	100	100	100	100	100	100	100	100	100
99.99	100	100	100	100	100	100	100	100	100	100	100	100	100	100	100	100
100.00	100	100	100	100	100	100	100	100	100	100	100	100	100	100	100	100

Table 111

EFFICIENCY OF TEST (IN PERCENT)
PREVALENCE=   4 PER 100,000

SENSITIVITY (%)

SPECIFICITY (%)	50	60	70	80	85	90	91	92	93	94	95	96	97	98	99	100
50.00	50	50	50	50	50	50	50	50	50	50	50	50	50	50	50	50
60.00	60	60	60	60	60	60	60	60	60	60	60	60	60	60	60	60
70.00	70	70	70	70	70	70	70	70	70	70	70	70	70	70	70	70
80.00	80	80	80	80	80	80	80	80	80	80	80	80	80	80	80	80
90.00	90	90	90	90	90	90	90	90	90	90	90	90	90	90	90	90
91.00	91	91	91	91	91	91	91	91	91	91	91	91	91	91	91	91
93.00	93	93	93	93	93	93	93	93	93	93	93	93	93	93	93	93
95.00	95	95	95	95	95	95	95	95	95	95	95	95	95	95	95	95
97.00	97	97	97	97	97	97	97	97	97	97	97	97	97	97	97	97
99.00	99	99	99	99	99	99	99	99	99	99	99	99	99	99	99	99
99.10	99	99	99	99	99	99	99	99	99	99	99	99	99	99	99	99
99.30	99	99	99	99	99	99	99	99	99	99	99	99	99	99	99	99
99.50	99	99	99	99	99	99	99	99	99	99	99	99	99	99	99	100
99.70	100	100	100	100	100	100	100	100	100	100	100	100	100	100	100	100
99.90	100	100	100	100	100	100	100	100	100	100	100	100	100	100	100	100
99.91	100	100	100	100	100	100	100	100	100	100	100	100	100	100	100	100
99.92	100	100	100	100	100	100	100	100	100	100	100	100	100	100	100	100
99.93	100	100	100	100	100	100	100	100	100	100	100	100	100	100	100	100
99.94	100	100	100	100	100	100	100	100	100	100	100	100	100	100	100	100
99.95	100	100	100	100	100	100	100	100	100	100	100	100	100	100	100	100
99.96	100	100	100	100	100	100	100	100	100	100	100	100	100	100	100	100
99.97	100	100	100	100	100	100	100	100	100	100	100	100	100	100	100	100
99.98	100	100	100	100	100	100	100	100	100	100	100	100	100	100	100	100
99.99	100	100	100	100	100	100	100	100	100	100	100	100	100	100	100	100
100.00	100	100	100	100	100	100	100	100	100	100	100	100	100	100	100	100

223

Table 112

EFFICIENCY OF TEST (IN PERCENT)
PREVALENCE=   5 PER 100,000

		SENSITIVITY (%)															
		50	60	70	80	85	90	91	92	93	94	95	96	97	98	99	100
	50.00	50	50	50	50	50	50	50	50	50	50	50	50	50	50	50	50
	60.00	60	60	60	60	60	60	60	60	60	60	60	60	60	60	60	60
	70.00	70	70	70	70	70	70	70	70	70	70	70	70	70	70	70	70
SPECI-	80.00	80	80	80	80	80	80	80	80	80	80	80	80	80	80	80	80
FICITY	90.00	90	90	90	90	90	90	90	90	90	90	90	90	90	90	90	90
(%)	91.00	91	91	91	91	91	91	91	91	91	91	91	91	91	91	91	91
	93.00	93	93	93	93	93	93	93	93	93	93	93	93	93	93	93	93
	95.00	95	95	95	95	95	95	95	95	95	95	95	95	95	95	95	95
	97.00	97	97	97	97	97	97	97	97	97	97	97	97	97	97	97	97
	99.00	99	99	99	99	99	99	99	99	99	99	99	99	99	99	99	99
	99.10	99	99	99	99	99	99	99	99	99	99	99	99	99	99	99	99
	99.30	99	99	99	99	99	99	99	99	99	99	99	99	99	99	99	99
	99.50	99	99	99	99	99	99	99	99	99	99	99	99	99	99	99	100
	99.70	100	100	100	100	100	100	100	100	100	100	100	100	100	100	100	100
	99.90	100	100	100	100	100	100	100	100	100	100	100	100	100	100	100	100
	99.91	100	100	100	100	100	100	100	100	100	100	100	100	100	100	100	100
	99.92	100	100	100	100	100	100	100	100	100	100	100	100	100	100	100	100
	99.93	100	100	100	100	100	100	100	100	100	100	100	100	100	100	100	100
	99.94	100	100	100	100	100	100	100	100	100	100	100	100	100	100	100	100
	99.95	100	100	100	100	100	100	100	100	100	100	100	100	100	100	100	100
	99.96	100	100	100	100	100	100	100	100	100	100	100	100	100	100	100	100
	99.97	100	100	100	100	100	100	100	100	100	100	100	100	100	100	100	100
	99.98	100	100	100	100	100	100	100	100	100	100	100	100	100	100	100	100
	99.99	100	100	100	100	100	100	100	100	100	100	100	100	100	100	100	100
	100.00	100	100	100	100	100	100	100	100	100	100	100	100	100	100	100	100

Table 113

EFFICIENCY OF TEST (IN PERCENT)
PREVALENCE=   10 PER 100,000

		SENSITIVITY (%)															
		50	60	70	80	85	90	91	92	93	94	95	96	97	98	99	100
	50.00	50	50	50	50	50	50	50	50	50	50	50	50	50	50	50	50
	60.00	60	60	60	60	60	60	60	60	60	60	60	60	60	60	60	60
	70.00	70	70	70	70	70	70	70	70	70	70	70	70	70	70	70	70
SPECI-	80.00	80	80	80	80	80	80	80	80	80	80	80	80	80	80	80	80
FICITY	90.00	90	90	90	90	90	90	90	90	90	90	90	90	90	90	90	90
(%)	91.00	91	91	91	91	91	91	91	91	91	91	91	91	91	91	91	91
	93.00	93	93	93	93	93	93	93	93	93	93	93	93	93	93	93	93
	95.00	95	95	95	95	95	95	95	95	95	95	95	95	95	95	95	95
	97.00	97	97	97	97	97	97	97	97	97	97	97	97	97	97	97	97
	99.00	99	99	99	99	99	99	99	99	99	99	99	99	99	99	99	99
	99.10	99	99	99	99	99	99	99	99	99	99	99	99	99	99	99	99
	99.30	99	99	99	99	99	99	99	99	99	99	99	99	99	99	99	99
	99.50	99	99	99	99	99	99	99	99	99	99	99	99	99	99	99	100
	99.70	100	100	100	100	100	100	100	100	100	100	100	100	100	100	100	100
	99.90	100	100	100	100	100	100	100	100	100	100	100	100	100	100	100	100
	99.91	100	100	100	100	100	100	100	100	100	100	100	100	100	100	100	100
	99.92	100	100	100	100	100	100	100	100	100	100	100	100	100	100	100	100
	99.93	100	100	100	100	100	100	100	100	100	100	100	100	100	100	100	100
	99.94	100	100	100	100	100	100	100	100	100	100	100	100	100	100	100	100
	99.95	100	100	100	100	100	100	100	100	100	100	100	100	100	100	100	100
	99.96	100	100	100	100	100	100	100	100	100	100	100	100	100	100	100	100
	99.97	100	100	100	100	100	100	100	100	100	100	100	100	100	100	100	100
	99.98	100	100	100	100	100	100	100	100	100	100	100	100	100	100	100	100
	99.99	100	100	100	100	100	100	100	100	100	100	100	100	100	100	100	100
	100.00	100	100	100	100	100	100	100	100	100	100	100	100	100	100	100	100

Table 114

EFFICIENCY OF TEST (IN PERCENT)
PREVALENCE=   20 PER 100,000

						SEN	SITI	VITY	(%)							
	50	60	70	80	85	90	91	92	93	94	95	96	97	98	99	100
50.00	50	50	50	50	50	50	50	50	50	50	50	50	50	50	50	50
60.00	60	60	60	60	60	60	60	60	60	60	60	60	60	60	60	60
70.00	70	70	70	70	70	70	70	70	70	70	70	70	70	70	70	70
SPECI- 80.00	80	80	80	80	80	80	80	80	80	80	80	80	80	80	80	80
FICITY 90.00	90	90	90	90	90	90	90	90	90	90	90	90	90	90	90	90
(%) 91.00	91	91	91	91	91	91	91	91	91	91	91	91	91	91	91	91
93.00	93	93	93	93	93	93	93	93	93	93	93	93	93	93	93	93
95.00	95	95	95	95	95	95	95	95	95	95	95	95	95	95	95	95
97.00	97	97	97	97	97	97	97	97	97	97	97	97	97	97	97	97
99.00	99	99	99	99	99	99	99	99	99	99	99	99	99	99	99	99
99.10	99	99	99	99	99	99	99	99	99	99	99	99	99	99	99	99
99.30	99	99	99	99	99	99	99	99	99	99	99	99	99	99	99	99
99.50	99	99	99	99	99	99	99	99	99	99	99	99	99	99	99	100
99.70	100	100	100	100	100	100	100	100	100	100	100	100	100	100	100	100
99.90	100	100	100	100	100	100	100	100	100	100	100	100	100	100	100	100
99.91	100	100	100	100	100	100	100	100	100	100	100	100	100	100	100	100
99.92	100	100	100	100	100	100	100	100	100	100	100	100	100	100	100	100
99.93	100	100	100	100	100	100	100	100	100	100	100	100	100	100	100	100
99.94	100	100	100	100	100	100	100	100	100	100	100	100	100	100	100	100
99.95	100	100	100	100	100	100	100	100	100	100	100	100	100	100	100	100
99.96	100	100	100	100	100	100	100	100	100	100	100	100	100	100	100	100
99.97	100	100	100	100	100	100	100	100	100	100	100	100	100	100	100	100
99.98	100	100	100	100	100	100	100	100	100	100	100	100	100	100	100	100
99.99	100	100	100	100	100	100	100	100	100	100	100	100	100	100	100	100
100.00	100	100	100	100	100	100	100	100	100	100	100	100	100	100	100	100

Table 115

EFFICIENCY OF TEST (IN PERCENT)
PREVALENCE=   30 PER 100,000

						SEN	SITI	VITY	(%)							
	50	60	70	80	85	90	91	92	93	94	95	96	97	98	99	100
50.00	50	50	50	50	50	50	50	50	50	50	50	50	50	50	50	50
60.00	60	60	60	60	60	60	60	60	60	60	60	60	60	60	60	60
70.00	70	70	70	70	70	70	70	70	70	70	70	70	70	70	70	70
SPECI- 80.00	80	80	80	80	80	80	80	80	80	80	80	80	80	80	80	80
FICITY 90.00	90	90	90	90	90	90	90	90	90	90	90	90	90	90	90	90
(%) 91.00	91	91	91	91	91	91	91	91	91	91	91	91	91	91	91	91
93.00	93	93	93	93	93	93	93	93	93	93	93	93	93	93	93	93
95.00	95	95	95	95	95	95	95	95	95	95	95	95	95	95	95	95
97.00	97	97	97	97	97	97	97	97	97	97	97	97	97	97	97	97
99.00	99	99	99	99	99	99	99	99	99	99	99	99	99	99	99	99
99.10	99	99	99	99	99	99	99	99	99	99	99	99	99	99	99	99
99.30	99	99	99	99	99	99	99	99	99	99	99	99	99	99	99	99
99.50	99	99	99	99	99	99	99	99	99	99	99	99	99	99	99	100
99.70	100	100	100	100	100	100	100	100	100	100	100	100	100	100	100	100
99.90	100	100	100	100	100	100	100	100	100	100	100	100	100	100	100	100
99.91	100	100	100	100	100	100	100	100	100	100	100	100	100	100	100	100
99.92	100	100	100	100	100	100	100	100	100	100	100	100	100	100	100	100
99.93	100	100	100	100	100	100	100	100	100	100	100	100	100	100	100	100
99.94	100	100	100	100	100	100	100	100	100	100	100	100	100	100	100	100
99.95	100	100	100	100	100	100	100	100	100	100	100	100	100	100	100	100
99.96	100	100	100	100	100	100	100	100	100	100	100	100	100	100	100	100
99.97	100	100	100	100	100	100	100	100	100	100	100	100	100	100	100	100
99.98	100	100	100	100	100	100	100	100	100	100	100	100	100	100	100	100
99.99	100	100	100	100	100	100	100	100	100	100	100	100	100	100	100	100
100.00	100	100	100	100	100	100	100	100	100	100	100	100	100	100	100	100

Table 116

EFFICIENCY OF TEST (IN PERCENT)
PREVALENCE=   40 PER 100,000

SENSITIVITY (%)

SPECI-FICITY (%)	50	60	70	80	85	90	91	92	93	94	95	96	97	98	99	100
50.00	50	50	50	50	50	50	50	50	50	50	50	50	50	50	50	50
60.00	60	60	60	60	60	60	60	60	60	60	60	60	60	60	60	60
70.00	70	70	70	70	70	70	70	70	70	70	70	70	70	70	70	70
80.00	80	80	80	80	80	80	80	80	80	80	80	80	80	80	80	80
90.00	90	90	90	90	90	90	90	90	90	90	90	90	90	90	90	90
91.00	91	91	91	91	91	91	91	91	91	91	91	91	91	91	91	91
93.00	93	93	93	93	93	93	93	93	93	93	93	93	93	93	93	93
95.00	95	95	95	95	95	95	95	95	95	95	95	95	95	95	95	95
97.00	97	97	97	97	97	97	97	9,7	97	97	97	97	97	97	97	97
99.00	99	99	99	99	99	99	99	99	99	99	99	99	99	99	99	99
99.10	99	99	99	99	99	99	99	99	99	99	99	99	99	99	99	99
99.30	99	99	99	99	99	99	99	99	99	99	99	99	99	99	99	99
99.50	99	99	99	99	99	99	99	99	99	99	99	99	99	99	99	100
99.70	100	100	100	100	100	100	100	100	100	100	100	100	100	100	100	100
99.90	100	100	100	100	100	100	100	100	100	100	100	100	100	100	100	100
99.91	100	100	100	100	100	100	100	100	100	100	100	100	100	100	100	100
99.92	100	100	100	100	100	100	100	100	100	100	100	100	100	100	100	100
99.93	100	100	100	100	100	100	100	100	100	100	100	100	100	100	100	100
99.94	100	100	100	100	100	100	100	100	100	100	100	100	100	100	100	100
99.95	100	100	100	100	100	100	100	100	100	100	100	100	100	100	100	100
99.96	100	100	100	100	100	100	100	100	100	100	100	100	100	100	100	100
99.97	100	100	100	100	100	100	100	100	100	100	100	100	100	100	100	100
99.98	100	100	100	100	100	100	100	100	100	100	100	100	100	100	100	100
99.99	100	100	100	100	100	100	100	100	100	100	100	100	100	100	100	100
100.00	100	100	100	100	100	100	100	100	100	100	100	100	100	100	100	100

Table 117

EFFICIENCY OF TEST (IN PERCENT)
PREVALENCE=   50 PER 100,000

SENSITIVITY (%)

SPECI-FICITY (%)	50	60	70	80	85	90	91	92	93	94	95	96	97	98	99	100
50.00	50	50	50	50	50	50	50	50	50	50	50	50	50	50	50	50
60.00	60	60	60	60	60	60	60	60	60	60	60	60	60	60	60	60
70.00	70	70	70	70	70	70	70	70	70	70	70	70	70	70	70	70
80.00	80	80	80	80	80	80	80	80	80	80	80	80	80	80	80	80
90.00	90	90	90	90	90	90	90	90	90	90	90	90	90	90	90	90
91.00	91	91	91	91	91	91	91	91	91	91	91	91	91	91	91	91
93.00	93	93	93	93	93	93	93	93	93	93	93	93	93	93	93	93
95.00	95	95	95	95	95	95	95	95	95	95	95	95	95	95	95	95
97.00	97	97	97	97	97	97	97	97	97	97	97	97	97	97	97	97
99.00	99	99	99	99	99	99	99	99	99	99	99	99	99	99	99	99
99.10	99	99	99	99	99	99	99	99	99	99	99	99	99	99	99	99
99.30	99	99	99	99	99	99	99	99	99	99	99	99	99	99	99	99
99.50	99	99	99	99	99	99	99	99	99	99	99	99	99	99	99	100
99.70	100	100	100	100	100	100	100	100	100	100	100	100	100	100	100	100
99.90	100	100	100	100	100	100	100	100	100	100	100	100	100	100	100	100
99.91	100	100	100	100	100	100	100	100	100	100	100	100	100	100	100	100
99.92	100	100	100	100	100	100	100	100	100	100	100	100	100	100	100	100
99.93	100	100	100	100	100	100	100	100	100	100	100	100	100	100	100	100
99.94	100	100	100	100	100	100	100	100	100	100	100	100	100	100	100	100
99.95	100	100	100	100	100	100	100	100	100	100	100	100	100	100	100	100
99.96	100	100	100	100	100	100	100	100	100	100	100	100	100	100	100	100
99.97	100	100	100	100	100	100	100	100	100	100	100	100	100	100	100	100
99.98	100	100	100	100	100	100	100	100	100	100	100	100	100	100	100	100
99.99	100	100	100	100	100	100	100	100	100	100	100	100	100	100	100	100
100.00	100	100	100	100	100	100	100	100	100	100	100	100	100	100	100	100

Table 118

```
                              EFFICIENCY OF TEST (IN PERCENT)
                                 PREVALENCE=  100 PER 100,000
```

	SENSITIVITY (%)															
	50	60	70	80	85	90	91	92	93	94	95	96	97	98	99	100
50.00	50	50	50	50	50	50	50	50	50	50	50	50	50	50	50	50
60.00	60	60	60	60	60	60	60	60	60	60	60	60	60	60	60	60
70.00	70	70	70	70	70	70	70	70	70	70	70	70	70	70	70	70
SPECI- 80.00	80	80	80	80	80	80	80	80	80	80	80	80	80	80	80	80
FICITY 90.00	90	90	90	90	90	90	90	90	90	90	90	90	90	90	90	90
(%) 91.00	91	91	91	91	91	91	91	91	91	91	91	91	91	91	91	91
93.00	93	93	93	93	93	93	93	93	93	93	93	93	93	93	93	93
95.00	95	95	95	95	95	95	95	95	95	95	95	95	95	95	95	95
97.00	97	97	97	97	97	97	97	97	97	97	97	97	97	97	97	97
99.00	99	99	99	99	99	99	99	99	99	99	99	99	99	99	99	99
99.10	99	99	99	99	99	99	99	99	99	99	99	99	99	99	99	99
99.30	99	99	99	99	99	99	99	99	99	99	99	99	99	99	99	99
99.50	99	99	99	99	99	99	99	99	99	99	99	99	99	99	99	100
99.70	100	100	100	100	100	100	100	100	100	100	100	100	100	100	100	100
99.90	100	100	100	100	100	100	100	100	100	100	100	100	100	100	100	100
99.91	100	100	100	100	100	100	100	100	100	100	100	100	100	100	100	100
99.92	100	100	100	100	100	100	100	100	100	100	100	100	100	100	100	100
99.93	100	100	100	100	100	100	100	100	100	100	100	100	100	100	100	100
99.94	100	100	100	100	100	100	100	100	100	100	100	100	100	100	100	100
99.95	100	100	100	100	100	100	100	100	100	100	100	100	100	100	100	100
99.96	100	100	100	100	100	100	100	100	100	100	100	100	100	100	100	100
99.97	100	100	100	100	100	100	100	100	100	100	100	100	100	100	100	100
99.98	100	100	100	100	100	100	100	100	100	100	100	100	100	100	100	100
99.99	100	100	100	100	100	100	100	100	100	100	100	100	100	100	100	100
100.00	100	100	100	100	100	100	100	100	100	100	100	100	100	100	100	100

Table 119

```
                              EFFICIENCY OF TEST (IN PERCENT)
                                 PREVALENCE=  200 PER 100,000
```

	SENSITIVITY (%)															
	50	60	70	80	85	90	91	92	93	94	95	96	97	98	99	100
50.00	50	50	50	50	50	50	50	50	50	50	50	50	50	50	50	50
60.00	60	60	60	60	60	60	60	60	60	60	60	60	60	60	60	60
70.00	70	70	70	70	70	70	70	70	70	70	70	70	70	70	70	70
SPECI- 80.00	80	80	80	80	80	80	80	80	80	80	80	80	80	80	80	80
FICITY 90.00	90	90	90	90	90	90	90	90	90	90	90	90	90	90	90	90
(%) 91.00	91	91	91	91	91	91	91	91	91	91	91	91	91	91	91	91
93.00	93	93	93	93	93	93	93	93	93	93	93	93	93	93	93	93
95.00	95	95	95	95	95	95	95	95	95	95	95	95	95	95	95	95
97.00	97	97	97	97	97	97	97	97	97	97	97	97	97	97	97	97
99.00	99	99	99	99	99	99	99	99	99	99	99	99	99	99	99	99
99.10	99	99	99	99	99	99	99	99	99	99	99	99	99	99	99	99
99.30	99	99	99	99	99	99	99	99	99	99	99	99	99	99	99	99
99.50	99	99	99	99	99	99	99	99	99	99	99	99	99	99	99	100
99.70	100	100	100	100	100	100	100	100	100	100	100	100	100	100	100	100
99.90	100	100	100	100	100	100	100	100	100	100	100	100	100	100	100	100
99.91	100	100	100	100	100	100	100	100	100	100	100	100	100	100	100	100
99.92	100	100	100	100	100	100	100	100	100	100	100	100	100	100	100	100
99.93	100	100	100	100	100	100	100	100	100	100	100	100	100	100	100	100
99.94	100	100	100	100	100	100	100	100	100	100	100	100	100	100	100	100
99.95	100	100	100	100	100	100	100	100	100	100	100	100	100	100	100	100
99.96	100	100	100	100	100	100	100	100	100	100	100	100	100	100	100	100
99.97	100	100	100	100	100	100	100	100	100	100	100	100	100	100	100	100
99.98	100	100	100	100	100	100	100	100	100	100	100	100	100	100	100	100
99.99	100	100	100	100	100	100	100	100	100	100	100	100	100	100	100	100
100.00	100	100	100	100	100	100	100	100	100	100	100	100	100	100	100	100

Table 120

EFFICIENCY OF TEST (IN PERCENT)
PREVALENCE= 300 PER 100,000

SENSITIVITY (%)

		50	60	70	80	85	90	91	92	93	94	95	96	97	98	99	100
	50.00	50	50	50	50	50	50	50	50	50	50	50	50	50	50	50	50
	60.00	60	60	60	60	60	60	60	60	60	60	60	60	60	60	60	60
	70.00	70	70	70	70	70	70	70	70	70	70	70	70	70	70	70	70
SPECI-	80.00	80	80	80	80	80	80	80	80	80	80	80	80	80	80	80	80
FICITY	90.00	90	90	90	90	90	90	90	90	90	90	90	90	90	90	90	90
(%)	91.00	91	91	91	91	91	91	91	91	91	91	91	91	91	91	91	91
	93.00	93	93	93	93	93	93	93	93	93	93	93	93	93	93	93	93
	95.00	95	95	95	95	95	95	95	95	95	95	95	95	95	95	95	95
	97.00	97	97	97	97	97	97	97	97	97	97	97	97	97	97	97	97
	99.00	99	99	99	99	99	99	99	99	99	99	99	99	99	99	99	99
	99.10	99	99	99	99	99	99	99	99	99	99	99	99	99	99	99	99
	99.30	99	99	99	99	99	99	99	99	99	99	99	99	99	99	99	99
	99.50	99	99	99	99	99	99	99	99	99	99	99	99	99	99	99	100
	99.70	100	100	100	100	100	100	100	100	100	100	100	100	100	100	100	100
	99.90	100	100	100	100	100	100	100	100	100	100	100	100	100	100	100	100
	99.91	100	100	100	100	100	100	100	100	100	100	100	100	100	100	100	100
	99.92	100	100	100	100	100	100	100	100	100	100	100	100	100	100	100	100
	99.93	100	100	100	100	100	100	100	100	100	100	100	100	100	100	100	100
	99.94	100	100	100	100	100	100	100	100	100	100	100	100	100	100	100	100
	99.95	100	100	100	100	100	100	100	100	100	100	100	100	100	100	100	100
	99.96	100	100	100	100	100	100	100	100	100	100	100	100	100	100	100	100
	99.97	100	100	100	100	100	100	100	100	100	100	100	100	100	100	100	100
	99.98	100	100	100	100	100	100	100	100	100	100	100	100	100	100	100	100
	99.99	100	100	100	100	100	100	100	100	100	100	100	100	100	100	100	100
	100.00	100	100	100	100	100	100	100	100	100	100	100	100	100	100	100	100

Table 121

EFFICIENCY OF TEST (IN PERCENT)
PREVALENCE= 400 PER 100,000

SENSITIVITY (%)

		50	60	70	80	85	90	91	92	93	94	95	96	97	98	99	100
	50.00	50	50	50	50	50	50	50	50	50	50	50	50	50	50	50	50
	60.00	60	60	60	60	60	60	60	60	60	60	60	60	60	60	60	60
	70.00	70	70	70	70	70	70	70	70	70	70	70	70	70	70	70	70
SPECI-	80.00	80	80	80	80	80	80	80	80	80	80	80	80	80	80	80	80
FICITY	90.00	90	90	90	90	90	90	90	90	90	90	90	90	90	90	90	90
(%)	91.00	91	91	91	91	91	91	91	91	91	91	91	91	91	91	91	91
	93.00	93	93	93	93	93	93	93	93	93	93	93	93	93	93	93	93
	95.00	95	95	95	95	95	95	95	95	95	95	95	95	95	95	95	95
	97.00	97	97	97	97	97	97	97	97	97	97	97	97	97	97	97	97
	99.00	99	99	99	99	99	99	99	99	99	99	99	99	99	99	99	99
	99.10	99	99	99	99	99	99	99	99	99	99	99	99	99	99	99	99
	99.30	99	99	99	99	99	99	99	99	99	99	99	99	99	99	99	99
	99.50	99	99	99	99	99	99	99	99	99	99	99	99	99	99	99	100
	99.70	100	100	100	100	100	100	100	100	100	100	100	100	100	100	100	100
	99.90	100	100	100	100	100	100	100	100	100	100	100	100	100	100	100	100
	99.91	100	100	100	100	100	100	100	100	100	100	100	100	100	100	100	100
	99.92	100	100	100	100	100	100	100	100	100	100	100	100	100	100	100	100
	99.93	100	100	100	100	100	100	100	100	100	100	100	100	100	100	100	100
	99.94	100	100	100	100	100	100	100	100	100	100	100	100	100	100	100	100
	99.95	100	100	100	100	100	100	100	100	100	100	100	100	100	100	100	100
	99.96	100	100	100	100	100	100	100	100	100	100	100	100	100	100	100	100
	99.97	100	100	100	100	100	100	100	100	100	100	100	100	100	100	100	100
	99.98	100	100	100	100	100	100	100	100	100	100	100	100	100	100	100	100
	99.99	100	100	100	100	100	100	100	100	100	100	100	100	100	100	100	100
	100.00	100	100	100	100	100	100	100	100	100	100	100	100	100	100	100	100

Table 122

EFFICIENCY OF TEST (IN PERCENT)
PREVALENCE= 500 PER 100,000

SENSITIVITY (%)

SPECI-FICITY (%)	50	60	70	80	85	90	91	92	93	94	95	96	97	98	99	100
50.00	50	50	50	50	50	50	50	50	50	50	50	50	50	50	50	50
60.00	60	60	60	60	60	60	60	60	60	60	60	60	60	60	60	60
70.00	70	70	70	70	70	70	70	70	70	70	70	70	70	70	70	70
80.00	80	80	80	80	80	80	80	80	80	80	80	80	80	80	80	80
90.00	90	90	90	90	90	90	90	90	90	90	90	90	90	90	90	90
91.00	91	91	91	91	91	91	91	91	91	91	91	91	91	91	91	91
93.00	93	93	93	93	93	93	93	93	93	93	93	93	93	93	93	93
95.00	95	95	95	95	95	95	95	95	95	95	95	95	95	95	95	95
97.00	97	97	97	97	97	97	97	97	97	97	97	97	97	97	97	97
99.00	99	99	99	99	99	99	99	99	99	99	99	99	99	99	99	99
99.10	99	99	99	99	99	99	99	99	99	99	99	99	99	99	99	99
99.30	99	99	99	99	99	99	99	99	99	99	99	99	99	99	99	99
99.50	99	99	99	99	99	99	99	99	99	99	99	99	99	99	99	100
99.70	99	100	100	100	100	100	100	100	100	100	100	100	100	100	100	100
99.90	100	100	100	100	100	100	100	100	100	100	100	100	100	100	100	100
99.91	100	100	100	100	100	100	100	100	100	100	100	100	100	100	100	100
99.92	100	100	100	100	100	100	100	100	100	100	100	100	100	100	100	100
99.93	100	100	100	100	100	100	100	100	100	100	100	100	100	100	100	100
99.94	100	100	100	100	100	100	100	100	100	100	100	100	100	100	100	100
99.95	100	100	100	100	100	100	100	100	100	100	100	100	100	100	100	100
99.96	100	100	100	100	100	100	100	100	100	100	100	100	100	100	100	100
99.97	100	100	100	100	100	100	100	100	100	100	100	100	100	100	100	100
99.98	100	100	100	100	100	100	100	100	100	100	100	100	100	100	100	100
99.99	100	100	100	100	100	100	100	100	100	100	100	100	100	100	100	100
100.00	100	100	100	100	100	100	100	100	100	100	100	100	100	100	100	100

Table 123

EFFICIENCY OF TEST (IN PERCENT)
PREVALENCE= 1000 PER 100,000

SENSITIVITY (%)

SPECI-FICITY (%)	50	60	70	80	85	90	91	92	93	94	95	96	97	98	99	100
50.00	50	50	50	50	50	50	50	50	50	50	50	50	50	50	50	50
60.00	60	60	60	60	60	60	60	60	60	60	60	60	60	60	60	60
70.00	70	70	70	70	70	70	70	70	70	70	70	70	70	70	70	70
80.00	80	80	80	80	80	80	80	80	80	80	80	80	80	80	80	80
90.00	90	90	90	90	90	90	90	90	90	90	90	90	90	90	90	90
91.00	91	91	91	91	91	91	91	91	91	91	91	91	91	91	91	91
93.00	93	93	93	93	93	93	93	93	93	93	93	93	93	93	93	93
95.00	95	95	95	95	95	95	95	95	95	95	95	95	95	95	95	95
97.00	97	97	97	97	97	97	97	97	97	97	97	97	97	97	97	97
99.00	99	99	99	99	99	99	99	99	99	99	99	99	99	99	99	99
99.10	99	99	99	99	99	99	99	99	99	99	99	99	99	99	99	99
99.30	99	99	99	99	99	99	99	99	99	99	99	99	99	99	99	99
99.50	99	99	99	99	99	99	99	99	99	99	99	99	99	99	99	100
99.70	99	99	99	100	100	100	100	100	100	100	100	100	100	100	100	100
99.90	99	100	100	100	100	100	100	100	100	100	100	100	100	100	100	100
99.91	99	100	100	100	100	100	100	100	100	100	100	100	100	100	100	100
99.92	99	100	100	100	100	100	100	100	100	100	100	100	100	100	100	100
99.93	99	100	100	100	100	100	100	100	100	100	100	100	100	100	100	100
99.94	99	100	100	100	100	100	100	100	100	100	100	100	100	100	100	100
99.95	99	100	100	100	100	100	100	100	100	100	100	100	100	100	100	100
99.96	99	100	100	100	100	100	100	100	100	100	100	100	100	100	100	100
99.97	99	100	100	100	100	100	100	100	100	100	100	100	100	100	100	100
99.98	99	100	100	100	100	100	100	100	100	100	100	100	100	100	100	100
99.99	99	100	100	100	100	100	100	100	100	100	100	100	100	100	100	100
100.00	99	100	100	100	100	100	100	100	100	100	100	100	100	100	100	100

Table 124

EFFICIENCY OF TEST (IN PERCENT)
PREVALENCE= 2000 PER 100,000

SENSITIVITY (%)

		50	60	70	80	85	90	91	92	93	94	95	96	97	98	99	100
	50.00	50	50	50	51	51	51	51	51	51	51	51	51	51	51	51	51
	60.00	60	60	60	60	60	61	61	61	61	61	61	61	61	61	61	61
	70.00	70	70	70	70	70	70	70	70	70	70	70	71	71	71	71	71
SPECI-	80.00	79	80	80	80	80	80	80	80	80	80	80	80	80	80	80	80
FICITY	90.00	89	89	90	90	90	90	90	90	90	90	90	90	90	90	90	90
(%)	91.00	90	90	91	91	91	91	91	91	91	91	91	91	91	91	91	91
	93.00	92	92	93	93	93	93	93	93	93	93	93	93	93	93	93	93
	95.00	94	94	94	95	95	95	95	95	95	95	95	95	95	95	95	95
	97.00	96	96	96	97	97	97	97	97	97	97	97	97	97	97	97	97
	99.00	98	98	98	99	99	99	99	99	99	99	99	99	99	99	99	99
	99.10	98	98	99	99	99	99	99	99	99	99	99	99	99	99	99	99
	99.30	98	99	99	99	99	99	99	99	99	99	99	99	99	99	99	99
	99.50	99	99	99	99	99	99	99	99	99	99	99	99	99	99	99	100
	99.70	99	99	99	99	99	100	100	100	100	100	100	100	100	100	100	100
	99.90	99	99	99	100	100	100	100	100	100	100	100	100	100	100	100	100
	99.91	99	99	99	100	100	100	100	100	100	100	100	100	100	100	100	100
	99.92	99	99	99	100	100	100	100	100	100	100	100	100	100	100	100	100
	99.93	99	99	99	100	100	100	100	100	100	100	100	100	100	100	100	100
	99.94	99	99	99	100	100	100	100	100	100	100	100	100	100	100	100	100
	99.95	99	99	99	100	100	100	100	100	100	100	100	100	100	100	100	100
	99.96	99	99	99	100	100	100	100	100	100	100	100	100	100	100	100	100
	99.97	99	99	99	100	100	100	100	100	100	100	100	100	100	100	100	100
	99.98	99	99	99	100	100	100	100	100	100	100	100	100	100	100	100	100
	99.99	99	99	99	100	100	100	100	100	100	100	100	100	100	100	100	100
	100.00	99	99	99	100	100	100	100	100	100	100	100	100	100	100	100	100

Table 125

EFFICIENCY OF TEST (IN PERCENT)
PREVALENCE= 3000 PER 100,000

SENSITIVITY (%)

		50	60	70	80	85	90	91	92	93	94	95	96·	97	98	99	100
	50.00	50	50	51	51	51	51	51	51	51	51	51	51	51	51	51	51
	60.00	60	60	60	61	61	61	61	61	61	61	61	61	61	61	61	61
	70.00	69	70	70	70	70	71	71	71	71	71	71	71	71	71	71	71
SPECI-	80.00	79	79	80	80	80	80	80	80	80	80	80	80	81	81	81	81
FICITY	90.00	89	89	89	90	90	90	90	90	90	90	90	90	90	90	90	90
(%)	91.00	90	90	90	91	91	91	91	91	91	91	91	91	91	91	91	91
	93.00	92	92	93	93	93	93	93	93	93	93	93	93	93	93	93	93
	95.00	94	94	94	95	95	95	95	95	95	95	95	95	95	95	95	95
	97.00	96	96	96	96	97	97	97	97	97	97	97	97	97	97	97	97
	99.00	98	98	98	98	99	99	99	99	99	99	99	99	99	99	99	99
	99.10	98	98	98	99	99	99	99	99	99	99	99	99	99	99	99	99
	99.30	98	98	98	99	99	99	99	99	99	99	99	99	99	99	99	99
	99.50	98	98	99	99	99	99	99	99	99	99	99	99	99	99	99	100
	99.70	98	99	99	99	99	99	99	99	99	100	100	100	100	100	100	100
	99.90	98	99	99	99	99	100	100	100	100	100	100	100	100	100	100	100
	99.91	98	99	99	99	99	100	100	100	100	100	100	100	100	100	100	100
	99.92	98	99	99	99	99	100	100	100	100	100	100	100	100	100	100	100
	99.93	98	99	99	99	99	100	100	100	100	100	100	100	100	100	100	100
	99.94	98	99	99	99	99	100	100	100	100	100	100	100	100	100	100	100
	99.95	98	99	99	99	100	100	100	100	100	100	100	100	100	100	100	100
	99.96	98	99	99	99	100	100	100	100	100	100	100	100	100	100	100	100
	99.97	98	99	99	99	100	100	100	100	100	100	100	100	100	100	100	100
	99.98	98	99	99	99	100	100	100	100	100	100	100	100	100	100	100	100
	99.99	98	99	99	99	100	100	100	100	100	100	100	100	100	100	100	100
	100.00	98	99	99	99	100	100	100	100	100	100	100	100	100	100	100	100

Table 126

EFFICIENCY OF TEST (IN PERCENT)
PREVALENCE= 4000 PER 100,000

SENSITIVITY (%)

SPECIFICITY (%)	50	60	70	80	85	90	91	92	93	94	95	96	97	98	99	100
50.00	50	50	51	51	51	52	52	52	52	52	52	52	52	52	52	52
60.00	60	60	60	61	61	61	61	61	61	61	61	61	61	62	62	62
70.00	69	70	70	70	71	71	71	71	71	71	71	71	71	71	71	71
80.00	79	79	80	80	80	80	80	80	81	81	81	81	81	81	81	81
90.00	88	89	89	90	90	90	90	90	90	90	90	90	90	90	90	90
91.00	89	90	90	91	91	91	91	91	91	91	91	91	91	91	91	91
93.00	91	92	92	92	93	93	93	93	93	93	93	93	93	93	93	93
95.00	93	94	94	94	95	95	95	95	95	95	95	95	95	95	95	95
97.00	95	96	96	96	97	97	97	97	97	97	97	97	97	97	97	97
99.00	97	97	98	98	98	99	99	99	99	99	99	99	99	99	99	99
99.10	97	98	98	98	99	99	99	99	99	99	99	99	99	99	99	99
99.30	97	98	98	99	99	99	99	99	99	99	99	99	99	99	99	99
99.50	98	98	98	99	99	99	99	99	99	99	99	99	99	99	99	100
99.70	98	98	99	99	99	99	99	99	99	99	100	100	100	100	100	100
99.90	98	98	99	99	99	100	100	100	100	100	100	100	100	100	100	100
99.91	98	98	99	99	99	100	100	100	100	100	100	100	100	100	100	100
99.92	98	98	99	99	99	100	100	100	100	100	100	100	100	100	100	100
99.93	98	98	99	99	99	100	100	100	100	100	100	100	100	100	100	100
99.94	98	98	99	99	99	100	100	100	100	100	100	100	100	100	100	100
99.95	98	98	99	99	99	100	100	100	100	100	100	100	100	100	100	100
99.96	98	98	99	99	99	100	100	100	100	100	100	100	100	100	100	100
99.97	98	98	99	99	99	100	100	100	100	100	100	100	100	100	100	100
99.98	98	98	99	99	99	100	100	100	100	100	100	100	100	100	100	100
99.99	98	98	99	99	99	100	100	100	100	100	100	100	100	100	100	100
100.00	98	98	99	99	99	100	100	100	100	100	100	100	100	100	100	100

Table 127

EFFICIENCY OF TEST (IN PERCENT)
PREVALENCE= 5000 PER 100,000

SENSITIVITY (%)

SPECIFICITY (%)	50	60	70	80	85	90	91	92	93	94	95	96	97	98	99	100
50.00	50	50	51	51	52	52	52	52	52	52	52	52	52	52	52	52
60.00	59	60	60	61	61	61	62	62	62	62	62	62	62	62	62	62
70.00	69	69	70	70	71	71	71	71	71	71	71	71	71	71	71	71
80.00	78	79	79	80	80	80	81	81	81	81	81	81	81	81	81	81
90.00	88	88	89	89	90	90	90	90	90	90	90	90	90	90	90	90
91.00	89	89	90	90	91	91	91	91	91	91	91	91	91	91	91	91
93.00	91	92	92	92	93	93	93	93	93	93	93	93	93	93	93	93
95.00	93	93	94	94	94	95	95	95	95	95	95	95	95	95	95	95
97.00	95	95	96	96	96	97	97	97	97	97	97	97	97	97	97	97
99.00	97	97	98	98	98	99	99	99	99	99	99	99	99	99	99	99
99.10	97	97	98	98	98	99	99	99	99	99	99	99	99	99	99	99
99.30	97	97	98	98	99	99	99	99	99	99	99	99	99	99	99	99
99.50	97	98	98	99	99	99	99	99	99	99	99	99	99	99	99	100
99.70	97	98	98	99	99	99	99	99	99	99	99	100	100	100	100	100
99.90	97	98	98	99	99	99	99	100	100	100	100	100	100	100	100	100
99.91	97	98	98	99	99	99	99	100	100	100	100	100	100	100	100	100
99.92	97	98	98	99	99	99	99	100	100	100	100	100	100	100	100	100
99.93	97	98	98	99	99	99	99	100	100	100	100	100	100	100	100	100
99.94	97	98	98	99	99	99	99	100	100	100	100	100	100	100	100	100
99.95	97	98	98	99	99	99	100	100	100	100	100	100	100	100	100	100
99.96	97	98	98	99	99	99	100	100	100	100	100	100	100	100	100	100
99.97	97	98	98	99	99	99	100	100	100	100	100	100	100	100	100	100
99.98	97	98	98	99	99	99	100	100	100	100	100	100	100	100	100	100
99.99	97	98	98	99	99	99	100	100	100	100	100	100	100	100	100	100
100.00	97	98	98	99	99	99	100	100	100	100	100	100	100	100	100	100

Table 128

EFFICIENCY OF TEST (IN PERCENT)
PREVALENCE=10000 PER 100,000

		SENSITIVITY (%)															
		50	60	70	80	85	90	91	92	93	94	95	96	97	98	99	100
SPECI- FICITY	50.00	50	51	52	53	53	54	54	54	54	54	54	55	55	55	55	55
	60.00	59	60	61	62	62	63	63	63	63	63	63	64	64	64	64	64
	70.00	68	69	70	71	71	72	72	72	72	72	72	73	73	73	73	73
	80.00	77	78	79	80	80	81	81	81	81	81	81	82	82	82	82	82
	90.00	86	87	88	89	89	90	90	90	90	90	90	91	91	91	91	91
(%)	91.00	87	88	89	90	90	91	91	91	91	91	91	91	92	92	92	92
	93.00	89	90	91	92	92	93	93	93	93	93	93	93	93	93	94	94
	95.00	90	91	92	93	94	94	95	95	95	95	95	95	95	95	95	95
	97.00	92	93	94	95	96	96	96	97	97	97	97	97	97	97	97	97
	99.00	94	95	96	97	98	98	98	98	98	98	99	99	99	99	99	99
	99.10	94	95	96	97	98	98	98	98	98	99	99	99	99	99	99	99
	99.30	94	95	96	97	98	98	98	99	99	99	99	99	99	99	99	99
	99.50	95	96	97	98	98	99	99	99	99	99	99	99	99	99	99	100
	99.70	95	96	97	98	98	99	99	99	99	99	99	99	99	100	100	100
	99.90	95	96	97	98	98	99	99	99	99	99	99	100	100	100	100	100
	99.91	95	96	97	98	98	99	99	99	99	99	99	100	100	100	100	100
	99.92	95	96	97	98	98	99	99	99	99	99	99	100	100	100	100	100
	99.93	95	96	97	98	98	99	99	99	99	99	99	100	100	100	100	100
	99.94	95	96	97	98	98	99	99	99	99	99	99	100	100	100	100	100
	99.95	95	96	97	98	98	99	99	99	99	99	99	100	100	100	100	100
	99.96	95	96	97	98	98	99	99	99	99	99	99	100	100	100	100	100
	99.97	95	96	97	98	98	99	99	99	99	99	99	100	100	100	100	100
	99.98	95	96	97	98	98	99	99	99	99	99	99	100	100	100	100	100
	99.99	95	96	97	98	98	99	99	99	99	99	99	100	100	100	100	100
	100.00	95	96	97	98	98	99	99	99	99	99	99	100	100	100	100	100

Table 129

EFFICIENCY OF TEST (IN PERCENT)
PREVALENCE=15000 PER 100,000

		SENSITIVITY (%)															
		50	60	70	80	85	90	91	92	93	94	95	96	97	98	99	100
SPECI- FICITY	50.00	50	51	53	54	55	56	56	56	56	57	57	57	57	57	57	57
	60.00	58	60	61	63	64	64	65	65	65	65	65	65	66	66	66	66
	70.00	67	68	70	71	72	73	73	73	73	74	74	74	74	74	74	74
	80.00	75	77	78	80	81	81	82	82	82	82	82	82	83	83	83	83
	90.00	84	85	87	88	89	90	90	90	90	91	91	91	91	91	91	91
(%)	91.00	85	86	88	89	90	91	91	91	91	91	92	92	92	92	92	92
	93.00	87	88	90	91	92	93	93	93	93	93	93	93	94	94	94	94
	95.00	88	90	91	93	93	94	94	95	95	95	95	95	95	95	96	96
	97.00	90	91	93	94	95	96	96	96	96	97	97	97	97	97	97	97
	99.00	92	93	95	96	97	98	98	98	98	98	98	99	99	99	99	99
	99.10	92	93	95	96	97	98	98	98	98	98	98	99	99	99	99	99
	99.30	92	93	95	96	97	98	98	98	98	99	99	99	99	99	99	99
	99.50	92	94	95	97	97	98	98	98	99	99	99	99	99	99	99	100
	99.70	92	94	95	97	97	98	98	99	99	99	99	99	99	99	100	100
	99.90	92	94	95	97	98	98	99	99	99	99	99	99	99	100	100	100
	99.91	92	94	95	97	98	98	99	99	99	99	99	99	99	100	100	100
	99.92	92	94	95	97	98	98	99	99	99	99	99	99	99	100	100	100
	99.93	92	94	95	97	98	98	99	99	99	99	99	99	99	100	100	100
	99.94	92	94	95	97	98	98	99	99	99	99	99	99	99	100	100	100
	99.95	92	94	95	97	98	98	99	99	99	99	99	99	100	100	100	100
	99.96	92	94	95	97	98	98	99	99	99	99	99	99	100	100	100	100
	99.97	92	94	95	97	98	98	99	99	99	99	99	99	100	100	100	100
	99.98	92	94	95	97	98	98	99	99	99	99	99	99	100	100	100	100
	99.99	92	94	95	97	98	98	99	99	99	99	99	99	100	100	100	100
	100.00	92	94	95	97	98	98	99	99	99	99	99	99	100	100	100	100

Table 130

EFFICIENCY OF TEST (IN PERCENT)
PREVALENCE=20000 PER 100,000

SENSITIVITY (%)

SPECI-FICITY (%)	50	60	70	80	85	90	91	92	93	94	95	96	97	98	99	100
50.00	50	52	54	56	57	58	58	58	59	59	59	59	59	60	60	60
60.00	58	60	62	64	65	66	66	66	67	67	67	67	67	68	68	68
70.00	66	68	70	72	73	74	74	74	75	75	75	75	75	76	76	76
80.00	74	76	78	80	81	82	82	82	83	83	83	83	83	84	84	84
90.00	82	84	86	88	89	90	90	90	91	91	91	91	91	92	92	92
91.00	83	85	87	89	90	91	91	91	91	92	92	92	92	92	93	93
93.00	84	86	88	90	91	92	93	93	93	93	93	94	94	94	94	94
95.00	86	88	90	92	93	94	94	94	95	95	95	95	95	96	96	96
97.00	88	90	92	94	95	96	96	96	96	96	97	97	97	97	97	98
99.00	89	91	93	95	96	97	97	98	98	98	98	98	99	99	99	99
99.10	89	91	93	95	96	97	97	98	98	98	98	98	99	99	99	99
99.30	89	91	93	95	96	97	98	98	98	98	98	98	99	99	99	99
99.50	90	92	94	96	97	98	98	98	98	98	99	99	99	99	99	100
99.70	90	92	94	96	97	98	98	98	98	99	99	99	99	99	100	100
99.90	90	92	94	96	97	98	98	98	99	99	99	99	99	100	100	100
99.91	90	92	94	96	97	98	98	98	99	99	99	99	99	100	100	100
99.92	90	92	94	96	97	98	98	98	99	99	99	99	99	100	100	100
99.93	90	92	94	96	97	98	98	98	99	99	99	99	99	100	100	100
99.94	90	92	94	96	97	98	98	98	99	99	99	99	99	100	100	100
99.95	90	92	94	96	97	98	98	98	99	99	99	99	99	100	100	100
99.96	90	92	94	96	97	98	98	98	99	99	99	99	99	100	100	100
99.97	90	92	94	96	97	98	98	98	99	99	99	99	99	100	100	100
99.98	90	92	94	96	97	98	98	98	99	99	99	99	99	100	100	100
99.99	90	92	94	96	97	98	98	98	99	99	99	99	99	100	100	100
100.00	90	92	94	96	97	98	98	98	99	99	99	99	99	100	100	100

Table 131

EFFICIENCY OF TEST (IN PERCENT)
PREVALENCE=25000 PER 100,000

SENSITIVITY (%)

SPECI-FICITY (%)	50	60	70	80	85	90	91	92	93	94	95	96	97	98	99	100
50.00	50	52	55	57	59	60	60	60	61	61	61	61	62	62	62	62
60.00	57	60	62	65	66	67	68	68	68	68	69	69	69	69	70	70
70.00	65	67	70	72	74	75	75	75	76	76	76	76	77	77	77	77
80.00	72	75	77	80	81	82	83	83	83	83	84	84	84	84	85	85
90.00	80	82	85	87	89	90	90	90	91	91	91	91	92	92	92	92
91.00	81	83	86	88	89	91	91	91	91	92	92	92	92	93	93	93
93.00	82	85	87	90	91	92	92	93	93	93	93	94	94	94	94	95
95.00	84	86	89	91	92	94	94	94	94	95	95	95	95	96	96	96
97.00	85	88	90	93	94	95	95	96	96	96	96	97	97	97	97	98
99.00	87	89	92	94	95	97	97	97	97	98	98	98	98	99	99	99
99.10	87	89	92	94	96	97	97	97	98	98	98	98	99	99	99	99
99.30	87	89	92	94	96	97	97	97	98	98	98	98	99	99	99	99
99.50	87	90	92	95	96	97	97	98	98	98	98	99	99	99	99	100
99.70	87	90	92	95	96	97	98	98	98	98	99	99	99	99	100	100
99.90	87	90	92	95	96	97	98	98	98	98	99	99	99	99	100	100
99.91	87	90	92	95	96	97	98	98	98	98	99	99	99	99	100	100
99.92	87	90	92	95	96	97	98	98	98	98	99	99	99	99	100	100
99.93	87	90	92	95	96	97	98	98	98	98	99	99	99	99	100	100
99.94	87	90	92	95	96	97	98	98	98	98	99	99	99	99	100	100
99.95	87	90	92	95	96	97	98	98	98	98	99	99	99	99	100	100
99.96	87	90	92	95	96	97	98	98	98	98	99	99	99	99	100	100
99.97	87	90	92	95	96	97	98	98	98	98	99	99	99	99	100	100
99.98	87	90	92	95	96	97	98	98	98	98	99	99	99	99	100	100
99.99	87	90	92	95	96	97	98	98	98	98	99	99	99	99	100	100
100.00	87	90	92	95	96	97	98	98	98	98	99	99	99	99	100	100

Table 132

EFFICIENCY OF TEST (IN PERCENT)
PREVALENCE=50000 PER 100,000

		SENSITIVITY (%)														
		50	6C	70	80	85	90	91	92	93	94	95	96	97	98	99	100
	50.00	50	55	60	65	67	70	70	71	71	72	72	73	73	74	74	75
	60.00	55	60	65	70	72	75	75	76	76	77	77	78	78	79	79	80
	70.00	60	65	70	75	77	80	80	81	81	82	82	83	83	84	84	85
SPECI-	80.00	65	70	75	80	82	85	85	86	86	87	87	88	88	89	89	90
FICITY	90.00	70	75	80	85	87	90	90	91	91	92	92	93	93	94	94	95
(%)	91.00	70	75	80	85	88	90	91	91	92	92	93	93	94	94	95	95
	93.00	71	76	81	86	89	91	92	92	93	93	94	94	95	95	96	96
	95.00	72	77	82	87	90	92	93	93	94	94	95	95	96	96	97	97
	97.00	73	78	83	88	91	93	94	94	95	95	96	96	97	97	98	98
	99.00	74	79	84	89	92	94	95	95	96	96	97	97	98	98	99	99
	99.10	75	8C	85	90	92	95	95	96	96	97	97	98	98	99	99	100
	99.30	75	80	85	90	92	95	95	96	96	97	97	98	98	99	99	100
	99.50	75	80	85	90	92	95	95	96	96	97	97	98	98	99	99	100
	99.70	75	8C	85	90	92	95	95	96	96	97	97	98	98	99	99	100
	99.90	75	80	85	90	92	95	95	96	96	97	97	98	98	99	99	100
	99.91	75	80	85	90	92	95	95	96	96	97	97	98	98	99	99	100
	99.92	75	80	85	90	92	95	95	96	96	97	97	98	98	99	99	100
	99.93	75	8C	85	90	92	95	95	96	96	97	97	98	98	99	99	100
	99.94	75	80	85	90	92	95	95	96	96	97	97	98	98	99	99	100
	99.95	75	8C	85	90	92	95	95	96	96	97	97	98	98	99	99	100
	99.96	75	80	85	90	92	95	95	96	96	97	97	98	98	99	99	100
	99.97	75	80	85	90	92	95	95	96	96	97	97	98	98	99	99	100
	99.98	75	80	85	90	92	95	95	96	96	97	97	98	98	99	99	100
	99.99	75	8C	85	90	92	95	95	96	96	97	97	98	98	99	99	100
	100.00	75	80	85	90	92	95	95	96	96	97	97	98	98	99	99	100

INDEX